Anesthesia and Pain Management for Veterinary Nurses and Technicians

T0272289

Tamara Grubb, DVM, MS, PhD, DACVAA
Mary Albi, LVT
Janel Holden, LVT, VTS (Anesthesia/Analgesia)
Shelley Ensign, LVT, CVPP (Certified Veterinary Pain Practitioner)
Shona Meyer, BS, LVT, VTS (Anesthesia/Analgesia)
Nicole Valdez, LVT, VTS (Anesthesia/Analgesia)

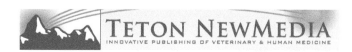

TETON NEWMEDIA
INNOVATIVE PUBLISHING OF VETERINARY & HUMAN MEDICINE

Executive Editor: Carroll C. Cann
Design and Production: www.fiftysixforty.com

Teton NewMedia
P.O. Box 4833
Jackson, WY 83001
1-888-770-3165
www.tetonnm.com

The author and publisher have made every effort to provide an
accurate reference text. However, they shall not be held responsible
for problems arising from errors or omissions, or from misunder-
standings on the part of the reader.

ISBN # 978-1-59161-050-2

Print number 5 4 3 2 1

Library of Congress Cataloging-in-Publication Data on file.

Preface

Our book was created to fill the need for a practical, 'hands-on' overview of anesthesia and analgesia for veterinary technicians and nurses. In the end, this book has become not only an excellent resource for the intended audience, but also for anyone who will use anesthesia equipment, administer anesthetics and analgesics, and manage patients. This audience includes veterinary and technician students studying the art and science of anesthesia and analgesia and practicing veterinarians wanting a review of the topic in an easy to use, easy to read resource.

We have made every effort to focus attention on important principles and clinical points within the text and have emphasized key information in call-out tips, boxes, figures, tables and photographs. Topics include anesthesia equipment, drugs, anesthetic techniques and protocols, monitoring, support and pain management. To make the information complete, we have included chapters not only on dogs and cats but also on horses and 'pocket pets'. Chapters 8, 9, and 10 are particularly strong reference and teaching features. Chapter 10 covers prevention and treatment of complications and emergencies. It should be one of the first chapters that you read if you are currently practicing anesthesia. Chapter 9 is a case-based review of anesthetic and analgesic protocols that we use every day in our hospital. We think Chapter 8 will be your favorite. It is a 'how to' chapter full of step-by-step instructions and 'tricks of the trade' wholly authored by practicing veterinary technicians.

Our editor stated, 'I believe that you, as a group, have done a wonderful job of creating a "hands on", focused and comprehensive guide' and we humbly agree with him. We hope you enjoy your copy of 'Anesthesia and Pain Management for Veterinary Nurses and Technicians' as much as we enjoyed creating it for you.

Finally, you might want to start by reading the appendix - it contains many tips and shortcuts that will make your day easier.

Acknowledgement/Dedication

Many thanks to our teachers and mentors that include not only our fellow technicians and veterinarians but also the patients who are, inadvertently, our best teachers. We are their advocates and their voices but so often they reciprocate and show us, through anesthesia/analgesia-associated physiologic and behavior changes, where we are doing a good job - and where we can do better. Our special thanks to Drs. Steve Greene, Rob Keegan, Lais Malavasi and Tania Perez who were working with us on clinics as we were writing this book.

We are grateful to Grant Meyer who worked with us throughout the process to provide the excellent photographs that are such a vital part of this presentation.

While You Sleep

Nicole Valdez, LVT, VTS (Anesthesia)

You don't know me,
I am silent.
Silently watching every breath you take.
Listening to every heartbeat you beat.
I stay by your side monitoring you as you sleep.
I'm there, the one giving you a voice.
I treat your pain while others are trying to put you back together.
You won't remember me when you wake, but I will remember you.
For you have touched my life in so many ways.
You're someone's beloved pet.
Even though you're not mine,
I feel as though you are a part of me.
It's more than just being there,
It's what I do because I care.

Table of Contents

Chapter 1
Principles of Anesthesia and Analgesia

Importance of Anesthesia

General anesthesia is achieved by depression of the central nervous system **(CNS)** to a point of loss of sensation. The sensation loss must be deep enough to allow invasive procedures to be performed without the patient being aware, yet not so deep that the CNS homeostatic functions (eg, maintenance of breathing and control of heart rate) are suppressed to a life-threatening level. The fact is that anesthesia causes some inherent risk of morbidity (compromised health) and mortality (death). Anesthesia-related mortality is higher in dogs and cats (0.05 TO 1.4%) [Brodbelt 2009] than in humans (0.02 TO 0.05%). It is up to the anesthetist to make anesthesia as safe as possible. Factors to consider for safety include the patient, anesthetic drugs, anesthesia equipment, analgesic drugs and techniques, monitoring equipment and techniques, and support drugs, equipment and techniques. By taking all of these factors into consideration, we should be able to not only decrease mortality but to actually IMPROVE the condition of the patient by enhancing oxygenation, stabilizing circulating volume and decreasing pain. Owners often ask how well their pet did during anesthesia before they ask about the surgical procedure. We want to be sure that we can say 'they did great!'

Importance of Analgesia

No matter what anesthetic protocol is chosen, the addition of adequate **analgesia** is **imperative for safe anesthesia** and **for enhanced patient outcomes.** Perioperative analgesia has three monumental advantages. 1) It improves our medical success rate because adequate analgesia improves healing and allows a decreased incidence of perioperative stress-related complications. Pain initiates a fairly profound stress response and a nervous system (parasympathetic vs sympathetic) imbalance. This can induce a cascade of adverse effects, including gastrointestinal **(GI)** ileus, GI ulceration, clotting dysfunction, hypertension, tachycardia, arrhythmias, and many others. Furthermore, stress and pain cause a fairly marked increase in cortisol release and a substantial increase in energy requirements, the latter of which may lead to a negative nitrogen balance and both of which impair healing. 2) Analgesia increases anesthetic safety by decreasing the necessary dosages of anesthetic drugs. Most anesthetic drugs, including the inhalant anesthetic drugs, block the brain's response to pain but don't actually block pain. If the pain is severe enough, the brain can still respond and make the animal appear to be inadequately anesthetized. The result is that the vaporizer is turned up and the brain ceases to respond, but the patient is now too deeply anesthetized and can be at a very dangerous physiologic plane. A more appropriate response is to decrease the pain with analgesic drugs and maintain a light, safe depth of anesthesia. 3) Adequate pain management at the time of intense pain (like surgery or trauma) decreases the potential that the patient will develop chronic pain postoperatively. Moderate to severe pain can create long-term pathologic changes in the pain pathway. Prevention of these changes can alleviate or eliminate the incidence of chronic pain syndromes related to the initial surgery, injury or disease. This can be vital because treatment of chronic pain can be difficult and is often ineffective.

In addition to the medical importance of treating pain, we have an ethical commitment to treat pain. All veterinarians and veterinary nurses are governed by the Veterinarian's Oath. Pain is described in Stedman's Medical Dictionary as, "**suffering**, either physical or mental; an impression on the sensory nerves causing distress or, when extreme, agony". The Veterinarian's Oath states that we pledge to '...use scientific knowledge and skills for the protection of animal health and welfare, the prevention and relief of animal **suffering**...' So, ethically, we committed to relieving pain when we joined this profession. This is not a new concept, in fact, the veterinarian's oath was adopted by the AVMA in August, 1961. Pain relief is both the ethically 'right thing to do', AND the medically 'right thing to do'.

Principles of Analgesia
Regardless of which analgesic drugs are chosen, 3 basic guidelines of pain management should always be followed: 1) analgesic drugs should be administered *preemptively* (i.e., BEFORE we cause pain) whenever possible; 2) *multimodal* analgesia (i.e., using more than one 'mode' of analgesia - like two or more drugs or a drug plus a nonpharmacologic modality like acupuncture) should be used whenever possible; and 3) analgesia should *continue* as long as pain affects the quality of life of the patient (i.e., pain does not generally stop just because the patient was discharged from the hospital).

Principles of Anesthesia
Anesthesia should always be provided using multimodal techniques, or 'balanced anesthesia'. Using a variety of drugs allows us to capitalize on the synergism between the drugs while decreasing the dose of each drug. With our current knowledge of pharmacology and the availability of safe, effective anesthetic and analgesic drugs, anesthetizing a patient with a single drug (ie, only an injectable drug or only an inhalant with no sedative/tranquilizers or analgesic drugs) is no longer appropriate. Nor is it safe. Anesthesia should be thought of as 4 distinct and equally important periods **(Figure 1-1):** 1) preparation/premedication; 2) induction; 3) maintenance and 4) recovery. We tend to diminish the importance of the phases of preparation/premedication and recovery and yet these phases contribute as much to successful anesthesia as the phases of induction and maintenance.

Preparation/Premedication
Preparation is patient specific. Some patients need nothing more than a physical exam while some may need extensive preoperative diagnostics and/or support like IV fluids or analgesia. Patient preparation is discussed in Chapters 2 and 9. Preparation includes checking all of the equipment (anesthesia machine, monitors, etc...) prior to use. Anesthetic equipment is discussed in Chapters 3 and 5. No matter what anesthetic protocol is chosen, safe and successful anesthesia will be enhanced by the use of *pre-anesthetic tranquilizers*. This is evidenced by two facts: 1) Stress in the perioperative period is extremely dangerous physiologically i.e. death can occur from stress. 2) Tranquilizers allow reduction in the dose of

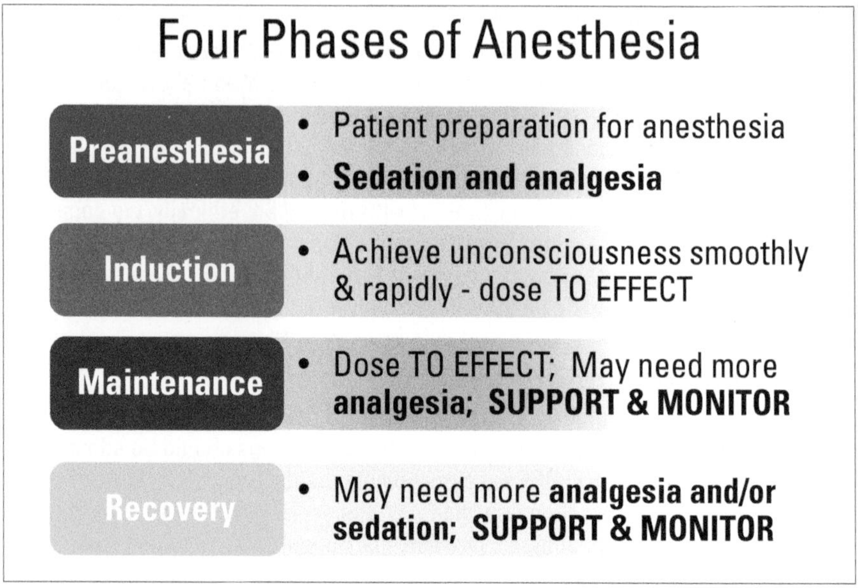

Four Phases of Anesthesia

Preanesthesia	• Patient preparation for anesthesia • **Sedation and analgesia**
Induction	• Achieve unconsciousness smoothly & rapidly - dose TO EFFECT
Maintenance	• Dose TO EFFECT; May need more **analgesia; SUPPORT & MONITOR**
Recovery	• May need more **analgesia and/or sedation; SUPPORT & MONITOR**

Figure 1-1. Anesthesia can be divided into four equally important phases: Preanesthesia/premedication, induction, maintenance and recovery.

both induction and maintenance drugs, thus increasing the margin between the 'effective dose' and 'dangerous or toxic dose' of drugs. Premedicant sedative/tranquilizers are discussed in Chapters 4 and 9 and include opioids, alpha-2 agonists, acepromazine and benzodiazepines. Analgesia should also be included as part of premedication. Premedicant analgesic drugs are discussed in Chapters 4, 7 and 9 and include opioids, alpha-2 agonists, and non-steroidal anti-inflammatory drugs **(NSAIDs)**. Other drugs that may be used as premedicants include maropitant, the anticholinergics **(atropine and glycopyrrolate)** and any stabilizing drugs required by the particular patient.

Induction
Induction must occur rapidly and smoothly so that the patient passes through the excitatory stage of anesthesia **(Table 1-1)** very quickly and so that control of the airway can be obtained as soon as possible (i.e., endotracheal intubation needs to occur quickly). Drugs should be dosed 'to effect'. Support like IV fluids, oxygen and infusions of support (eg, dopamine) or analgesic drugs may need to start at induction. Monitoring like ECG and blood pressure measurement may need to be started at induction. Drugs used for induction include propofol, ketamine, tiletamine/zolazepam, etomidate, thiobarbiturates and alfaxalone.

Maintenance
Anesthesia can be maintained using inhalant drugs (isoflurane, sevoflurane, desflurane). Anesthesia can be maintained using injectable drugs (e.g., ketamine

Table 1-1
Stages and Planes of Anesthesia
(Based on 'Guedel's Classification' of Anesthetic Drugs)

Stage	Description
I	Defined as stage from beginning of induction of general anesthesia to loss of consciousness. Some 'disorientation' may occur during this phase
II	Defined as stage from loss of consciousness to onset of automatic breathing. Also called the 'stage of excitement or delirium'. This is the stage to pass through QUICKLY. A prolonged time in Stage II often occurs with mask or chamber induction, which is one reason that this method of induction is not recommended. Patients recovering from anesthesia will also pass through this phase, which explains some of the dysphoria in recovery. However, this should be brief and, if not, analgesic and sedative drugs should be administered to the patient. Struggling, coughing, vomiting and other excitatory responses can occur if Stage II lasts too long.
III	This is the stage of surgical anesthesia and is divided into four planes: • Plane 1 - very light anesthesia. Palpebral reflex is light to nonexistent, swallowing reflex is absent, some eye movement may occur. • Plane 2 - generally an adequate but not too deep plane of anesthesia. This plane is best achieved with a low-dose of inhalant anesthesia with analgesics. Eye movement stops, secretion of tears increases and breathing is generally automatic and regular. • Plane 3 - slightly deep plane of anesthesia. The plane is often achieved if analgesic drugs are not used. Pupils are dilated and light reflex disappears. If tidal volume is measured, a decrease will likely be noted as breathing starts to become impaired. • Plane 4 - excessively deep plane of anesthesia. Intercostal (rib) muscles and the diaphragm become completely relaxed and apnea is likely.
IV	Stage from total apnea to death. The patient is WAY TOO DEEP. Avoid this stage!!

combinations, tiletamine/zolazepam, and propofol infusions). Drugs, regardless of whether they are inhalant or injectable, should be dosed 'to effect'. Monitoring (eg, anesthetic depth, heart rate, respiratory rate, ECG, blood pressure and oxygen-hemoglobin saturation) and support (eg, supplemental oxygenation, IV fluids and warming) are imperative during the maintenance phase. Analgesia should be re-addressed and might include repeat boluses of opioids, local/regional anesthetic blockade and constant rate infusions **(CRIs)**.

Recovery

This is often the most critical part of the anesthetic period. Unfortunately, most unexpected deaths occur in the recovery phase of anesthesia (Brodbelt 2009). Factors that contribute to death include; 1) excessive anesthetic depth during the maintenance phase which leads to excessive anesthetic depth in recovery, and 2) insufficient patient support and monitoring during recovery. Both support and monitoring should continue in recovery, especially if the patient is compromised. Drugs that might be used during recovery include; sedative/tranquilizers for patients having a 'rough' recovery, analgesic drugs for painful patients and reversal drugs for patients that are excessively deep or that need to be aroused quickly. Drugs whose effects can be reversed include the opioids (full reversal with naloxone, partial reversal with butorphanol), alpha-2 agonists (atipamezole, yohimibine and tolazoline) and benzodiazepines (flumazenil).

How to use this Book

The chapters in this book are designed to guide the anesthetist through the 4 phases of anesthesia in the logical order of your anesthesia day. Every time that you prepare to anesthetize a patient you should follow these steps (which correspond to the numbered chapters in the book):

1. Be sure you understand the principles of anesthesia and analgesia.
2. Check your patients: Physical exam, history, serum chemistry analysis, etc. Stabilize any patients that need it. Make sure your patients are ready!
3. Check and diligently maintain your anesthetic equipment.
4. Choose drugs for the patients. Drugs include those for premedication (sedative/ tranquilizers, analgesic drugs, etc.), induction (single drug or combination of drugs), maintenance (inhalant or injectable drugs, analgesic drugs, support drugs, etc…) and recovery (sedatives/tranquilizers, analgesic drugs, reversal drugs, etc.).
5. Make sure the monitoring equipment is ready, that you know what to monitor and that you know the significance of changes in physiologic parameters.
6. Make sure support 'agents' (e.g., oxygen, IV fluids, warming blankets, etc.) and drugs are ready and that you know how to respond to patient problems.
7. Understand the importance of good pain management and have a plan for analgesia.
8. Anesthetize your patient Step-by-Step. Don't take any shortcuts!
9. Be ready for specific cases.
10. Be ready to prevent, or treat, emergencies, including cardiac arrest.
11. Be prepared to anesthetize horses (if your practice includes horses).
12. Be prepared to anesthetize 'pocket pets' (if your practice includes pocket pets).

Now it is your turn. Be the best anesthetist that you can be!

Reference

Brodbelt D. Perioperative mortality in small animal anesthesia Vet J 2009; 182:152-161.

Chapter 2
Preparing the Patient for Anesthesia

Nicole Valdez, LVT, VTS (Anesthesia/Analgesia)

Introduction

Although this chapter is short, it may be one of the most important chapters in the book because safe anesthesia is preceded by appropriate patient assessment, preparation and stabilization (when necessary).

> **IMPORTANT NOTE**
>
> **More information on preparation for anesthesia is presented in Chapter 8 and includes not only patient preparation, but also preparation of equipment and drugs. All of this information should be understood BEFORE the patient is anesthetized.**

Preoperative patient assessment is critical for anesthetic safety. The patient should be assessed using physical examination and medical history. 'Blood work' (serum chemistry analysis and complete blood count **[CBC]**) and urinalysis are also commonly recommended. More advanced assessment (e.g., radiographs, ultrasound, and specialized serum chemistry tests) may be necessary for some patients. Once the initial assessment is complete, an American Society of Anesthesiologists **(ASA)** physical status score should be assigned to the patient **(Table 2-1)**. Further diagnostics and patient stabilization/support will be determined by the ASA score.

Table 2-1
Adapted American Society of Anesthesiologists (ASA) Physical Status Scores

I	Healthy patient with no anesthetic risk beyond the normal expected risk from anesthesia
II	Patient with localized disease or systemic disease that is unlikely to have a major impact on anesthetic risk (a patient with a fracture but no other injuries, a patient that is febrile but not systemically ill or a patient with uncomplicated hypothyroidism are examples)
III	Patient with moderate to severe systemic disease that is likely to have an impact on anesthetic risk unless the patient is stabilized (patients with untreated but not immediately life-threatening cardiovascular disease, moderate electrolyte imbalances or endocrine abnormalities are examples). These patients should be stabilized prior to anesthesia, if possible, to decrease anesthetic risk.
IV	Patient with severe systemic disease that is a threat to life and that will have a major impact on anesthetic risk (a septic patient or a patient with profound hyperkalemia are examples). These patients are very likely to die if they are not stabilized prior to anesthesia.
V	Patient that will die from its disease if not anesthetized but is also likely to die if it is anesthetized (a patient that is actively hemorrhaging from a ruptured splenic mass or a patient in septic shock are examples). These patients are at extreme risk and should be stabilized as much as possible but emergency anesthesia is often required.

If the patient must undergo emergency anesthesia, an 'E' (for emergency) should be placed next to the ASA category in the record.

Physical Exam
A Thorough Physical Examination And History Are Required For Every Patient Prior To Anesthesia

The physical exam **(Table 2-2)** should include assessment or measurement of:

Overall Health Status
Is the patient alert and active? Is the patient in good body condition? Are the eyes clear and bright? Is there any discharge from nostrils or other orifices? Does the hair coat look healthy? If 'no' is the answer to any of these questions, a more extensive physical exam and other diagnostic tests (like serum chemistry analysis) should be done to determine the cause before the patient is anesthetized. Many illnesses can cause these abnormalities.

Body Weight
Is the patient too thin, appropriate, or too fat? This is important for both assessment of overall health and for dosing of drugs. Drugs should be dosed on lean body weight.

Heart and Respiratory Rates
Are the rates normal for species, body size, health status and level of stress from being in the hospital? These may be elevated due to the stress of being in the hospital so these 'normal' elevations need to be differentiated from elevations due to disease.

Mucous Membrane Color and Capillary Refill Time (CRT)
Is the mucous membrane pink to pale pink and is the CRT < 2 seconds? Capillary refill time is one of the best 'simple' monitors to evaluate perfusion. CRT is evaluated by pressing firmly with a finger on an area of pink mucous membrane, generally the area just above the canine tooth, for several seconds. This forces the blood out of the capillaries in the area under pressure and 'blanches' the mucous membrane site, which makes it look white. The finger is then removed. The number of seconds for the blood to return to the compressed capillaries and return the membrane to its normal color is the CRT.

A prolonged CRT indicates poor perfusion and a patient that definitely requires further diagnostics and supportive stabilization (like warming and IV fluids or blood) prior to anesthesia. The cause can be anything from hypothermia or dehydration to severe hemorrhage or shock. A very rapid CRT is less common than a prolonged CRT. It may occur with pyrexia (i.e., fever), heat stroke, or early onset of some forms of shock.

Table 2-2
Sample Form for Physical Examination and Patient History

YOUR VETERINARY CLINIC

Patient Name:	Owner Name:	Date:

Reason for visit:

Weight	Heart Rate	Resp. Rate	Body Temp
MM color	Cap Refill Time	Hydration	
Attitude (anxious, excited, alert, sedate calm, lethargic)		Body Condition (over, normal, under weight)	

Indicate N for normal or describe any abnormalities in the organ systems listed below

General Appearance	
Skin	
Eyes/ears	
Cardiovascular System	
Respiratory System	
GI System	
Renal System	
Lymphatics	
Other Systems	

Pain Score 0 (no pain) 1   2   3   4   5   6   7   8   9   10 (severe pain)

History

Description of problem:

Onset of problem	Duration of problem
Changes in problem	
Appetite	Urinating normally?
Sleep/Activity levels normal?	Feces normal?
Current treatment/Response to treatment	
Other medications	
Other pets or people ill?	
Any history of illness in pet's family?	
Other information	

HISTORY CAN BE CONTINUED ON BACK OF PAGE

Mucous membrane color can be used to assess vascular (vessel) tone and abnormalities in color can indicate direct changes in the vessels or changes in the sympathetic nervous system that impact the vessel tone. Blood volume can also impact mucous membrane color. Pale mucous membranes can indicate vasoconstriction from conditions such as hypothermia, hypotension, and shock. Drugs that cause vasoconstriction, like the alpha-2 agonists, can cause pale mucous membranes. Severe anemia and hemorrhage can also cause pale mucous membranes. Red mucous membranes (also called 'injected' mucous membranes) often occur with septic or endotoxic shock but dark pink mucous membranes can be caused by vasodilation from other causes, such as administration of high dosages of acepromazine or some of the alpha-2 antagonists, particularly yohimbine and tolazoline. Bluish mucous membranes are caused by hemoglobin desaturation (profound hypoxemia) or profound sludging of blood in patients with severe circulatory compromise. These patients need stabilization prior to anesthesia.

Auscultation of the Heart and Lungs

Abnormalities in either of these systems can significantly impact the safety of anesthesia and warrant further diagnostics prior to anesthesia. Auscultation of the heart for murmurs and while simultaneously feeling for a pulse to make sure that every ausculted heart beat is associated with a pulse is important. Pulse deficits (or ausculted heart beat that does not result in a palpable pulse) can indicate severe cardiac disease and warrant further diagnostics prior to anesthesia. Respiratory disease can cause the lung sounds like 'crackles' and 'wheezes'. The presence of these sounds warrants further diagnostics prior to anesthesia.

Breathing

Assess movement of air through the airways by watching chest excursions (i.e., movement of the chest with each breath) and feeling for movement of air from the nostrils and/or mouth. Failure to move air normally can indicate severe respiratory disease which can significantly impact the safety of anesthesia. Further diagnostics are required prior to anesthesia.

Body Temperature

Is the temperature within the normal range? Either pyrexia or hypothermia can indicate the presence of disease that will impact the safety of anesthesia and both conditions should be investigated prior to anesthesia.

History

A thorough history that includes information on the patient's current condition and treatments, previous medical conditions and treatments, and any abnormalities in daily function (like eating and urinating) is important. The history should also include information on health conditions in the patient's family.

Recent Health Issues
Why has the patient been presented (if the patient is presented for a health concern) or has the patient been ill recently (if the patient is presented for an elective procedure and seems currently healthy)?

Current Medications
Especially medications that could affect anesthesia (like medications for cardiac disease) or analgesia (like nonsteroidal anti-inflammatory drugs **[NSAIDs]**). Also ask the client if the patient is on any herbal compounds as some of these can impact anesthesia.

Appetite, Urination and Defecation
Any recent changes in these daily functions can indicate changes in health status that may not have been recognized by the owner.

Familial Health Issues
Do any siblings have health issues that need to be considered?

Other Tests
Other Tests may be Recommended or even Required for Specific Patients Prior to Anesthesia

Although preoperative serum chemistry analysis and complete blood count (or 'blood work') may not be necessary for all patients, preoperative blood work is often recommended to fully assess the health of the patient and because the scheduled anesthetic procedure may be the only time or first time the patient has been seen by a veterinarian. Thus, the preoperative blood work can provide a baseline not only for anesthesia but also for general patient health. Preoperative blood work should be required for geriatric & neonatal patients and patients that have systemic disease. Urinalysis should be considered in these patients and required in those with renal disease. The following tests should be considered and/or required, depending on the patient:
- Packed cell volume **(PCV)** and total protein **(TP)**, which is also called total solids **(TS)**.
- Renal enzymes (blood urea nitrogen **[BUN]** and creatinine).
- Hepatic enzymes (alkaline phosphatase **[ALP]**, alanine transaminase **[ALT]**).
- Electrolytes (sodium, chloride, potassium and calcium).
- Glucose, especially in neonate/pediatric patients and in diabetic patients.
- Urinalysis (urine specific gravity, perhaps protein, blood, glucose, electrolytes).

Other diagnostic tests may be appropriate for selected patients. Examples include:
- Thoracic radiographs or ultrasound for patients with respiratory or cardiovascular disease.
- Abdominal radiographs or ultrasound for patients with gastrointestinal or genitourinary disease.

- Abdominocentesis for patients with abdominal trauma or some forms of gastrointestinal disease.
- Neurologic exams for patients with central nervous system **(CNS)** disease or head trauma.
- Specific serum chemistry analysis tests, for example bile acids for liver disease and T4 for thyroid disease.
- Blood gas analysis for oxygenation for patients with severe respiratory disease.
- White blood cell count **(WBC)** in patients with suspected bacterial or viral diseases (such as parvovirus or feline immunodeficiency virus),
- Fecal analysis and blood smear for detection of parasites, which should be considered for assessment of overall health.

Patient Preparation and Stabilization
Appropriate Preparation is Required for every Patient Prior to Anesthesia and Stabilization may be Required for Specific Patients

Preparation is very patient specific. For healthy patients anesthetized for short, elective procedures, preparation may be nothing more than a thorough physical exam and history with, perhaps, PCV and TP. On the other end of the spectrum, preparation for critically ill patients likely means stabilization prior to anesthesia. Stabilization can occur over several days to weeks (e.g., stabilizing glucose levels using insulin in diabetics or controlling heart disease with drugs like pimobendin, enalapril and furosemide). Stabilization may also need to occur within minutes to hours (e.g., fluid loading a patient with an intestinal foreign body and perforated intestine) but it **SHOULD OCCUR**.

Increasing ASA status increases the risk for anesthetic adverse events (Brodbelt 2009). Thus, **DECREASING ASA** status should **DECREASE** anesthetic risk for morbidity and even mortality. The ASA status can be decreased by using patient-appropriate preparation and stabilization. For example, an anorexic, vomiting cat with a linear foreign body that is severely dehydrated and has electrolyte imbalances is an ASA status of IV. If intravenous fluids are administered to the cat, correcting dehydration and electrolyte balance prior to surgery, the ASA status decreases to III and the cat is at a lower risk for anesthetic morbidity/mortality.

Reference
Brodbelt D. Perioperative mortality in small animal anaesthesia Vet J 2009; 182:152-161.

Chapter 3
Anesthesia Machines and Equipment

Shona Meyer, BS, LVT, VTS (Anesthesia/Analgesia)

"To be prepared is half the victory" Miguel de Cervantes

Introduction

A thorough knowledge of anesthesia equipment and breathing systems, along with appropriate maintenance and trouble-shooting techniques, is vital. This is best expressed by this quote: "The integrity of the anesthesia system is a critical part of the entire anesthesia process. If you consider that the job of the anesthesia machine is to supply every life giving breath to a patient while intentionally maintaining the animal in a comatose state, you will understand the need for these units to function properly" (Harvey 2010).

An effective way to organize the understanding of all of the components of anesthesia equipment is to trace the flow of oxygen through the system. Oxygen is supplied by an oxygen supply source (usually a compressed gas cylinder or 'tank'), makes its way through a variety of hoses and pressure regulators and then enters the anesthesia machine where the flow is divided with part going to the oxygen 'flush' button (or flush 'valve') and part to the flow meter control knob. It continues to move through the flowmeter, vaporizer, and the fresh gas outlet, into the breathing system and to the patient. Excess oxygen and inhalant gases, along with carbon dioxide, then move from the patient back through the breathing system to the waste anesthetic gas scavenging system. The main components of the anesthesia machine will be discussed in this chapter. A checklist to help you through the daily process of checking the machine is presented in **Table 3-6** at the end of the chapter.

The Anesthesia Machine

The anesthesia machine, along with the oxygen source and the vaporizer, is designed to deliver a precise, but changeable, mixture of anesthetic gas and oxygen at a safe pressure and flow to a breathing system, which in turn delivers anesthetic gas and oxygen to a patient. Although there are quite a variety of machines in use in veterinary medicine, they all have the same function and the components are similar for almost all of the machines that might be encountered. This information will be applicable to a machine in any practice, even if your machine does not look like those in these photos.

Anesthesia machines, like those in **Figure 3-1 A and B**, look like a lot of hardware. The anesthesia machine, however, only includes the connection between the oxygen source and oxygen regulator(s) on the back of the machine (not pictured here), the gas flow meter(s) *(Figure 3-2 A)*, the emergency oxygen 'flush' valve *(Figure 3-2 B)*, a scavenger connection *(Figure 3-2 K)*, and a common or "fresh" gas outlet (See **Figure 3-3**). The vaporizer *(Figure 3-2 C)* is added to the machine to supply inhalant anesthetics. All the rest of the components are actually part of the breathing system *(Figure 3-2 D through J)*.

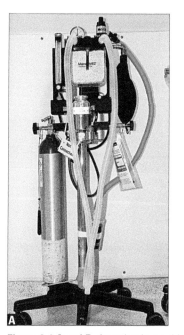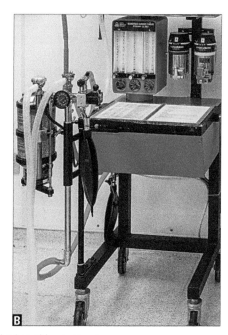

Figure 3-1 A and B. Anesthesia machines and rebreathing systems.

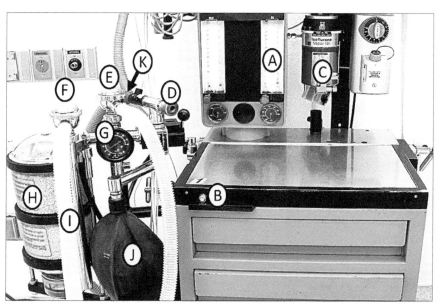

Figure 3-2. The anesthesia machine only includes the connection between the oxygen source and oxygen regulator(s) on the back of the machine (not shown), the gas flow meter(s) *(A)*, the oxygen 'flush button' *(B)*, a scavenger connection *(K)*, and a common or "fresh" gas outlet (see figure 3-3). The vaporizer *(C)* is added to the machine to supply inhalant anesthetics. All the other components shown are part of the rebreathing system *(D-J)*.

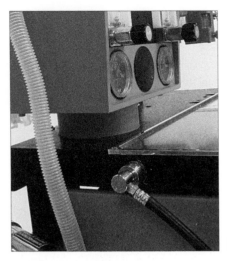

Figure 3-3. The common or "fresh "gas outlet.

Pressure Circuits

The machine is divided into three pressure circuits, named according to the amount of pneumatic (air) pressure within each circuit. Many of these components go relatively unnoticed because we don't change them, open/close them, etc... However, understanding all of these components will allow trouble shooting if the need arises.

High-Pressure Circuit

Consists of components which receive gas at high cylinder pressure (2200 pounds per square inch or 'psi'). These include the hanger yoke (including filter and unidirectional valve), yoke block, cylinder pressure gauge and cylinder pressure regulators **(Figure 3-4)**. We deal with this circuit when we place an oxygen tank onto a machine (into the hanger yoke) and when we check the pressure in the tank by looking at the cylinder pressure gauge (See Figure 3-9).

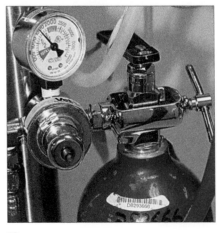

Figure 3-4. The hanger yoke, at the top of the green cylinder, is the metal portion that holds the tank to the machine and connects with the pin system to allow oxygen to flow from the tank to the machine.

Intermediate Pressure Circuit

This circuit receives gases at intermediate, relatively constant pressures (37 to 55 psi), which is pipeline pressure, or the pressure 'downstream'- meaning closer to the patient - from a cylinder regulator. The components of this circuit include the pipeline inlets and pressure gauges, ventilator power inlet, flowmeter valves, second-stage regulators and oxygen flush valve. We deal with this circuit often because we adjust the oxygen flowing through the flowmeter by turning the flow meter valve and we sometimes use the oxygen flush valve **(Figure 3-5)**. Now you understand why we have to be careful using the oxygen flush valve [or 'button'] - flow from here is at a higher pressure than in any other part of the circuit that is in direct contact with the patient!

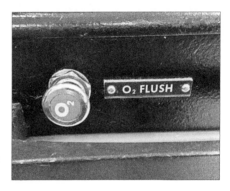

Figure 3-5. The oxygen "flush" or emergency oxygen flush button.

Low-Pressure Circuit

These are components downstream from the flowmeter needle, including valves, flowmeter tubes, vaporizers **(Figure 3-6)** and the common (fresh) gas outlet (See figure 3-3). Clearly, this is the circuit that we will interact with the most since all of the components listed are used to deliver oxygen and fresh gas directly to the patient and most are components that we adjust during anesthesia.

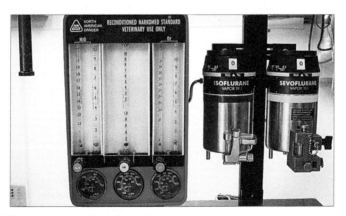

Figure 3-6. Flow meters and Vaporizers. These and the fresh gas outlet are the components of the low pressure system that we most commonly deal with.

Important Components

Familiarity with all machine components is ideal but perhaps not critical. However, a thorough understanding of the components that are most commonly used or whose misuse is most likely to result in danger to the patient is critical.

Oxygen Source

Oxygen is generally supplied as compressed gas in metal cylinders (or 'tanks'). One of the most common sources of oxygen is the E-cylinder or tank **(Figure 3-7)** which is the small, portable tank generally attached to the anesthesia machine. The E tank contains about 700 liters of oxygen. H-cylinders or tanks are also used but H tanks are generally stationary and are used with a hospital line that ends in a ceiling drop or wall mount connection **(Figure 3-8)**. The H tank is larger and holds about 7000 liters of oxygen. Larger tanks or oxygen concentrators or even liquid oxygen are other sources of oxygen that are sometimes utilized. The content of the oxygen tanks should be checked every morning (for the H tanks) and before every surgery (for the E tanks).

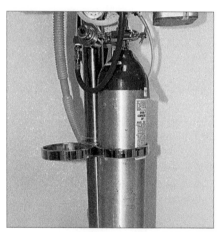

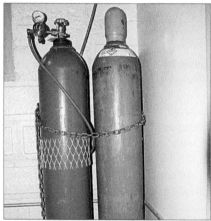

Figure 3-7. A machine- mounted 'E tank' or 'E cylinder'. This tank holds approximately 700 liters of oxygen when full. Note the green color (specific for oxygen) around the top of the tank.

Figure 3-8. An 'H tank' or 'H cylinder'. Oxygen lines from the tank can deliver oxygen to oxygen connections throughout the hospital. This tank holds approximately 7000 liters of oxygen when full. Note the green color.

How to: Determine how much Oxygen is Left in the Cylinder

The amount of oxygen in the cylinders in liters can be estimated by multiplying the pressure seen on the cylinder gauge **(Figure 3-9)** by 3 for the H tanks and by 0.3 for the E tanks.

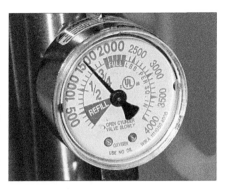

Figure 3-9. Pressure gauge on an oxygen tank. There are 450 liters of oxygen remaining in this E tank (1500 psi x 0.3 = 450). To determine how long the oxygen in the tank will last, divide the liters in the tank by the current oxygen flow on the oxygen flow meter.

IMPORTANT TIP
Oxygen cylinders should definitely be changed when the pressure gauge indicates that the pressure is below 200 psi. A pressure of below 500 psi may be grounds for changing the tank if the tank will be used heavily. If 500 psi is multiplied by 0.3 (E tank), we know that 150 liters are left in the cylinder. If the patient is on a non-rebreathing system with a 3 liter per minute flow, this tank will only last 50 minutes (150 L divided by 3 L/min = 50 minutes)!

For safety, all medical gases are housed in color-specific tanks or are supplied from a central source by color-specific lines **(Table 3-1)**. Tanks and lines also have a 'pin-index' safety system. In this system, the pins (meaning the parts that protrude) on the gas line or hanger yoke fit into the holes that are 'indexed' or specifically configured for each individual gas. Therefore, only the tank or line with the correct pin-index system can be attached in the specific position that is designed for that gas.

Table 3-1
Cylinders/Lines are Color Coded for Safety Purposes

Gas	Formula	United States	State in Cylinder
Oxygen	O_2	Green	Gas
Nitrous oxide	N_2O	Blue	Gas + Liquid (below 98°F)

CRITICAL TIP!
Medical gas equipment is color coded. The color for oxygen equipment in the US is green. Make sure that only tanks or lines colored green are connected to the oxygen port on the anesthesia machine.

The color for oxygen equipment in the US is green and the pin-index safety system for oxygen can be seen in **Figure 3-10**. The small pin holes for oxygen are linear and centered, whereas those for nitrous oxide are slightly off-center **(Figure 3-11)**.

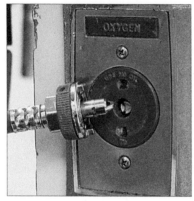

Figure 3-10. Pin-index safety system. The pins (parts that protrude) on the gas line fit into the holes that are specifically located for each individual gas. This is the pin index configuration for oxygen. This connection is for oxygen lines, the exact same configuration of pins and holes is present on an oxygen tank and the hanger yoke on the back of the anesthesia machine.

Although not part of every machine and not commonly used in veterinary medicine, nitrous oxide **(N_2O)** deserves mention because it is also supplied in a cylinder and is delivered as an inhaled gas along with oxygen. The color in the US for nitrous oxide is blue. Nitrous oxide is present as both a liquid and a gas in a cylinder (oxygen is present only as a gas), but the pressure gauge reads only the gas state. Thus, the pressure gauge is not completely indicative of the amount of nitrous oxide left in the cylinder since liquid continues to evaporate as the gas leaves the tank and the pressure in the tank will not change until all of the liquid has evaporated.

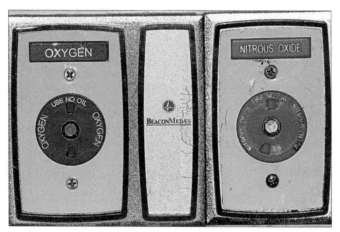

Figure 3-11. In the pin index safety system, the small pin holes for oxygen are linear and centered, while those for nitrous oxide are slightly off-center so that the lines for oxygen will not fit into the connection for nitrous oxide. The connections are colored green (for oxygen) and blue (for nitrous oxide).

How to: Determine how much Nitrous Oxide is Left in the Cylinder

Vaporized nitrous oxide leaves the tank and more vapor is produced from the liquid. The pressure in the tank remains the same as long as there is any liquid remaining.

Generally, when the pressure reaches approximately 745 psi, the cylinder is less than one-fourth full (approximately 400 L of nitrous oxide) and there is no liquid remaining. The pressure will start to decrease rapidly at this point and the tank should be changed when the pressure gauge reads less than 500 psi. The contents can also be measured by weighing the tank and subtracting the empty weight (which should be stamped on the neck of the tank).

CRITICAL TIP!

Nitrous oxide takes the place of some of the oxygen in the inhaled gas. To prevent hypoxemia in the patient, the nitrous oxide should never be more than 75% of the inhaled gas. So, for instance, a flow of 250 ml of oxygen + 750 ml of nitrous oxide would result in 75% of the inhaled gas being nitrous oxide. In most patients, a 50:50 mixture of oxygen and nitrous oxide is preferred.

Because cylinders of compressed gas (oxygen, nitrous oxide, etc.) are highly pressurized, they can cause severe damage if they fall and break at the neck. The compressed gas will immediately exit the cylinder and the cylinder will be rapidly and forcefully propelled in a direction away from the neck. ALL STANDING TANKS MUST BE SECURED SO THEY CANNOT FALL. Alternatively, tanks can be stored in a laying rather than a standing position **(Figure 3-12)**. Be extremely careful when handling cylinders of compressed gas that you do not drop them or put them in a position from which they could fall. Also, cylinders should never be subjected to temperatures above 54°C (130°F) or below -7°C (20°F). Pressure (and liquid volume for N_2O) will change as the environmental temperature changes.

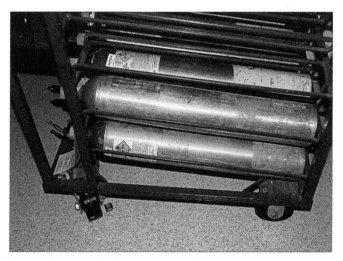

Figure 3-12. Oxygen tanks are highly pressurized and become extremely dangerous projectiles if they fall and break. Tanks should be secured if standing, or stored on their sides.

Oxygen Flush Button
(Figure 3-13)

The oxygen flush button, or 'emergency oxygen flush button', is a part of the intermediate pressure system and is a machine component that everyone should be extremely familiar with. The oxygen flush is designed to rapidly fill the entire breathing system with oxygen in the event of an anesthetic emergency. Oxygen flow from the flush button bypasses the vaporizer, and does not deliver inhalant, therefore diluting the inhalant anesthetic concentration that is in the breathing system. Rapidly decreasing the inhalant anesthetic concentration is useful in an emergency since a light plane of anesthesia - or even a quick return to consciousness - may be the goal. But for most anesthetized patients, rapid return to consciousness in the middle of a surgical procedure is probably not the goal. In these patients, flow through the oxygen flowmeters should be increased if more oxygen is needed. This flow is delivered at a clinically appropriate pressure through the vaporizer, causing neither excessive pressures in the breathing system nor dilution of anesthetic gas.

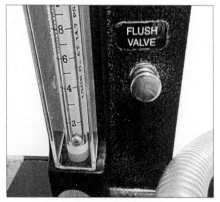

Figure 3-13. The oxygen "flush" or emergency 'flush' button is designed to rapidly fill the entire breathing system with oxygen in an emergency. Oxygen delivered when pressing this button is at high flow (35-75 liters/min) and high pressure (50-60 psi), which can be very dangerous for the patient. The button is placed in a very obvious or protected spot so that it is never accidentally pushed.

Because the objective is a rapid filling of the system, the flush generates high flows (usually somewhere between 35 and 75 liters per minute) at fairly high pressures (generally 50 to 60 psi). This flow can be quite excessive and flushing the anesthetic system can easily lead to barotrauma (damage to the lungs from high pressure) if used inappropriately. Thus, the flush button is generally protected so that it cannot accidentally be pushed and it should never be used in small patients (less than 5 kg) or in patients on non-rebreathing systems or in systems in which the pressure reducing valve, or 'pop-off valve' is closed. In any of these scenarios, the pressure in the entire system will increase dangerously fast and can cause serious injury to the patient.

CRITICAL TIP!
The oxygen flush button delivers a high volume of oxygen in a very short period of time and the pressure produced by this action can easily lead to barotrauma. DO NOT USE THE FLUSH BUTTON IN SMALL PATIENTS OR IN PATIENTS ON A NONREBREATHING SYSTEM.

CRITICAL TIP!
Using the oxygen flush button will dilute the anesthetic gas in the breathing system and can lead to rapid awakening of the patient. ONLY USE THE FLUSH VALVE IF YOU WANT THE PATIENT TO WAKE UP QUICKLY.

IMPORTANT POINT
Oxygen flow from the flowmeters is delivered at a clinically appropriate pressure through the vaporizer, therefore adjusting the flowmeter should be used to safely increase oxygen flow in a system when increased oxygen is needed but dilution of the inhalant is not desirable.

Flowmeters

Flowmeters adjust the higher pressures and flows from the intermediate pressure system to low pressures and flows that are clinically appropriate for the patient. This allows safe delivery of oxygen (also called the 'carrier gas') and anesthetic gases to the patient. Because each gas (e.g., oxygen, nitrous oxide, air) has physical properties that will affect its flow, each gas has a dedicated flowmeter that allows calibrated delivery of that gas. Oxygen flowmeters are the most commonly used in veterinary medicine and they are colored green. Nitrous oxide is also sometimes used in veterinary medicine and the flow meter is colored blue. Other gases, like air, may be used in some machines. For oxygen flow, some machines have one flowmeter that goes from 0 to 10 liters **(Figure 3-14 A)** and some have two flowmeters, one of which goes from 0 to 1 liters and the other which goes from 1 to 10 liters **(Figure 3-14 B)**. It is crucial for safe and appropriate oxygen flow to the patient that the type of flowmeter on your machine be identified and that everyone in the practice be taught to read the scale accurately. To determine the precise flow from either type of flowmeter, look at the 'float' in the flowmeter. Except for the ball float, which is the most common type of float in veterinary machines, read the flow at the top of the float. For the ball float read the flow at the middle of the ball **(Figure 3-15)**.

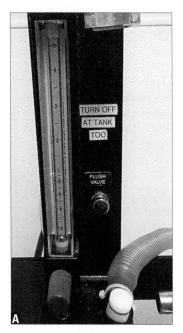

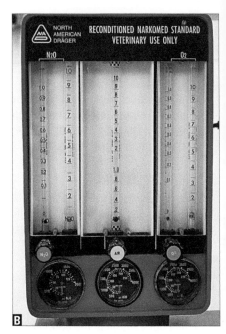

Figure 3-14. Oxygen flowmeters can be calibrated as one flowmeter that provides flows of 0-1 and then 1+ liters/min on the same flowmeter. Note that the lower end of the flowmeter indicates 200 mls-1 liter/min and the upper end indicates 1-4 liters/min **(A)**. Flowmeters can also be calibrated as a dual system, with one flowmeter providing flows of 0-1 liters/min and one providing flows of 1+ (usually 10) liters/min **(B)**.

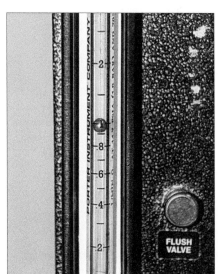

Figure 3-15. To determine the precise flow, read the flow at the middle of the ball. The flow in this photo is slightly less than 1 liter/min. If the flowmeter has a 'bobbin' or rectangular shaped float, read the flow at the top of the float.

Vaporizers
(Figure 3-16)

The vaporizer is not really part of the anesthesia machine. It is added to the machine in order to supply inhalant anesthetic gas. Modern vaporizers, like those used in most veterinary practices are precision vaporizers, meaning that they deliver an exact percentage of anesthetic gas. They are variable bypass vaporizers, meaning that, based on the dial setting of the vaporizer, a variable amount of the oxygen flow will bypass the vaporizing chamber inside the vaporizer. This alters the amount of anesthetic gas that is vaporized and subsequently delivered to the patient when the dial setting on the vaporizer is altered. The vaporizers are flow and temperature compensated so that reasonable changes in oxygen flow or ambient temperature will not affect the vaporizer output. However, many vaporizers will not deliver an accurate concentration of gas below a minimum oxygen flow of 500 ml/min and extremes of temperature can affect vaporizer output (too hot = increased output, too cold = decreased output). They are gas (or 'agent') specific, requiring a separate vaporizer for each anesthetic inhalant gas (e.g., isoflurane, sevoflurane). If the incorrect gas is used in a vaporizer, an unpredictable amount of gas concentration is delivered to the patient and this can be extremely dangerous as the concentration may result in an overdose. If the vaporizer, is filled with an incorrect inhalant liquid, the vaporizer must be completely drained and all liquid discarded. Oxygen should flow through the vaporizer (5 L/min for 45 minutes) then the vaporizer should be filled with the correct inhalant liquid or the vaporizer should be sent in for servicing.

Vaporizers should not be tilted or tipped. If tipped more than 45°, liquid inhalant may have entered the bypass chamber/outlet which could dangerously increase the output concentration of inhalant gas. This must be fixed before the vaporizer can be used.

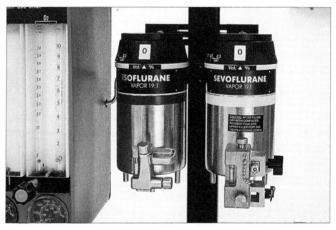

Figure 3-16. Vaporizers are added to the machine to provide inhalant anesthesia. All oxygen, except that delivered by using the oxygen flush valve, flows through the vaporizers if they are turned on. A variable amount of oxygen, controlled by the vaporizer dial, is moved through the vaporizing chamber (the location of the liquid inhalant) to produce a variable percent of inhalant gas (isoflurane on the left, sevoflurane on the right).

How to: Fix a Vaporizer that has been Tipped

The liquid must be removed from the bypass chamber before the vaporizer can be used on a patient. To remove the liquid place a rebreathing bag on the end of the breathing hoses, turn on the vaporizer and set a fresh gas flow of 5 L for ten minutes. Be sure that the scavenging system is connected. Alternatively, do not use the vaporizer for 24hrs while the vaporizer is left standing upright.

Vaporizers should not be overfilled - this may lead to liquid anesthetic leaking out of the filling chamber and contaminating the room with vapor. Vaporizers should be cleaned, and recalibrated every 1 to 3 years depending on recommendations from the manufacturer and actual use of the equipment. At the very least a calibration/inspection should be performed whenever a sudden or major change in dial settings is consistently required to maintain the desired level of anesthesic depth.

CRITICAL TIP!

Treat your vaporizers very carefully or they may deliver the wrong gas concentration to the patient! Don't use the wrong drug in the vaporizer, do not tip the vaporizer and do not overfill the vaporizer.

Common or 'Fresh' Gas Outlet and Inlet
(See Figure 3-3)

The common or fresh gas outlet is where fresh gas - which is defined as oxygen alone or oxygen PLUS anesthetic inhalant gas - will exit the machine and enter the breathing system. All of the oxygen from the flow meter will pass through the vaporizer and some oxygen will mix with anesthetic gases if the vaporizer is on. The amount of oxygen and anesthetic vapor - or 'fresh gas' - exiting the machine will depend on the oxygen flow and the vaporizer setting. Remember, as discussed previously, oxygen from the emergency flush valve does not flow through the vaporizer but instead will join the fresh gas flow further downstream. The fresh gas inlet is on the other end of the tubing that exits at the fresh gas outlet. The fresh gas inlet is where the gas enters the breathing system.

CRITICAL TIP!

If you are changing between rebreathing and nonrebreathing systems, MAKE SURE that the common gas outlet is connected to the breathing system that you are using.

Waste Anesthetic Gas Scavenging System

Although the interface between the anesthetic machine and the scavenging system is part of the machine, the actual scavenging system is not technically a part of the machine. However, this is an important component of any anesthetic system.

Scavenging of waste anesthetic gases is required, REGARDLESS of which breathing system is used. This is because human exposure to high concentrations of waste gases is unacceptable and can result in health issues.

There are three main ways to scavenge waste anesthetic gases. 1) Active scavenging utilizing a light vacuum, or negative pressure, from a central hospital line **(Figure 3-17 A)**, 2) passive scavenging which allows waste gases to passively move through a long tube to the outside of the building or to a well-ventilated, low-traffic area, and 3) use of a charcoal canister to filter inhalant gases (e.g., Omincom f/air®) **(Figure 3-17 B)**. The charcoal canister is probably the most commonly used system in veterinary medicine. The canister should be weighed frequently and should be changed when its weight has increased by 50 grams or after 12 hours of use with inhalant anesthetics.

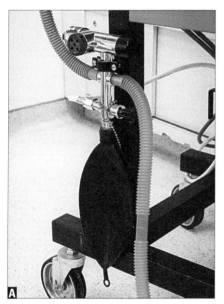 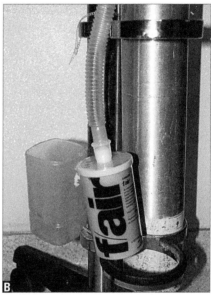

Figure 3-17. The waste gas scavenging system. This photo demonstrates active scavenging utilizing a light vacuum, from a central hospital line **(A)** and a charcoal canister to filter inhalant gases (Omincom f/air) **(B)**.

How to: Choose an Anesthesia Machine

Because almost all of the anesthesia machines in veterinary medicine function similarly, almost any machine that works for your practice is a good choice. Our recommendation is to choose based on: 1) customer service of the company that sells the machine since follow-up service is critical; and 2) components that are useful to your practice, e.g., do you need a movable machine? Or maybe a table-top machine? Do you need a machine that fits into a very small space? Or a big machine with a work table and shelves for monitors and other equipment? Whatever your needs are, you can find a machine to fit! Then take care of your machine!

Breathing Systems

Breathing circuits or systems move the oxygen and inhalant gas from the fresh gas inlet through a hose to the patient, and then carry 'waste' anesthetic gases (i.e., inhalant anesthetic that was exhaled from the patient or was never inhaled and just circulated through the breathing system) and carbon dioxide (CO_2) back through a hose away from the patient to the waste gas scavenging outlet. Breathing systems are classified as rebreathing (**Figure 3-18**) or non-rebreathing (**Figure 3-19**). Both of these systems include common components from the fresh gas inlet to the scavenging outlet, but there are some major differences between the two systems, including the system-specific components, the mechanism to eliminate CO_2 and the rate of oxygen flow.

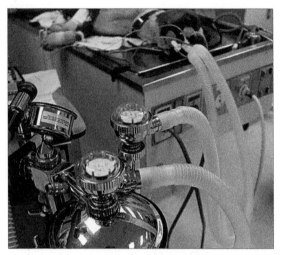

Figure 3-18. A rebreathing or 'circle' system on an anesthetized dog. Note typical components of the rebreathing system including the unidirectional valves, the carbon dioxide absorbent canister, (at bottom of this photo) and the inspiratory and expiratory breathing hoses.

REMINDER
'Fresh gas' is any gas that enters the breathing system from the anesthetic machine and has not yet been breathed by the patient. It is usually a mix of oxygen and inhalant gas but could be oxygen alone.

Rebreathing System
The most commonly used breathing system is called a **'rebreathing system'** (often called a 'circle' system). In this system, some fresh gas enters the circuit but the exhaled gases are also partially recirculated & rebreathed by the patient and partially evacuated into the scavenging system. Because the exhaled gases contain CO_2, there must be a mechanism to remove the CO_2 before the gas is re-delivered to the patient. The components in the system that prevent rebreathing of CO_2 (the CO_2 absorbent and the unidirectional valves) also create resistance to breathing, which

30

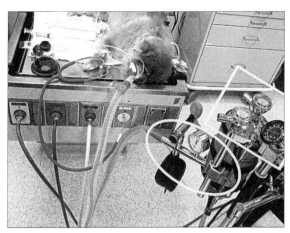

Figure 3-19. A nonrebreathing system on an anesthetized dog. Note the coaxial breathing tube and the Bain mount (in the oval) attached to the pole of the rebreathing system by a bracket (the component with the red paint). The Bain mount has a pressure gauge, pressure relief valve and bag for giving the patient a breath. Note the components of the rebreathing system on the machine (in the square). The one-way valves, pressure gauge, pressure relief valve and carbon dioxide absorbent are all clearly visible and it is obvious that no breathing hoses are connected to the ports near the one-way valves.

increases the work of breathing. This increase has minimal impact on medium to large patients but can decrease respiratory efficiency in small patients. Thus, this system is most appropriate for patients that weigh MORE than 5 kg.

IMPORTANT POINT
Although a rebreathing (circle) system is not ideal for patients less than 5 kg, a pediatric circle system can be used if a non-rebreathing circuit is not available. The pediatric circle system has a much smaller volume than the standard adult system and can be used for small patients to increase respiratory efficiency.

Oxygen Flow in the Rebreathing System
The oxygen flow is typically 20 to 40 ml/kg/min, allowing what is technically called 'partial rebreathing' because some of the gas is rebreathed but some of the gas is fresh gas delivered directly from the machine. Total rebreathing of all exhaled gases can be achieved with a lower oxygen flow of 3 to 10 ml/kg/min and this is called 'low flow' anesthesia. This flow will meet, but not exceed, the patient's metabolic oxygen consumption rate so there is only a minimal amount of wasted gas. However, many vaporizers may not deliver accurate concentrations of inhalant gas at flows below 500ml/minute, thus flows below this rate are not recommended.

With either partial or total rebreathing, higher oxygen flow rates, for example 2 to 3 liters per minute, should be used at induction to rapidly fill the entire system, including the patient's airways, with oxygen. This is often called 'denitrogenation' because the nitrogen from room air is replaced with oxygen in the lungs, allowing the patient to oxygenate more effectively. Denitrogenation takes about 5 minutes (up to 10 in large patients) and then the oxygen flow should be turned down to the level described above to reduce oxygen/inhalant waste. Higher gas flows can be used again in recovery with a rebreathing system to help speed the clearance of exhaled gases.

Rebreathing System Advantages
Low gas flows in this system are more economical & minimize environmental contamination. Rebreathed gas is warmer and more humid than fresh gas, which is better for the patient's airways and for maintenance of adequate body temperature.

Rebreathing System Disadvantages
Low gas flows reduce the speed at which a change in anesthesia depth will occur. The components of this system are numerous, making the system bulky and somewhat expensive. The carbon dioxide absorbent adds to the cost and the absorbent can sometimes introduce dust to the breathing system. The absorbent canister is a common site for leaks in the anesthesia circuit. Both the carbon dioxide absorbent and the unidirectional valves cause an increase in resistance to breathing making the system less ideal for very small patients.

Components of the Rebreathing System
The components of the rebreathing system in the order that they are encountered by the fresh gas flow circulating through most systems are: the inspiratory unidirectional (or 'one-way') valve, the inspiratory breathing hose, the Y piece, the expiratory breathing hose, the expiratory unidirectional (or 'one way valve'), the carbon dioxide absorbent and canister, the reservoir bag and the scavenging system.

Unidirectional Valves: There are two unidirectional valves **(Figure 3-20)**, the inspiratory valve opens on inspiration (or inhalation) and is closed during exhalation. The expiratory valve opens on expiration (or exhalation) and is closed during inhalation. These valve movements create a unidirectional flow of gases and prevents rebreathing of exhaled gases prior to their exposure to carbon dioxide absorbent. The valves on all machines are almost always located near the carbon dioxide absorbent canister, and the expiratory valve is generally closest to the pressure relief valve (or 'pop off' valve) and the rebreathing bag. Fortunately, these valves are labeled on most machines.

The valves can create a few problems. They increase resistance to breathing, thus, are absent in non-rebreathing systems. The valves must be movable. Sometimes the valves can stick in the closed, or even the open, position and this can drastically alter respiratory function.

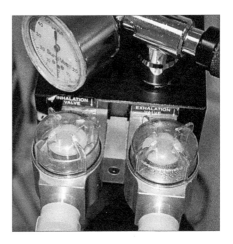

Figure 3-20. Unidirectional valves. There are two unidirectional valves in the rebreathing system. The valves on all machines are usually located near the absorbent canister, and the expiratory valve is generally closest to the pressure relief valve and the rebreathing bag.

CRITICAL TIP!

Appropriate valve maintenance is critical to normal function of the rebreathing system. The dome housing that covers the valve should be opened and the valves dried and then carefully replaced, to avoid them sticking open or closed. Then the dome housing should be tightly screwed back on. The frequency of valve maintenance depends on your surgery case load. Certainly it should be done anytime that you see condensation build up on the domes. If you have a high case load, the valves should be dried at the end of each surgery day. Also, the valves should be checked during pressure checking of the machine to insure that they move (Figure 3-21 A & B).

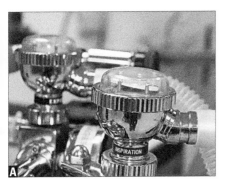 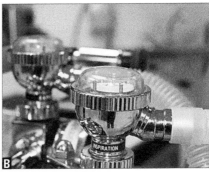

Figure 3-21. The inspiratory unidirectional valve opens on inspiration (the white disc or 'valve' is slightly elevated) **(A)** and is closed during exhalation (the white disc is flat) **(B)**. The expiratory valve (in the background of the photo) opens on expiration and closes during inhalation. These valve movements create a unidirectional flow of gases and prevents rebreathing of exhaled gases prior to their exposure to carbon dioxide absorbent.

Breathing Hoses: The breathing hoses consist of an inspiratory limb, the 'Y piece' between the two limbs, and an expiratory limb **(Figure 3-22)**. The inspiratory limb of the hoses runs from the inspiratory valve to the Y-piece and the expiratory limb of

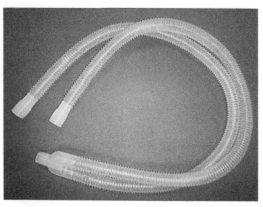

Figure 3-22. In a rebreathing system, the breathing hoses consist of an inspiratory limb, the 'Y piece' between the two limbs, and an expiratory limb. The 'Y piece' (at the bottom left) attaches to the endotracheal tube and the ends of the breathing hoses (at the top left) attach to the ports for the inspiratory and expiratory unidirectional valves.

the hoses runs from the Y-piece to the expiratory valve. The patient's endotracheal tube (ET) is connected to the system at the Y-piece. Breathing hoses are generally made of light, flexible rubber or plastic and are corrugated to prevent kinking. They are often clear so that the internal surfaces can be observed for cleanliness and accumulation of condensation. Ideally, the hoses and Y-piece should be rinsed with clean water daily and sterilized or discarded if contaminated with any material that could be hazardous to other patients. Breathing hoses come in pediatric, standard adult, and large animal versions. The hoses can be as long as necessary keeping in mind that as the length of the hoses increases so does the work of breathing (because of increased resistance) and the overall volume of the breathing system, which increases the amount of time required for a change in anesthetic depth following a change in vaporizer setting. As the diameter of the hoses increases, the resistance to breathing decreases and the internal diameter of the breathing tubes should always be larger than the internal diameter of the patient's ET tube. The Y-piece (or Y-connector) between the inhalation and exhalation hoses should contain a septum to decrease deadspace and keep the gas flow unidirectional, which decreases the potential for rebreathing of carbon dioxide **(Figure 3-23)**.

REMINDER
'Deadspace' is space in the breathing system where inhaled gases and exhaled gases mix, forcing the patient to rebreathe carbon dioxide (CO_2). The breathing system should have minimal dead space.

Carbon Dioxide Absorbent Granules and Canister(s): The carbon dioxide absorbent granules and canister(s) **(Figure 3-24)** are critical components of the rebreathing system because they remove CO_2 from the breathing system, thereby preventing rebreathing of CO_2. The granules are able to remove CO_2 because the CO_2 is an acid

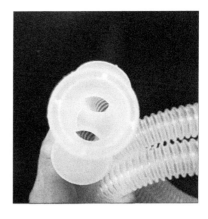

Figure 3-23. The Y-piece (or Y-connector) between the inhalation and exhalation hoses should contain a septum to keep the flow unidirectional and decrease the potential for rebreathing carbon dioxide. This is the view looking directly into the Y-piece. The septum is in the middle of the photo and corrugated tubing from the inspiratory and expiratory limbs of the breathing hoses are on either side of the septum.

that can be buffered by a base, and the absorbent is a base. This chemical reaction creates moisture, heat and a pH change - and the color indicators in the absorbent granules are pH sensitive so the pH change causes the blue or purple color to appear (or it may turn another color depending on the type of absorbent).

CRITICAL TIP!
When ⅔ of the granules in the canister have changed color, the absorbent should be changed. Remember that the color of the granules may revert to white if the machine is not being used but this does NOT mean that efficacy of the absorbent has returned. The absorbent is still exhausted and ineffective and must be changed.

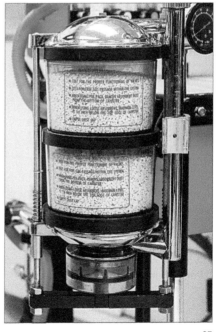

Figure 3-24. The carbon dioxide absorbent granules, here in a dual canister, remove carbon dioxide (CO_2) from the rebreathing system. The canister should be filled to about 70% of capacity and a small space of 1 to 3 inches should be left between the top of the canister and the absorbent granules for initial distribution of air flow. Note the space at the top of the canister in this photo and in Figure 3-26).

CRITICAL TIP!

It is the presence of effective absorbent granules that insures that only exhaled oxygen and anesthetic gas are rebreathed by the patient on the next inspiration. Ineffective or 'exhausted' (in other words, 'used') granules will allow carbon dioxide to build up in the system and may result in a hypercarbic (high CO_2) patient with respiratory acidosis.

If in doubt, check the consistency of the absorbent granules. Fresh absorbent is very brittle and 'crumbly' but exhausted granules are hard. Better yet, keep a log for each canister and change the canister after 10 to 12 hours of use. Another good way to determine the efficacy of the absorbent is to measure carbon dioxide in the system with an end-tidal carbon dioxide monitor (see Chapter 5) and change the absorbent when the inspired carbon dioxide in the system starts to increase. Normally, there is no inspired carbon dioxide in an appropriately functioning rebreathing system. Finally, the CO_2 absorbent should also be changed if unused for longer than 30 days.

CRITICAL TIP!

If the anesthesia machine is not being used but the oxygen flow is left on, the absorbent will be desiccated (dry), not able to absorb exhaled gases, and carbon monoxide may have formed. This is very dangerous! Change the granules before using the machine.

The total volume of the absorbent canister that holds the granules should be at least twice the patient's tidal volume, which is 10 to 15 mls/kilogram. This is because the capacity of the canister must be large enough to allow a patient to inhale or exhale a maximum tidal volume.

The canister or the canister attachment on the machine is generally constructed with screens (Figure 3-25) to prevent dust and granules from entering the breathing system and with baffles (Figure 3-26) to prevent channeling. An excessive amount of dust in the granules will cause an increase in airway resistance as well as causing

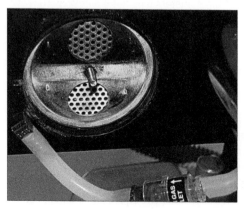

Figure 3-25. The canister or the canister attachment on the machine is generally constructed with screens to prevent dust and granules from entering the breathing system.

36

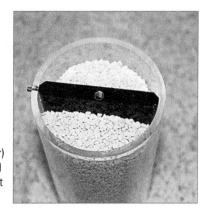

Figure 3-26. Most canisters have 'baffles' or partitions (the black object in the middle of the canister) to prevent channeling which occurs when exhaled gas follows set routes through the canister without dissipating throughout the absorbent granules.

dust to accumulate in the breathing circuit and potentially breathed by the patient. If your absorbent is excessively 'dusty' or powdery, pour it very slowly into the canister and consider buying a different brand for future use. Return excessively dusty absorbent to the manufacturer.

Channeling occurs when exhaled gas follows set paths or 'channels' through the canister without dissipating throughout all of the granules in the canister. This causes rapid exhaustion of the absorbent along the path of the exhaled gases and leaves the rest of the granules unused and wasted. Unfortunately, channeling is often undetected and carbon dioxide can begin to build up in the system. To prevent channeling, the absorbent canister must be filled correctly. It should be gently tapped as it is filled to allow the granules to spread uniformly throughout the canister and should be shaken lightly from side to side before being placed on the machine. Also, a small space of 1 to 3 inches should be left between the top of the canister and the absorbent granules for initial distribution of air flow (See Figures 3-24 and 3-26). The gap at the top should result in a canister that is filled approximately 70% of its capacity with granules.

If a double-chamber absorbent canister is used (See Figure 3-24), canisters can be rotated once by reversing the positions of the canisters (i.e., put the bottom canister on top) when ⅔ of the granules in the top canister have turned blue, then replace all of the absorbent when the granules in the canister that you moved turn blue.

Reservoir Bag: The reservoir bag or 'rebreathing bag' has several functions in the system.

The bag is a reservoir of gases to be inhaled so that a patient that takes a maximum inspiratory breath (i.e., very deep breath) won't totally empty the entire breathing system. The bag is also a safety reservoir for exhaled gases and excess volume of gases that could over-pressurize the system, as when the oxygen flush button is used. Finally, the bag provides a means of delivering positive pressure ventilation to the patient - simply by closing the pressure relief valve and squeezing the bag. For small animals, 0.5, 1, 2, 3 and 5 L bags are commonly used **(Figure 3-27)**. A guideline for size: the bag volume should be 4 to 6 times the patient's tidal volume (10 to 15 ml/kg). Some approximate bag sizes can be seen in the chart **(Table 3-2)**. If the bag is too small, inspiratory demand (i.e., a deep breath) may exceed bag capacity and the patient will empty the entire breathing system, causing the potential for the development of extreme negative pressures in the respiratory system, which can cause damage to the patient's lungs. If the bag is too large, the anesthetist cannot easily visualize respirations or estimate tidal volume because the small tidal volume of the patient will not make the bag move appreciably. Also, the anesthetic depth cannot be changed quickly without emptying the bag and starting over. This is because the capacity of the bag far exceeds the capacity of the patient's respiratory system.

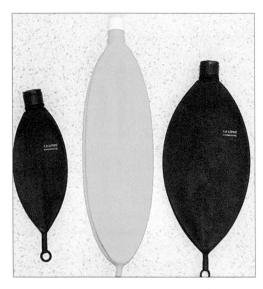

Figure 3-27. Different sized rebreathing bags, from left to right, one liter, five liter and three liter.

Table 3-2
Approximate Reservoir Bag Sizes by Weight of Patient

Body Weight in Kgs ('size' of patient)	Recommended volume of rebreathing bag in liters
1 to 8 (toy dog or cat)	0.5
9 to 16 (small to medium dog, large cat)	1
17 to 33 (medium to large dog)	2
34 to 50 (large to giant dog)	3
51 to 83 (giant dog)	5

How to: Choose a Reservoir Bag Size: A good guideline is to use reservoir bags with a volume of 4 to 6 times the patient's maximum tidal volume, or, an easier calculation is to choose a bag that has a volume of approximately 60 ml/kg of patient body weight. Bags with a larger volume than this will not allow for rapid change of anesthetic depth and may waste anesthetic gas, but bags with less volume may not provide an adequate reservoir for a large breath. If a patient is in-between bag sizes, round up to the next biggest size.

The Pressure Relief or 'Pop-Off' Valve (Figure 3-28): This is technically called the **APL or 'adjustable pressure-limiting' valve,** and is used to control the pressure in the breathing system and the release of gases exhaled from the breathing system.

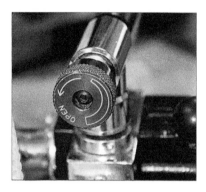

Figure 3-28. The Pressure Relief or 'Pop-Off' Valve. This is technically called the **APL** or 'adjustable pressure-limiting' valve.

CRITICAL TIP!

It is important to remember that the 'pop-off' or APL valve is a safety valve that allows escape of excess gases from the breathing system so that the system does not become over-pressurized and cause barotrauma (i.e., damage to the patient's lungs due to excess pressure in the airway). The valve should remain open during spontaneous ventilation and should only be closed during positive pressure ventilation or when pressure checking the machine. The valve can be PARTIALLY closed to assist in keeping the reservoir bag open during lower flows of oxygen but the pressure manometer (Figure 3-29) MUST BE WATCHED CAREFULLY to insure that pressure is not building up in the system.

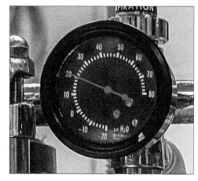

Figure 3-29. The airway pressure manometer. The pressure indicated on this manometer is 20 cm H_2O, which is the pressure used for checking that the endotracheal tube cuff is not leaking.

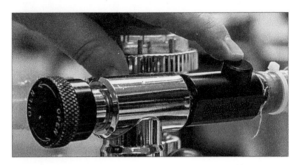

Figure 3-30. To avoid inadvertently leaving the valve closed, a 'button type' attachment to the pop-off valve is recommended.

The Airway Pressure Manometer: The airway pressure manometer **(Figure 3-29)** is usually located near the pop-off valve. The manometer is used to continuously monitor airway pressure and to insure that excessive pressure is not applied when manually ventilating the patient.

Types of Rebreathing Systems

There are two types of **rebreathing systems,** the **circle system** and the **Universal F system**. The previous discussion covered the circle system (See Figure 3-18). The Universal F system **(Figure 3-31)** functions just like a circle system so all components and considerations just discussed are the same for the F system as for the circle system. This system includes a carbon dioxide absorber, rebreathing bag, unidirectional valves, pressure relief valve, and pressure manometer. The main difference is that the F system breathing hose design is 'co-axial' or tube within a tube. Standard adult and pediatric sizes are available. The inspiratory limb of the breathing hose is inside the expiratory limb of the breathing hose. The advantage of the coaxial system is the ability to warm and humidify fresh gas above and beyond the warming and humidification provided by the regular circle system. This helps the patient retain body heat and provides a more normal atmosphere for the respiratory tract. Another advantage is that the coaxial tubing is lighter weight and less bulky than the traditional circle system tubing.

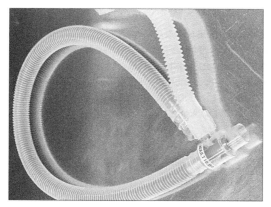

Figure 3-31. The Universal-F breathing system is a coaxial system with the inspiratory breathing hose inside the expiratory breathing hose (the blue inspiratory hose inside the clear expiratory hose).

TIP

To properly connect the Universal F system to the rest of the rebreathing system, insure that the inner tube is connected to the inspiratory valve and outer tubing is connected to the expiratory valve (Figure 3-32). However, since the inspiratory tube size is only slightly narrower than the expiratory tube size, a reverse connection would probably not create a problem, but the system would not function to warm and humidify gases.

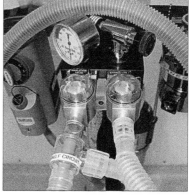

Figure 3-32. To properly connect the Universal-F system to the rest of the rebreathing system, insure that the inner tube (left) is connected to the inspiratory valve and the outer tubing is connected to the expiratory valve. Most systems are clearly labled.

TIP

Check the F system for damage before each use. If the end of the inspiratory hose pulls away from the end of the expiratory hose it will allow the patient to rebreathe carbon dioxide.

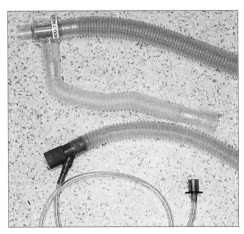

Figure 3-33. Both the Universal-F rebreathing system (top) and many nonrebreathing sytems (Bains system on the bottom) are coaxial. They are easily distinguished from each other. The Universal-F system is a rebreathing system. The inspiratory hose (green hose) is within the expiratory hose (clear hose). The expiratory hose separates from the coaxial system at the level of attachment to the anesthesia machine. This is the clear hose that is attached to the coaxial system in the upper left portion of the photo. It attaches to the expiratory valve on the anesthesia machine, making a circle system. For the nonrebreathing system, there is no separate expiratory hose but there is inlet tubing (long thin tube entering the nonrebreathing system on the left) for fresh gas flow.

Non-Rebreathing Systems

A non-rebreathing system (See Figure 3-19) delivers fresh gas to the patient and prevents rebreathing of exhaled gases. There is no CO_2 absorbent in this system so high fresh gas flows are required to eliminate carbon dioxide and prevent rebreathing. This higher fresh gas flow pushes all expired gas to the scavenger. The lack of a carbon dioxide absorber and unidirectional airway valves decreases the resistance to breathing, thereby reducing the work of breathing through the system and making it more functional for patients that are less than 5 kg body weight.

Oxygen Flow in the Non-Rebreathing System

Different non-rebreathing systems have slightly differing flow recommendations from 150 to 300 ml/kg/min but an average flow of 200 ml/kg/min will be appropriate for all commonly used systems. Because flow is already high in the non-rebreathing system, a higher flow than the 200 ml/kg/min to "denitrogenate" the system is not necessary at induction, nor is an increased flow necessary to increase the rate of elimination of inhalant gases at recovery.

TIP

As with the non-rebreathing systems, the absolute minimum flow is generally 500 ml/min due to vaporizer requirements - the output of many commonly used vaporizers is not totally accurate at oxygen flows lower than 500 ml/min.

Non-Rebreathing System Advantages

There are no airway valves or a carbon dioxide absorbent canister, thus there is less airway resistance and increased likelihood that the small patients will adequately ventilate under anesthesia. Increased flow rate means that anesthetic depth can be changed very quickly following an adjustment to the vaporizer. The tubing is lightweight, and will be less likely to cause trauma to the trachea or accidental extubation from pulling on the endotracheal tube.

Non-Rebreathing System Disadvantages

There is an increased use of oxygen and inhalant because of the high gas flows. The system depends on the high gas flows to remove carbon dioxide, so an accidental decrease in oxygen flow rate can create accumulation of carbon dioxide, hypercarbia and respiratory acidosis. Increased gas flows increase the likelihood of pollution of the operating room air. High flow rates can directly affect patient airway pressure (so don't use the oxygen flush button!), potentially causing barotrauma to the patient if any occlusion of the outflow system occurs. High flow rates can also contribute to chilling and drying of the airway and, unfortunately, the small patients using the nonrebreathing systems are already more prone to hypothermia.

Components of the Non-Rebreathing System

The non-rebreathing system is very simple and consists only of a fresh gas inlet, inspiratory and expiratory breathing hoses that are usually coaxial or 'tube within a tube' **(Figure 3-34)** and sometimes a bag similar to a reservoir bag **(Figure 3-35)**. The bag, however, is not a true reservoir bag and may even be open at one end, but the end can be occluded and the bag allowed to fill so that a breath can be delivered to the patient. The scavenging system can also be loosely connected to the end of the bag.

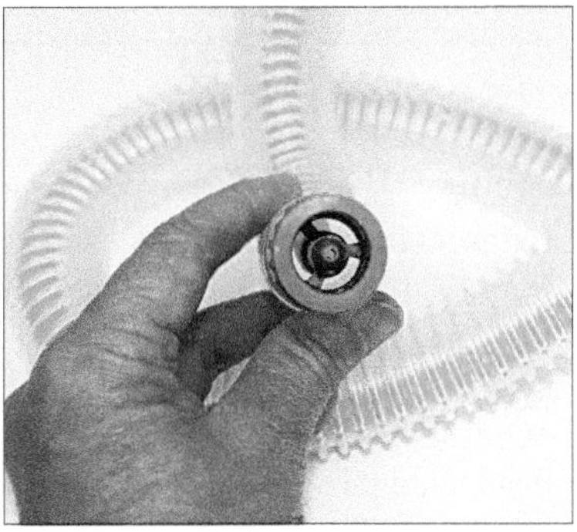

Figure 3-34. The nonrebreathing system is a coaxial system with the green inspiratory breathing hose inside the clear expiratory breathing hose.

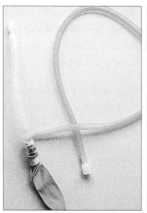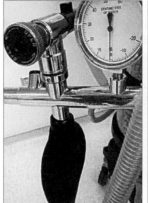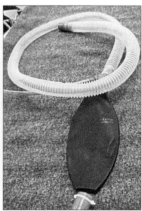

Figure 3-35. Three types of reservoir bag configurations for use in non-rebreathing systems are shown here. The bag is not a true reservoir bag but can be used to give the patient a breath. The scavenging system can also be loosely connected to the end of the bag (right) or to the specialized mounting block (middle photo).

A pressure relief or 'pop-off' valve can be used with the non-rebreathing system by using a Bain mount **(Figure 3-36)**, which allows the non-rebreathing system to be attached to a reservoir bag, airway pressure manometer, pop off valve and attachment for scavenging anesthetic waste gas. The pop off valve may cause a slight increase in resistance but the advantage of enhancing the ability to manually ventilate the patient (if necessary) outweighs the slight increase in resistance. The inclusion of an airway pressure manometer improves safety because the manometer can be used to monitor airway pressure when manually ventilating the patient.

Types of Non-Rebreathing Systems
There are several types of non-rebreathing systems but the Bain's circuit, or sometimes called the modified Mapleson D circuit, is a co-axial design (inspiration

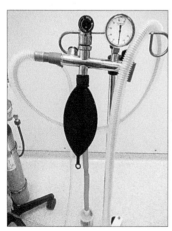

Figure 3-36. A **Bain mount** is used to attach the non-rebreathing system (the coaxial hoses) to a reservoir bag, airway pressure manometer, pop off valve and scavenging systems, all of which are components of the Bain mount. The Bain mount can be clamped to a stand, to the anesthesia machine or to the surgery table. Note the fresh gas line (small clear tubing) coming from the anesthesia machine (left).

tube inside expiration tube) and is the most common non-rebreathing system used in veterinary medicine (See Figure 3-19) Other non-rebreathing systems include the modified Jackson Rees, Ayres T-piece and Norman Elbow.

▌TIP
Check the non-rebreathing system for damage before each use. If the end of the inspiratory hose pulls away from the end of the expiratory hose or if there are any holes in the interior tube, the patient will rebreathe carbon dioxide.

How to: Choose a Breathing System

For patients over 5 kg or 10 lbs, use a rebreathing (circle) system. For patients less than 5 kg or 10 lbs, use a non-rebreathing system or a pediatric circle system. Some people use 7.5 kg patient body weight as the cut-off between non-rebreathing and rebreathing systems and this is also appropriate.

How to: Set up a Breathing System

The set up for both rebreathing and nonrebreathing systems is similar. For either system, the set up should be done in a step-wise fashion and in the same order each time to avoid accidentally forgetting a component. Here is a recommended order for set-up for both rebreathing and nonrebreathing systems with differences between the systems clearly indicated **(Figure 3-37)**.

Figure 3-37

1. BOTH SYSTEMS (rebreathing and nonre-breathing): First, connect the oxygen supply to the hospital source (left) OR open the oxygen tank to insure that the amount of oxygen in the tank is adequate (> 500 psi (right).

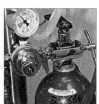

2. BOTH SYSTEMS: Briefly turn on the flow meter to make sure that the oxygen is connected correctly and that the flowmeter float does not stick. Turn the flowmeter off.

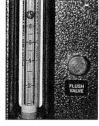

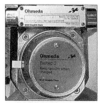

3. BOTH SYSTEMS: Check the vaporizer connections, the inlet tubing should come from the flowmeter to the vaporizer and the outlet tubing should leave the vaporizer and go to the fresh gas outlet. This is a photo of the top of the vaporizer with the inlet port on the left and the outlet port on the right. Both ports are clearly marked.

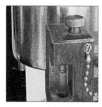

4. BOTH SYSTEMS: Check that the vaporizer is full. This vaporizer is just a little less than completely full, note the fluid line just below the black fill line.

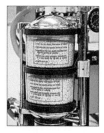

5. REBREATHING SYSTEMS: Insure that the carbon dioxide absorbent is fresh and that the canister is sealed tightly. Change the absorbent if necessary. Nonrebreathing systems do not include carbon dioxide absorbent.

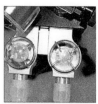

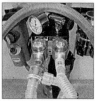

6. REBREATHING SYSTEMS: Attach the breathing hoses to the unidirectional valves on the machine. The circle system is composed of open hoses so it does not matter which side of the hose goes onto which valve (top). For the Universal F system make sure that the inner tube is connected to the inspiratory valve and the outer tube is connected to the expiratory valve (bottom). The inhalation (inspiratory) and exhalation (expiratory) valves are clearly marked. Nonrebreathing systems do not include unidirectional valves.

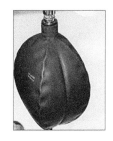

7. REBREATHING SYSTEMS: Attach the appropriately sized reservoir bag.

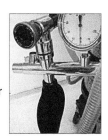

8. NONREBREATHING SYSTEMS USING A BAIN MOUNT: Place a 1-liter bag on the port at the bottom of the mount. This is not a reservoir bag as it is in a rebreathing system but it will allow the anesthetist to breathe for the patient when necessary.

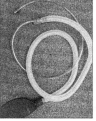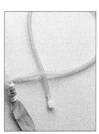

9. NONREBREATHING SYSTEMS WITH NO BAIN MOUNT: For the Bain system (left), a bag with an open end should be attached to the end of the system (Figure 3-35, photo on right). Others, like a 'Jackson-Rees' system (right), will accommodate a normal 1-liter bag. This system has a valve that can be opened to relieve pressure in the system.

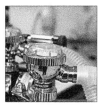

10. REBREATHING SYSTEMS: Breathe through the breathing tubes and make sure that the unidirectional valves open and close as you inhale and exhale. The valve pictured here is slightly open. If they do not open, unscrew the unidirectional valve domes and make sure that the one-way valves are dry and movable, then close the domes tightly.

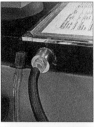

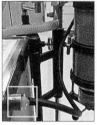
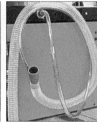

11. BOTH SYSTEMS: Connect the fresh gas line from the machine to the breathing system. The top photo shows a common site for the fresh gas line to exit a machine. The black tubing is connected to the fresh gas port and is part of the rebreathing system. It would have to be disconnected and the clear line on the left connected to the fresh gas port for a nonrebreathing system. The photo on the bottom left shows the fresh gas line exiting the fresh gas port (in the middle of the square) in a rebreathing system. The photo on the bottom right shows the nonrebreathing system connected to the fresh gas port.

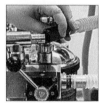

12. FOR REBREATHING SYSTEMS (left) AND NONREBREATHING SYSTEMS USING A BAIN MOUNT (right): Attach the scavenge hose to the scavenge system port, which is generally near the pressure limiting or 'pop off' valve.

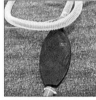

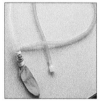

13. FOR NONREBREATHING SYSTEMS WITH NO BAIN MOUNT: For some nonrebreathing systems (top), the scavenging system is simply placed LOOSELY near the open end of the bag on the nonrebreathing hose. This is less than ideal because 1) attaching the vacuum line to the bag can evacuate all of the air in the system (with active scavenging) or increase resistance to breathing (if using a charcoal canister) AND 2) will cause some anesthetic gas to leak into the room. The system on the bottom can be attached directly to the scavenging system using a small diameter corrugated hose (blue hose in photo).

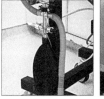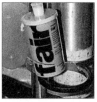

14. BOTH SYSTEMS: Check the attachment of the scavenging hose to the scavenging system (left) or charcoal canister (right).

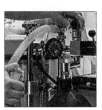

15. BOTH SYSTEMS: Pressure or 'leak' test the system (rebreathing pressure check on left and nonrebreathing pressure without Bain mount check on right). This is a very important step!

How to: Pressure Check the Machine and Breathing System (Figure 3-38)
Reasons to Pressure Check

• Pressure checking the machine and breathing system is a crucial step that should be done before every single patient - a lot can happen to the system between patients. The test is very quick and performing it will not greatly affect the outcome of the day with regards to how many patients you have time to anesthetize, but skipping it could greatly affect the outcome for any particular patient.

• Gas leaking from an anesthesia machine is a significant source of personnel exposure. By the time the smell of a gas leak can be detected, the dose that could be inhaled by personnel is often dangerous and above OSHA (Occupational Safety and Health Administration) recommended levels.

• The plane of anesthesia for the patient will be inconsistent if the anaesthesia machine leaks.

• Prevention of leaks will ensure that the patient is receiving 100% oxygen.

CRITICAL TIP!
DO NOT FORGET TO OPEN THE PRESSURE RELIEF (OR POP-OFF) VALVE.

Checking Patency of the Inner Tube
There is one more step that should occur with coaxial (tube-in-a-tube) nonre-breathing systems and that is a check for leaks of the inner tube (to make sure it doesn't have any holes or cracks):
1. Connect the breathing system as described above
2. Set the flow meter at 2 L/min
3. Occlude the small inner tube **(Figure 3-39)** with something small like a small syringe plunger or your thumb or a finger.

Figure 3-38 Pressure Check Step-by-Step

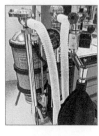 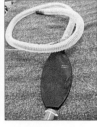

1. BOTH SYSTEMS: Set up all the equipment, including the machine and breathing system. A rebreathing circle system (left) and a nonre-breathing system with no mount (right) are shown here.

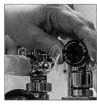 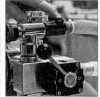

2. FOR REBREATHING SYSTEMS AND NONRE-BREATHING SYSTEMS USING A BAIN MOUNT: Close the pressure relief or 'pop-off' valve using the valve (left) or a button valve (right).

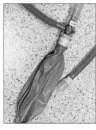 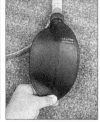

3. FOR NONREBREATHING SYSTEMS WITHOUT A BAIN MOUNT: Close the open end of the bag by pinching (right) or close the valve at the neck of the bag (left).

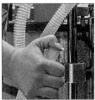

4. BOTH SYSTEMS: Occlude the end of the breathing tube at the patient end with a cork, your thumb, or anything that makes a complete seal of the tube. Rebreathing system (left); Nonre-breathing system (right).

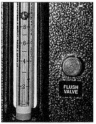

5. BOTH SYSTEMS: Inflate the reservoir bag by pressing the flush button or by turning up the oxygen flow meter until the pressure on the manometer reaches 20 cm H_2O (FOR REBREATHING SYSTEMS OR NONREBREATHING SYSTEMS USING A BAIN MOUNT) or the reservoir bag is full enough to be tight (FOR NONREBREATHING SYSTEMS WITH NO BAIN MOUNT). Stop the flow of oxygen into the system by releasing the flush button or turning off the flow meter. Some experts recommend pressure checking to 30-40 cm H_2O.

6. FOR REBREATHING SYSTEMS OR NONREBREATHING SYSTEMS USING A BAIN MOUNT: Watch the manometer, the system should hold the 20 cm H_2O pressure for 15 seconds or longer. A very slight drop in pressure might occur, this is normal and due to compliance of the breathing tubes and reservoir bag. The pressure should only drop by a few centimeters of water and should NOT continue to drop after the initial fall.

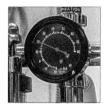

7. FOR NONREBREATHING SYSTEMS NOT USING A BAIN MOUNT: Watch the bag, it should stay tight for 15 seconds or longer. There may be a slight drop in pressure, due to compliance of the breathing tubes and reservoir bag. This is normal. The pressure should only drop enough to cause a very slight loss in the fullness of the bag and should NOT continue to drop after the initial fall.

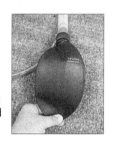

8. BOTH SYSTEMS: If the pressure drops, turn on the oxygen flow meter until the pressure stabilizes at 20 cm H_2O or until the nonrebreathing bag stays full and read the level on the flowmeter. If more than 250 ml/min of oxygen is required to maintain the pressure at 20 cm H_2O, the leak MUST BE LOCATED BEFORE USING THE SYSTEM. Any leak, regardless of how many mls are leaking, should eventually be located using the soapy water test (Figures 3-40 and 3-41).

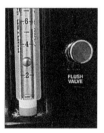

9. REBREATHING SYSTEMS AND NONRE-BREATHING SYSTEMS USING A BAIN MOUNT: IF A PRESSURE RELIEF VALVE IS IN THE SYSTEM: Perform this absolutely imperative step: OPEN THE PRESSURE RELIEF VALVE (left). If using a pressure relief valve button (right), just lift your finger.

 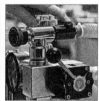

10. REBREATHING SYSTEMS: When releasing the pressure in the system, open the pressure relief valve first, then remove the occlusion from the end of the breathing tubes. This will prevent dust contamination from the absorbent from entering the breathing circuit, and confirm the patency of the scavenging system. If the system remains pressurized after the pressure relief valve is open, the scavenging system is obstructed or the pressure relief valve is faulty.

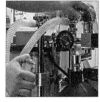

4. If the inner tube is intact, the flowmeter ball will drop in the flow tube because of the increased back pressure.

5. Immediately let off the pressure! Maintaining excess pressure can damage the system.

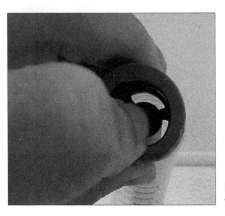

Figure 3-39. Checking the patency of the inner tube.

How to: Trouble-Shoot Leaks in the System

• When a leak is discovered it should be located and fixed as soon as possible. Make up a bowl or bottle of dilute soapy water and, with the patient end of the breathing system occluded and oxygen flowing through the system, start dabbing or spraying the water on the possible leak sites described below **(Figure 3-40)**. Escaping air will make bubbles!

• Once you find the bubbles, you have found the leak **(Figure 3-41)**.

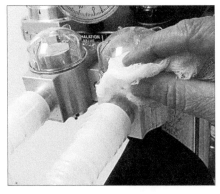

Figure 3-40. Dabbing soapy water on suspected leak sites.

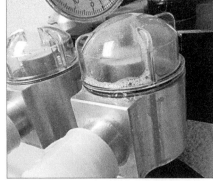

Figure 3-41. Bubbles escaping from a leak at the one-way valve housing.

- The most common leak sites are located at parts of the machine and breathing system that are changed, moved or disconnected **(Figure 3-42 A-E)**, starting in the upper left hand corner:
  - The connections between breathing tubes and the valve ports of the unidirectional valves **(Figure 3-42 A)**;
  - The connection between the reservoir bag and the bag port **(Figure 3-42 B)**;
  - The seals at the top and bottom of absorbent canisters **(Figure 3-42 C)**;
  - The domes of the unidirectional valves **(Figure 3-42 D)**;
  - Holes in the reservoir bag and breathing tubes **(Figure 3-42 E)**

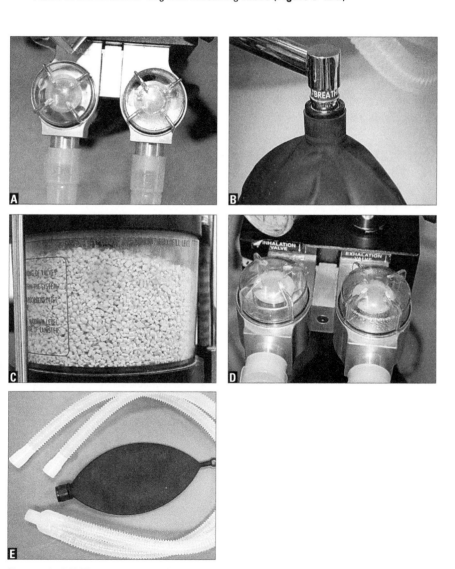

Figure 3-42 A-E. The most common leak sites on anesthesia machines and breathing systems.

Another common leak site when a patient is attached to the machine is the connection between breathing tubes and the endotracheal tube.

Troubleshooting Anesthesia Equipment

Here are some more trouble shooting tips and a chart of the most common trouble 'spots' (Table 3-3).

Consistently Empty Reservoir Bag
(Figure 3-43)

A leak in the anesthetic circuit or insufficient oxygen flow into the system are the most likely problems.

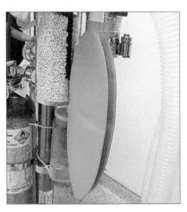

Figure 3-43. A consistently empty reservoir bag could be due to leaks or a lack of oxygen flow into the system.

Make sure that:
• The oxygen source is connected and that there is oxygen in the tank (Figure 3-44 A & B).
• Oxygen is flowing through the flowmeter (Figure 3-45).
• The oxygen flow is adequate for the patient's size (REMEMBER, the recommended oxygen flow is 20 to 40 ml/kg for rebreathing systems and 200 mls/kg for non-rebreathing systems). If your machine requires an excessively high oxygen flow to keep oxygen in the reservoir bag, it is time to have your machine checked by a machine maintenance person.

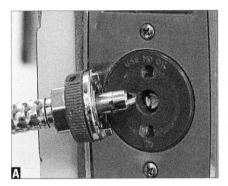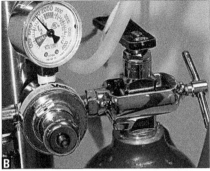

Figure 3-44 A&B. The oxygen source connection and the oxygen level in the tank should be checked if the reservoir bag remains empty.

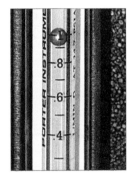

Figure 3-45. The flow meter should be checked to insure that oxygen is flowing in the breathing system.

• The fresh gas supply is connected to the breathing system, especially when switching between rebreathing and non-rebreathing systems. **Figure 3-46 A** shows the fresh gas supply hooked up to a rebreathing system and **Figure 3-46 B** shows the fresh gas supply hooked up to a non-rebreathing system.

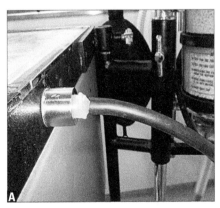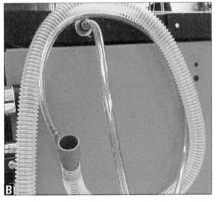

Figure 3-46. The fresh gas supply should be connected to the breathing system being used on the patient. The fresh gas connection to a rebreathing system **(A)** and a non-rebreathing system **(B)**.

Table 3-3
Most Common Equipment Trouble 'Spots'

Trouble spot	Consequence	Fix
Closed pressure relief or 'pop off' valve	Rapid increase in pressure in the breathing system and in the patient's lungs. This is critically dangerous!	QUICKLY open the valve and squeeze the reservoir bag (Figure 3-49) to relieve the pressure and to make sure that the gas can now flow out of the valve. If the valve can't be opened, remove the bag immediately (this will relieve pressure in the system but will allow inhalant to escape into the room) and then switch the patient to another machine.
Esophageal intubation	The patient is likely to become hypoxemic and may regain consciousness	Reanesthetize with injectable anesthetics and quickly reintubate. Ideally, use a laryngoscope so that intubation can be confirmed as you see the tube pass through the arytenoids. Can also confirm intubation by using a capnograph (esophageal intubation would not provide a normal capnograph tracing), by watching the tube 'steam up' as the patient exhales and by watching the reservoir bag move as the patient's thorax moves. (See Chapter 5).
Leaking endotracheal tube cuff	Room air can be inhaled around the tube, diluting the oxygen and the inhalant. The patient is likely to get hypoxemic and to get 'too light' or regain consciousness	Inflate the cuff to a pressure that prevents a leak at 20 cm H_2O on the pressure manometer. DO NOT INFLATE MORE THAN THIS. Excessive pressure can cause tracheal damage. If the tube continues to leak, replace the tube with a tube that has a cuff that is not leaking and/or a larger tube. Sometimes the leak occurs because the tube is too small and, no matter how much the cuff is inflated, it cannot completely seal the trachea.
Disconnected fresh gas flow between the machine and the breathing system	The patient is getting no oxygen or inhalant so will get hypoxemic and will regain consciousness.	This occurs because the fresh gas line is not connected to the breathing system (rebreathing vs nonrebreathing) being used. If the breathing system is changed and the fresh gas line is not moved, the patient will not be receiving oxygen or inhalant. Find the line and connect it to the breathing system!

Empty vaporizer	The patient will wake up.	This happens fairly commonly in practices where the machine is not checked in between patients. Don't forget to run through the check-lists in this chapter for every patient. Fill the vaporizer! May need to reanesthetize the patient with injectable anesthetic drugs.
Exhausted carbon dioxide absorbent	Hypercarbia and respiratory acidosis, which are very dangerous conditions, will occur. The patient may seem too lightly anesthetized at first as ventilation and heart rate increase in an attempt to remove the excessive carbon dioxide.	Once hypercarbia reaches a critical level, it will contribute to anesthetic depth and the patient can no longer respond by trying to eliminate the carbon dioxide and the problem will continue to get worse. IMMEDI-ATELY change the CO_2 absorbent and start breathing for the patient to help eliminate the CO_2. The oxygen flow rate can be increased so that the high flow eliminates the CO_2 (this makes a rebreathing system function like a non-rebreathing system). Be sure to check the absorbent regularly and change it before this problem occurs!
Excessive use of oxygen flush valve	This rapidly pressurizes the breathing system and can cause severe barotrauma, especially in patients on small volume breathing systems (like non-rebreathing systems or pediatric circles) because these small systems will rapidly fill. The flush valve also by-passes the vaporizer and dilutes the inhalant concentration in the reservoir bag so the patient receives less inhalant and will get light.	**DO NOT USE THE FLUSH VALVE UNLESS YOUR GOAL IS TO RAPIDLY DECREASE ANESTHETIC DEPTH.** **DO NOT USE THE FLUSH VALVE IN PATIENTS ON SMALL VOLUME BREATHING SYSTEMS (nonrebreathing or pediatric circle systems).**
Unidirectional valves stuck closed	If inspiration valve is stuck, oxygen and inhalant will not enter the system so the patient may become hypoxemic and/or may regain consciousness. If the exhalation valve is stuck, pressure will rapidly build up in the system, just as occurs with a closed pressure relief (pop-off) valve.	One-way valve movement should be checked when the machine is pressure-checked. If they are not moving, the valve domes should be unscrewed and the valves should be unstuck, cleaned and normal movement should be verified.

- The reservoir bag is not too small for the patient's tidal volume. This would cause the patient to empty the bag with a large breath (REMEMBER, the volume of the reservoir bag should be approximately 60 mls/kg of patient body weight).
- The inspiratory unidirectional valve is not stuck in the closed position - this would mean that fresh gas was not actually entering the system **(Figure 3-47)**.
- The scavenging system is not set at an excessively high vacuum pressure. This technically should not impact the breathing system but frequently does.

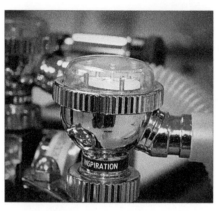

Figure 3-47. The inspiratory unidirectional valve (front of photo) contains a plastic or metal disc (the little white disk under the dome) that should open on inhalation. If it is stuck in the closed position, no fresh gas can enter the system. The valve should be checked DAILY as part of the routine machine set up.

Consistently full Reservoir Bag
(Figure 3-48)
Start looking for some occlusion in the exhalation limb of the system.

Make sure that:
- **THE 'POP-OFF' VALVE IS NOT CLOSED (Figure 3-49).**
- There is no occlusion between the rebreathing bag and the scavenging system.

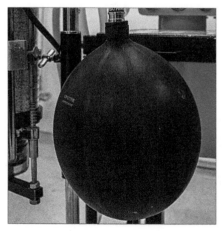

Figure 3-48. A consistently full reservoir bag could be due to excessive input (flow) or blocked output to the scavenging system. An overly full, tight reservoir bag could be an emergency - relieve pressure immediately! (See Figure 3-49 and Table 3-3)

• The oxygen flow rate is not too high for the patient. An extra high flow does not improve anesthetic safety. The patient will still consume a low percentage of the supplied oxygen so there is no need to provide more than the patient needs.

• The scavenging system is not set at an excessively low pressure. Technically, the scavenging system interface should keep the vacuum from impacting the reservoir bag but the interface could be faulty, causing a consistently over-distended reservoir bag.

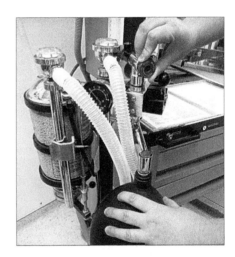

Figure 3-49. When pressure builds up in the breathing system due to a closed pressure relief valve, quickly open the valve AND squeeze air out of the rebreathing bag to rapidly decrease the pressure in the system and in the patient's lungs.

Problems that SEEM to be Patient Problems but may Actually be Equipment Problems

The two most common items on the list would be a patient that seems continuously too light - or one that seems continuously too deep - in spite of normal trouble shooting techniques for these issues.

If the Patient seems too Lightly Anesthetized
• First **CHECK THE PATIENT!** Patients that are hypoxic (low in oxygen) and/or hypercarbic (high CO_2) can initially appear 'light' because the heart rate and respiratory rate will increase and the patient may even have exaggerated reflexes - like the palpebral reflex - for a short time. If hypoxia is expected, start searching for any oxygen flow interruption, and if hypercarbia is expected, first check the integrity of your carbon dioxide absorbent.

• If the patient is okay, start checking your equipment. Look for:
  • a leak, the system may be entraining room air and diluting the concentration of inhalant gas
  • an empty vaporizer
  • an inadequate setting on the vaporizer
  • a faulty vaporizer - the latter is unlikely if the vaporizer receives regular maintenance, but can happen.

If the Patient seems too Deeply Anesthetized
• First CHECK THE PATIENT and TURN DOWN THE VAPORIZER - maybe the patient really IS too deep. Remember that the response to anesthesia is highly variable between patients and that anesthesia should ALWAYS be administered 'to effect' and NOT merely by the number on the vaporizer dial.

• If the patient is not too deep but physiologic changes are occurring that seem like excessive anesthetic depth, start checking your equipment for causes of severe hypoxia or hypercarbia, like:
  • Problems with the oxygen source or flow (tanks, connections, flow meters).
  • Exhausted carbon dioxide absorbent.
  • Problems with oxygen delivery (fresh gas line not connected, inspiratory unidirectional valve closed, blockage of the inspiratory limb of breathing hoses, etc.).
  • Anything that might cause excessive rebreathing (inspiratory unidirectional valve closed, blockage of the expiratory limb of the breathing hoses (rebreathing system), inside tube of the coaxial breathing system disconnected or leaking (nonrebreathing system), etc.).
  • Exhausted carbon dioxide absorbent.

• Hypothermia can also make patients 'deeper' because a decrease in body temperature causes a decrease in anesthetic requirements (See Chapter 6).

Mechanical (Intermittent Positive Pressure [IPPV]) Ventilation
NOTE: There is an overview of how to use IPPV at the end of this chapter (Table 3-5). This is a checklist that is designed for daily use in your practice.

Mechanical ventilators deliver breaths using intermittent positive pressure ventilation (IPPV) to prevent or treat hypoventilation, which can lead to hypercapnia (excessively high carbon dioxide, also called hypercarbia), decreased oxygenation (hypoxemia or hypoxia) and acid-base disturbances (mainly respiratory acidosis from the hypercapnia). Patients that are hypoventilating have not only inadequate gas exchange (decreased carbon dioxide out and oxygen in), they may also have inadequate uptake of anesthetic gases. Ventilators are useful in maintaining a consistent depth of anesthesia since they deliver a consistent 'dose' of the inhalant anesthetic each time an IPPV breath is delivered.

TERMINOLOGY NOTE
Of course, intermittent positive pressure ventilation (IPPV) doesn't have to be delivered by a machine - a person intermittently squeezing the reservoir bag will also deliver positive pressure ventilation. We tend to call mechanical ventilation with a ventilator IPPV, but don't forget that you can deliver IPPV without a mechanical ventilator!

The main cause of hypoventilation is excessive anesthetic depth so merely turning down the vaporizer often solves the problem. But some patients have difficulty breathing due to other factors and might benefit from IPPV. Patients that could benefit from IPPV include:

• Patients with a distended abdomen (obesity, pregnancy or gastric dilatation), diaphragmatic hernia, thoracic wall abnormalities (fractured ribs) or those undergoing laparotomy (abdominal surgery).

• Patients that may not respond to increasing levels of CO_2 (hypercapnia; which is normally the main stimulant of respiration), like neonatal, geriatric and critically ill patients.

• Patients in which a normal CO_2 (normocapnia) is critical (patients with increased intracranial pressure (ICP) like head trauma patients, and those with brain tumors).

• Patients undergoing intrathoracic surgery and patients receiving neuromuscular blocking agents (atracurium) cannot breathe on their own and REQUIRE IPPV (from a ventilator or from a person squeezing the reservoir bag).

Disadvantages of Mechanical Ventilation
Mechanical ventilation creates a loss of contact between the anesthesia provider and the patient. The "feel" of squeezing a reservoir bag ('rebreathing bag') to administer a breath can reveal such things as disconnections, changes in resistance or compliance, and spontaneous respiratory movements. The intra-thoracic positive pressure created by IPPV impedes venous return of blood to the heart (because the veins are compressed by the intra-thorax pressure), thus decreasing diastolic ventricular filling, stroke volume, cardiac output, and arterial blood pressure. The use of high airway pressures/volumes can cause alveolar damage.

Mechanical Ventilator Types

Oddly, ventilators are named by what the ventilator bellows does in exhalation rather than inhalation. A ventilator bellows that descends in exhalation after ascending to deliver a breath is called a 'descending bellows' **(Figure 3-50)**. A bellows that ascends in exhalation after descending to deliver a breath is called an 'ascending bellows' **(Figure 3-51)**. The latter type of bellows is preferred because:

• A disconnect, leak or interruption in oxygen supply is easy to determine since the bellows will descend to deliver a breath and then won't be able to ascend again because it isn't filling. The descending bellows may fall and rise regardless of content or connection.

• The patient can be connected to the ventilator even if the ventilator isn't on and the ventilator bellows can serve as a rebreathing bag without increasing work of breathing because the bellows will simply descend as the patient inhales. If the ventilator is off with a descending bellows, the patient actually has to breathe hard enough to make the bellows ascend (so the patient is literally 'picking up' the bellows with a breath!) - that is a big increase in the work of breathing!

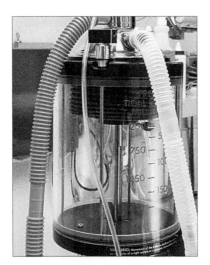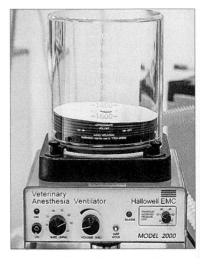

Figure 3-50 & Figure 3-51. Mechanical ventilators. A ventilator bellows that descends on exhalation after ascending to deliver a breath is called a 'descending bellows' (Figure 3-50, left). A bellows that ascends on exhalation after descending to deliver a breath is called a 'ascending bellows' (Figure 3-51, right).

How to: Set up the Ventilator:

This is a generic procedure for initiating ventilation (mechanical IPPV) **(Figure 3-52, Tables 3-4 and 3-5)**. Always read specific manufacturer's operating manuals before ventilator use.

Figure 3-52

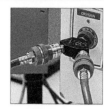

1. Connect the ventilator to oxygen. You will need an oxygen hose splitter since oxygen needs to be supplied into the bellows to reach the patient but also needs to be delivered to the ventilator housing to 'push' the bellows on inspiration.

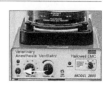

2. Turn the ventilator power on and make sure it starts normally.

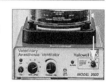

3. Insure that the maximum working pressure limit is set appropriately (to 20 cm H_2O or less for most patients). This is an important safety feature that limits the amount of pressure delivered to the patient, thereby avoiding barotrauma.

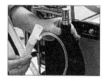

4. The bellows of the ventilator is basically a mechanical reservoir or, 'rebreathing' bag, that takes the place of the rebreathing bag on the anesthesia machine. Remove the rebreathing bag and connect the corrugated tube from the ventilator to the port that the bag came from.

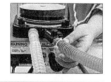

5. Move the scavenge hose from the location near the pressure relief valve ('pop-off' valve) to the ventilator.

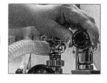

6. Close the anesthesia machine's pop-off valve or pressure-limiting valve. The ventilator has an internal pressure release valve so **this is the ONE TIME that the pop off valve on the anesthesia machine should remain closed.** The ventilator will not be able to deliver a breath if this valve is not closed.

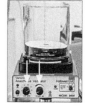

7. Set initial parameters as described in **Table 3-4**.

Table 3-4
General Guidelines for Ventilator Settings for Patients with Normal Lungs

1.	If the ventilator allows the tidal volume to be set, set at 10 to 15 ml/kg (maybe up to 20 ml/kg in larger patients).
2.	Set the respiratory rate at 6 to 20 breaths/minute. The goal is to deliver a minute ventilation (tidal volume × respiration rate) of about 150 to 250 ml/kg/minute (see more in Chapter 6).
3.	If the ventilator allows the inspiration time to expiration time (I:E) ratio to be set, set at 1:2 or higher (i.e., 1:3, 1:4, etc). Inspiration time= positive pressure time. Using a higher ratio (shorter inspiration time) decreases the likelihood that IPPV will cause a decrease in blood pressure. Long inspiratory times (i.e., low ratio of 1:1) are especially detrimental in patients with high abdominal pressure (e.g., GDV) that are prone to be hypotensive. 1:3 or 1:4 is usually ideal. Any higher than this often does not allow enough time for a normal inspiration.
4.	Check the end expiratory pressure (the pressure on the manometer at the end of an exhaled breath) and make sure that it is 0 to +2 cm H_2O. The peak end-expiratory pressure (PEEP) may be increased using PEEP valves in some patients (see Chapter 10).

TIPS for Using Ventilators
1. Double check that mechanical ventilation is moving the chest by visualizing normal chest excursions with minimal abdominal movement.
2. The initial ventilator settings may not meet the ventilation and oxygenation needs of the patient throughout the procedure and may need to be adjusted.
3. Carbon dioxide monitoring using capnography or blood gas analysis can be used to perfect the ventilator settings.

How to: Troubleshoot the Ventilator
To use the ventilator appropriately and safely, familiarity with the ventilator's various alarms is necessary.

Low Breathing System Pressure Alarm
This alarm is activated at the end of inspiration if there is not enough pressure to deliver a breath (5 cm H_2O for most ventilators). Use the settings in Table 3-4 to make sure that the tidal volume is adequate and that the peak inspiratory pressure is being reached. Causes of inadequate pressure include:
• Gas leaking out of the system, which is the most common cause. Make sure the pressure relief valve is closed and the endotracheal cuff is inflated. Check all other sources of leaks - carbon dioxide canister seal, one-way valve dome housing, etc.
• Excessively low oxygen flow. Insure that the oxygen flow is adequate.
• Loss of driving gas delivered to the ventilator. Ensure the ventilator is appropriately hooked up to a driving gas (generally meaning the oxygen delivered by the

Table 3-5
Step-By-Step Checklist for Using the Ventilator

Check list for using the mechanical ventilator	
1. Connect the driving gas for the bellows. Use a splitter if necessary.	
2. Turn the ventilator power on. Does it start normally?	
3. Set the maximum working pressure limit to 20 cm H_2O.	
4. Disconnect the rebreathing bag and connect the bellows hose at the bag port.	
5. Move the scavenge hose from the breathing system to the ventilator.	
6. Close the 'pop-off' valve on the anesthesia machine.	
7. Set the initial parameters that will produce a minute volume of 150-250 ml/kg/min a. Tidal volume 10-15 ml/kg b. Respiratory rate 6-20 breaths/min c. I:E ratio 1:2 or higher (1:3 or 1:4 is usually ideal)	
8. Connect the patient and turn on ventilator.	
9. Watch for appropriate chest movement.	
10. Double check that the parameters are indeed correct.	
11. Check that peak inspiratory pressure is no greater than 10-20 cm H_2O	
12. Check that the end-expiratory pressure is no greater than 2 cm H_2O.	

This table is a checklist for using IPPV. It is designed to be copied and used in your practice. We recommend that you use it on every patient!

splitter in the oxygen line), and that the line is not kinked.
• If trouble shooting fails to determine the cause of the problem, assume that a leak is causing the problem. Disconnect the patient from the ventilator, reattach the rebreathing bag, and make sure that the breathing system is not leaking, then look at the ventilator as the source of the leak.

High Pressure Alarm
This alarm is activated when the airway pressure reaches the maximum working pressure limit. Use the settings in Table 3-4 to insure that tidal the volume is not set too high.
• Make sure that the oxygen flow is not excessive.
• Check for any obstructions in the system. Obstructions would cause a rapid build-up of pressure.
• Make sure that the maximum working pressure limit is set at a reasonable pressure. If it is too low, the ventilator cannot deliver a breath.
• Make sure that the patient is not breathing out of phase with the ventilator (see below) since this can cause momentary excessive pressure.

If the source of the high pressure cannot be rapidly detected, disconnect the patient from the ventilator and ventilate manually using the reservoir bag until the trouble can be corrected. Allowing excessive pressure to build up in the system can lead to barotrauma.

Patient Breathing out of Phase with the Ventilator

This is also called 'bucking' the ventilator or 'breathing against' the ventilator. This may be normal for 1-2 minutes after starting the ventilator but should be corrected quickly if it lasts longer than that since it can interrupt ventilation and cause rapid deterioration of oxygenation.

1. Correct settings as described in Table 3-4. Make sure tidal volume, respiratory rate and peak inspiratory pressure are adequate;
2. Check for technical problems with the ventilator;
3. Check for worsening pulmonary disease (pneumothorax);
4. Check for an excessively light level of anesthesia/ painful stimulus;
5. Make sure that the breathing system is holding pressure;
6. Check patient for hypoxia or hypercapnia using end-tidal carbon dioxide and oxygen-hemoglobin saturation (SpO_2 on the pulse oximeter), or arterial blood gases if available.
7. If all parameters are normal, you may have to synchronize the ventilator to the patient. Adjust the ventilation rate to match that of the patient. Adjust the I:E ratio so that a full tidal volume can be completed within the time preferred by the patient.

How to: Wean (Remove) the Patient from the Ventilator

When weaning (or removing) the patient from the ventilator, decrease the minute volume (Table 3-4) to allow carbon dioxide levels to increase slightly to stimulate the patient to breathe spontaneously. This can be done by either decreasing the respiratory rate or the tidal volume. When you are ready to take the patient off the ventilator replace the reservoir bag in place of the corrugated tubing from the ventilator, **open the pressure relief valve,** and reconnect the scavenging hose from the ventilator to the rebreathing system. WATCH the patient's breaths and support as needed until the patient is breathing on its own. Expect to manually ventilate the patient for several minutes - this usually does not mean completely controlling breathing but only supplementing the breaths taken by the patient. Don't over support the patient - the carbon dioxide has to increase to stimulate breathing. If the patient is still too deeply anesthetized or very sick, it will take longer to wean it from the ventilator. High carbon dioxide may not stimulate breathing in old, sick or excessively deep patients and they will require ventilatory support to avoid hypercarbia.

Table 3-6
Daily Checklist for Setting up Anesthesia Equipment

Basic Check list for Anesthesia Equipment, Supplies and Drugs	
1. Check the oxygen level in the tanks, change if < 500 psi	
2. Check the patency of the carbon dioxide absorbent, change if necessary	
3. Make sure the vaporizer is full of liquid	
4. Assess the scavenge system, change the charcoal canister if necessary	
5. Choose a breathing system and appropriate reservoir bag for the patient and attach them to the machine	
6. Turn on the oxygen to make sure it is flowing normally, then turn off the oxygen.	
7. Close the pressure relief valve ('pop-off' valve) and leak test the machine. Watch that the valves on the breathing system (if a rebreathing system) move appropriately. Fix any leaks.	
8. OPEN THE PRESSURE RELIEF VALVE	

Reference
Harvey 2010,http.abbotanimalhealth.com/docs/AAHA-160R1anestheticequ

Chapter 4

Anesthesia Drugs

Nicole Valdez, LVT, VTS (Anesthesia/Analgesia)

Janel Holden, LVT, VTS (Anesthesia/Analgesia)

Tamara Grubb, DVM, PhD, DACVAA

Introduction

Anesthetic drugs include tranquilizers/sedatives, analgesics, and drugs used for induction, maintenance, and recovery. Although technically not anesthetic drugs, support drugs like anticholinergics and positive inotropes are an integral part of anesthesia.

Choosing Drugs

Regardless of the phase of anesthesia (preparation/premedication, induction, maintenance, recovery), drugs should be chosen primarily based on the health of the patient and the expected duration of and pain level produced by the procedure. The demeanor of the patient (i.e., excited, calm, nervous, etc...) will have a bearing on the drug selection and/or drug dose, primarily for drugs used for premedication and potentially for those used in recovery. The expected duration of the procedure may have a bearing on whether or not to use reversible drugs and/or inhalant vs injectable drugs for maintenance.

Administering Drugs

For all phases of anesthesia, drugs can be administered intravenously (IV). Premedications and postoperative drugs are often administered intramuscularly (IM) and occasionally subcutaneously (SQ), orally (PO), oral transmucosally (OTM) or transdermally. Inhalant drugs for maintenance, of course, must be administered by inhalation. Specific guidelines for administering drugs are provided in Chapter 8.

Specific Drug Considerations

Drug Enforcement Agency (DEA) Controlled Drugs

Some anesthesia drugs are Drug Enforcement Agency (DEA) controlled, meaning that their use has to be carefully recorded in the patient's record and in a controlled drug log. For anesthesia, most opioids, ketamine, alfaxalone, benzodiazepines and tiletamine/zolazepam are DEA controlled **(Table 4-1)**. Some practices feel that handling Class II drugs (morphine, hydromorphone, fentanyl, and methadone) is too difficult but Class II drugs require only one extra form (DEA 222 form). Storage (i.e., a locked box with limited access) and recording in patient records and drug logs is required for all controlled drugs so handling Class II drugs is not really all that difficult. In addition, Class II drugs are very potent, inexpensive analgesics whose effects are reversible, making them ideal for almost all patients experiencing pain.

Food & Drug Administration (FDA)-Approved Drugs vs Generics vs Compounded Drugs

Drugs that are approved by the FDA have been proven to be safe and efficacious when used at the approved dose for the approved condition in the approved species. We often use 'off label' dosages when we don't want the exact effect

Table 4-1
DEA Drug Classifications

DEA Class	Class Description	Drug Examples
I	Drugs with no currently accepted medical use and a high potential for abuse. Considered dangerous.	heroin, lysergic acid diethylamide (LSD), marijuana
II	Drugs with a high potential for abuse, but less abuse potential than Schedule I drugs, and strong potential for severe psychological or physical dependence.	Morphine, methadone, hydromorphone, fentanyl, codeine
III	Drugs with a moderate to low potential for physical and psychological dependence.	Ketamine, Telazol, buprenorphine, codeine + acetaminophen
IV	Drugs with a low potential for abuse and low risk of dependence.	Diazepam, midazolam, butorphanol, tramadol, alfaxalone
V	Drugs with lower potential for abuse than Schedule IV. Primarily consists of preparations containing limited quantities of certain narcotics.	Some cough suppressants with a very low dose of codeine

offered by the drug or when we combine the drug with other drugs that produce the same effect. For instance, we may use less than the label-approved dose of dexmedetomidine if we only want light sedation or if we are combining the dexmedetomidine with an opioid, both of which produce sedation. It is important to use drugs that are FDA approved for veterinary species whenever possible since drugs approved for humans are not always safe or efficacious in our species. However, there are many drugs that have only a formulation for humans and nothing for our veterinary patients. For these drugs, look for published data on their safety and efficacy in the species you want to treat before administering them to any animal.

Generic drugs are also FDA approved but the companies that make generics are not required to provide safety and efficacy data of the same rigor as that provided by the company that made the parent drug. Thus, generic drugs are less expensive but companies that make generic drugs rarely develop new drugs.

Compounded drugs have little or no regulatory oversight and pharmacies can compound drugs and sell them without efficacy or safety studies. Thus, compounded drugs should be our last choice. However, some drugs do not come in a formulation or concentration that is useful in our patients so compounded drugs are used fairly commonly in veterinary medicine. For instance, many drugs are too concentrated for accurate dosing in cats and drugs can be compounded at lower concentrations for this species. Because there is no oversight for compounded drugs, your practice should choose a compounding pharmacy that they trust and should assess the safety and efficacy of the drug by monitoring the patient for signs of improvement of disease symptoms and for absence of adverse effects.

Basic Drug Information

Everyone that administers drugs should understand at least a little bit about pharmacokinetics (or what the body does to the drug - like metabolism and clearance) and pharmacodynamics (what the drug does to the body - the effects and adverse effects).

Important Pharmacokinetic Points

Most drugs are removed from the body by hepatic (liver) metabolism and/or renal (kidney) clearance. If drugs are metabolized or cleared primarily by one route and the patient has disease that affects that route, the drug may need to be avoided or administered at a very low dose. In patients with hepatic disease, drugs that are metabolized primarily by the liver may be metabolized slowly, creating prolonged or exaggerated effects. An example is acepromazine. In patients with renal disease, drugs that are cleared primarily by the kidney may be cleared slowly, creating prolonged or exaggerated effects. An example is ketamine in cats.

Some drugs are cleared by other routes. The inhalant anesthetic drugs are primarily exhaled without undergoing any metabolism at all. Propofol is metabolized by the liver and cleared by the kidney but is also metabolized by the lung and by enzymes in plasma. Thus clearance of inhalants and propofol are less impacted by renal or hepatic disease.

The effects of some drugs are reversible. These drugs will still undergo hepatic metabolism or renal clearance but the effects of the drug can be reversed. This increases the safety of these drugs since adverse effects can be quickly decreased or eliminated. Examples of reversible drugs include the alpha-2 agonists (e.g., dexmedetomidine [Dexdomitor®], medetomidine [Domitor®], xylazine, romifidine and detomidine), opioids (e.g., morphine, hydromorphone, methadone, fentanyl, butorphanol and buprenorphine) and the benzodiazepines (diazepam and midazolam).

The degree that drugs bind to protein is important because the non-protein bound 'free fraction' of the drug is the active portion. If the patient has low protein, more of the drug is 'free', resulting in greater activity, which could result in an increased likelihood of dose-dependent adverse effects. If other drugs that bind to the same proteins are administered, either the new drug will not be able to bind to proteins already bound to the first drug, or the new drug will replace the first drug at the binding site. In either scenario, one of the drugs could potentially reach concentrations that lead to an increased likelihood of dose-dependent adverse effects. This situation is more common in drugs that are highly protein bound because a very small free fraction is responsible for the drug's effects and even a minimal competition for binding sites can cause a dramatic increase in the free fraction. For instance most non-steroidal anti-inflammatory drugs (NSAIDs) are around 98% protein bound. Protein binding is not covered in this book but that information is available on the product insert (the information sheet that comes with the drug).

Important Pharmacodynamic Points

The desired *effects* of all drugs are offset by *side effects* and *adverse effects*. For instance, the primary effect of opioids is analgesia and a side effect is sedation (at least in dogs). This isn't necessarily an adverse effect because we want sedation when using these drugs for anesthesia premedication. However, the opioids also can cause vomiting and this is usually an adverse effect, meaning an unwanted side effect. For all drugs, the benefit of the effects should be weighed against the potential side or adverse effects of that drug in that particular patient. Using opioids as an example, the profound analgesia produced generally far outweighs the fact that vomiting occurs since vomiting is an annoying, but not generally life-threatening, adverse effect.

Drugs used in the Premedication Phase of Anesthesia

The choice of premedication drugs should be based on: patient health; species and breed; patient temperament; level of pain expected from the procedure; and type and duration of the procedure. Choosing the correct premedications for your patient will decrease the dosages of drugs needed for induction, maintenance, and recovery from anesthesia (which increases anesthetic safety) and will make the entire anesthetic period run more smoothly.

Drugs that are commonly used for premedication include analgesic drugs (e.g., opioids and alpha-2 agonists) and tranquilizer/sedatives (e.g., acepromazine, alpha-2 agonists and benzodiazepines). Note that opioids and alpha-2 agonists fit into both the analgesic and tranquilizer/sedative categories. Although not truly anesthetic drugs, NSAIDs are often administered as a premedication as part of the analgesic protocol. Ketamine and tiletamine/zolazepam are most commonly considered to be induction drugs but may be used as premedications, primarily as tranquilizers for extremely excited or aggressive patients. Anticholinergics may be administered in the premedication period, not as part of the anesthetic drugs per se, but to support heart rate. In compromised patients, other support drugs may be administered. Premedication is important in all species but this chapter will focus on dogs and cats. All dosages in this chapter are for both dogs and cats unless otherwise specified. All drugs are supplied as injectable solutions unless otherwise specified.

Also, all routes of drug administration are listed for completeness but premedications are generally administered IM, SQ or IV. The SQ route is not recommended for most premedications since absorption from this site is very slow and results in a lower peak serum concentration of the drug. Thus, premedications administered SQ take a long time to work and have unpredictable absorption and drugs administered by this route are often not as effective as if administered IM or IV.

> **IMPORTANT POINT**
> **Don't forget that the premedication phase of anesthesia entails more than just choosing and administering drugs. For other patient and equipment considerations for this phase of anesthesia, read Chapters 2 and 8.**

Premedication: Analgesic Drugs
Opioids
General Information: The opioids are the most potent, and among the safest, systemically administered analgesic drugs. Opioids fit both in the analgesic and sedative/tranquilizer category in dogs and ruminants but can be excitatory in cats and horses. Thus, opioids can be used alone as premedications in dogs, especially sick dogs, but are usually administered with a sedative in healthy dogs, cats and horses. The incidence of serious adverse effects is low and the benefits of the opioid class are numerous. It is an excellent class for compromised, geriatric and neonatal patients, especially when dosed at the low end of the clinical dosing range. Also, the effects are reversible, and this adds to the safety of the drug class since adverse effects can be eliminated. Opioids can be used to treat both chronic and acute pain. Opioids are among the most commonly used premedications and there are more opioids to choose from than with any other class of premedications.

Mechanism of Action: Opioids provide analgesia by binding to mu and/or kappa opioid receptors in the central and peripheral nervous systems. Opioids that bind to both mu and kappa receptors (e.g., morphine, hydromorphone, fentanyl and methadone) are the most potent drugs, and they provide the most profound analgesia. Agonist-antagonists (butorphanol) and partial agonists (buprenorphine) provide less potent analgesia, but also have a slightly lower incidence of side/adverse effects **(Table 4-2)**.

Metabolism/Clearance: Opioids are metabolized primarily by the liver and the metabolites (and sometimes the unmetabolized portion of the parent drug) are cleared by the kidneys. However, opioids do not exacerbate hepatic or renal disease and are safe for patients with disease of either organ system. These diseases may cause exaggerated and/or prolonged opioid-mediated effects, but this can be minimized by using the low end of the dosing range in diseased patients and can be eliminated using reversal drugs, if necessary.

Reversal Drugs: Effects are reversed by naloxone and naltrexone (the latter is rarely used in veterinary medicine and not covered in this book). Butorphanol and buprenorphine can be used to partially reverse (buprenorphine) the mu receptor-mediated effects of the full opioid agonists or to reverse the mu effects but not the kappa receptor-mediated effects (butorphanol). This allows reversal of some effects but not total reversal of analgesia. In most instances, reversal with butorphanol or buprenorphine is adequate and naloxone can be reserved for opioid-overdose or opioid-mediated emergencies.

Routes of Administration: Opioids may be administered IV (as boluses or infusions), IM, SQ, transdermally, epidurally, intraarticularly, and transmucosally (e.g., buccal or 'oral transmucosal' [OTM] administration).

Species Used: All mammals; birds; reptiles, etc.

FDA Approval: Few opioids are FDA approved for use in veterinary medicine. Exceptions include the specific 24-hour duration buprenorphine for cats (Simbadol®). Oxymorphone is approved for use in dogs but is rarely used because it is hard to get. A specific dose of butorphanol (0.4 mg/kg) is approved in cats. Despite few FDA approved products, the opioids have been studied in-depth in dogs and cats. There are numerous publications on both safety and efficacy of the opioids used in these species, and most all species that we treat in veterinary medicine. This is true for all of the opioids described in this book.

DEA Control: All opioids except for nalbuphine are Drug Enforcement Agency (DEA) controlled drugs.

Effects: The full mu and kappa opioid agonists and butorphanol provide analgesia in all patients, and dose-dependent sedation in dogs and ruminants (a beneficial effect when used as a premedication and sedation is desired). Buprenorphine provides long-lasting analgesia but minimal sedation.

Side/Adverse Effects: Most of the adverse effects are mild with minimal to no clinical significance. Not all opioids cause all of these adverse effects and not all patients will experience the same adverse effects. Common effects include sedation (which is only an adverse effect if sedation wasn't the goal), panting (usually only with the mu opioid agonists and not really a problem but sometimes annoying), and vagally-mediated bradycardia (which can be treated or prevented with the use of anticholinergics if the bradycardia causes hypotension). Nausea and vomiting often occur in nonpainful patients (e.g., when the opioid is used as a premedication in a healthy patient that does not have existing pain) but will rarely cause these effects in painful patients (e.g., when the opioid is used postoperatively or in a patient that has just experienced some painful traumatic injury). Excitement, rather than sedation, can occur in horses and cats - but, as with adverse effects in dogs, is much more likely to occur in nonpainful patients and rarely occurs when opioids are used postoperatively or in traumatized patients. Constipation may occur with long-term use (e.g., treatment of chronic pain). Hyperthermia may occur in cats (see more information under hydromorphone). Respiratory depression was long reported to be a major adverse effect of opioids but this is much more likely to occur in humans than in animals. Some mild respiratory depression may occur, but it is generally related to the degree of sedation in animals. Urinary retention may occur when opioids are used epidurally, but this is uncommon (Chapter 7). Histamine release may occur with rapid IV injection of morphine. Gastrointestinal (GI) motility can be slowed but this is rarely clinically significant and ileus (total cessation of GI motility) is extremely unlikely. They may cause myosis (constricted pupils) in dogs and mydriasis (dilated pupils) in cats.

Clinical Use: For analgesia in all 4 phases of anesthesia and as a mild sedative in dogs (more sedating in sick or old dogs). Opioids commonly used for premedication include morphine, hydromorphone, methadone, butorphanol or buprenorphine. Fentanyl is often used as a bolus at induction and transdermal fentanyl patches can be used postoperatively. Intraoperatively and postoperatively opioids are commonly administered as boluses or infusions. Opioids (particularly morphine) can be administered in the epidural or intra-articular (joint) space intraoperatively.

Precautions

• Vomiting may be beneficial since it empties anything that might be in the stomach, but it can be detrimental in some patients such as those with esophageal foreign bodies and those with specific upper airway dysfunction which prevents the epiglottis from completely covering the laryngeal opening (e.g., brachycephalic dogs with severe epiglottic hypoplasia), which could predispose the patient to aspiration pneumonia if it vomited and then aspirated the vomitus.

• Also, vomiting can cause an increase in intracranial and intraocular pressure and would be undesirable in patients with head trauma, brain lesions and some ocular diseases like glaucoma.

• Opioids may be detrimental in patients with moderate to severe head trauma since even mild respiratory depression can cause elevated carbon dioxide levels, which increases cerebral blood flow and intracranial pressure.

• If cats appear agitated after receiving an opioid, check their body temperature since the agitation may be due to hyperthermia.

• Morphine can cause histamine release if administered rapidly IV but can be administered IM or slowly IV (a slow bolus or an infusion) without causing this effect.

Absolute Contraindications: None for the class.

IMPORTANT TIP:
Opioid-induced vomiting can be reduced or eliminated by:
1. Premedicating the patient with maropitant.
2. Administering the opioid IV instead of IM or SQ.
3. Administering the opioid after induction to anesthesia (but before pain is induced!).
4. Using lesser potent opioids like butorphanol or buprenorphine (don't forget to use multimodal analgesia [Chapter 7] in this case).
5. Using methadone. It is the least likely of the potent opioids to cause vomiting.

KEY POINTS
• Opioids provide moderate to potent analgesia, depending on the specific drug.

• Opioids are generally very safe drugs and should be considered for sedation and analgesia in all patients, including critical patients, geriatrics and neonates.

• Most opioids can cause vomiting, which is generally not a clinically significant problem.

• There are numerous opioids to choose from so the opioid can be tailored to the patient and to the degree of expected pain.

• Some opioids can cause excitement in horses and cats, but this effect is easily and commonly controlled with the concurrent administration of a sedative.

• The effects of opioids are reversible with the drug naloxone. Remember that reversing the opioids reverses analgesia so be sure to address pain relief with other drug classes.

Specific Opioids
(In alphabetical order; Table 4-2)

Buprenorphine
Receptor Binding: Partial agonist at the mu receptor.
DEA Class: 3
Products: An injectable solution (which is the same solution that is used OTM) and a long duration (Simbadol®) injectable solution. There are a variety of compounded oral products with no research on efficacy.
FDA Approval: The long duration (24-hours) injectable buprenorphine (Simbadol®) is FDA approved for use in cats. This is not to be confused with the compounded sustained release injectable that is not FDA approved nor with the injectable from human medicine that most people are familiar with which is used for injection and OTM administration.
Routes of Administration: IV, IM, SQ, and buccal/OTM. In general, SQ administration leads to low serum concentrations and is not recommended (See Chapter 8 for more information in injection routes). The extended release formula (Simbadol®) is the exception and must be administered SQ since it is the SQ administration along with

the high concentration of the drug that provides the 24-hour duration analgesia. Buccal or OTM administration was originally thought to provide very high serum levels of buprenorphine but recent research shows that the serum concentration is actually lower after OTM administration than after IV or IM administration. Thus, IV or IM should be used for moderate pain in hospitalized patients but OTM administration is still a good choice for pet owners to utilize at home or when pain is mild, but the dose now recommended is higher than the IV/IM dose. The OTM route was once thought to be ineffective in dogs but this was incorrect - this route works for dogs, cats, rabbits and probably most small mammals.

Species: Primarily dogs, cats, and other small mammals. Also birds and reptiles. Some use in large animals but cost usually limits use in these species.

Dose: 0.01 to 0.03 mg/kg; IV, IM but 0.03-0.05 mg/kg may be required for adequate analgesia when administered OTM. The dose is 0.03-0.1 mg/kg IV, IM or SQ in rabbits. Dosing is usually BID-QID depending on the severity of the pain.

Onset of Action: Slow compared to other opioids, 10 to 30 minutes for full effects. Onset is prolonged regardless of route of administration. The onset of Simbadol® is one hour so be sure to administer one hour before surgery or supplement with rapidly acting drugs (e.g., dexmedetomidine) if the patient is already painful.

Duration of Action: 4 to 8 (maybe up to 12 if pain is MILD) hours depending on route of administration, dose and intensity of pain. Simbadol® has a 24 hour duration.

Drug Specific Information: Buprenorphine binds very tightly to opioid receptors and, because opioid reversal drugs (or 'antagonists') work by competing for binding at the receptor, the effects of buprenorphine can be hard to reverse. Fortunately, buprenorphine rarely causes effects that need to be reversed. If reversal is needed, use the high end of the naloxone dose and repeat naloxone up to two times, if necessary. This should provide at least partial reversal of the buprenorphine effects.

Clinical Use: Patients with mild to moderate pain; cats (not likely to cause excitement like other opioids, can easily be administered OTM, Simbadol® is approved for cats only); patients in which sedation is not desired; patients in which vomiting is contraindicated. Just remember that buprenorphine-mediated analgesia is mild to moderate so be sure to use multimodal analgesia if pain is severe (see Chapter 7).

KEY POINTS

- **Buprenorphine is appropriate for mild to moderate pain.**
- **Provides analgesia for 4-8 hours with minimal to no sedation.**
- **Can be used therapeutically to reverse the adverse effects of pure mu opioids.**
- **Binds very tightly to opioid receptors so effects are hard to reverse.**
- **Commonly used in cats because it is unlikely to cause excitement or hyperthermia (like some mu receptor opioids occasionally do) and the small volume required for dosing cats is more cost effective than volumes required for dosing medium to large dogs.**
- **Absorbed from the oral mucosa, which is generally an easy place for owners to administer drugs, making buprenorphine a good drug for at-home analgesia.**
- **Moderately expensive in most countries.**

Butorphanol

Receptor Binding: Antagonist at the mu receptor, agonist at the kappa receptor.

DEA Class: 4.

Products: Available as an injectable solution and tablets, which are really used as antitussives (i.e., cough suppressants). Analgesia provided by the tablets is highly questionable.

FDA Approval: Approved as an antitussive in the dog but not approved for sedation or analgesia. Approved for analgesia in cats when administered at 0.4 mg/kg.

Routes of administration: IV, IM, SQ.

Dose: 0.2 to 0.4 mg/kg, as needed. Should be administered very frequently (frequency based on reported duration) if used for analgesia.

Onset of action: 3 to 5 minutes IV; 5 to 15 minutes IM; 10+ SQ.

Duration of action: 45 to 90 minutes. Duration may be as short as 20 minutes (and up to 60 minutes) in dogs but is probably closer to 90 minutes in cats.

Clinical Use: Commonly used as a mild sedative (alone for mild sedation, with acepromazine or an alpha-2 agonist for more profound sedation). Should not routinely be used alone for analgesia since the duration of action is so short.

KEY POINTS

- **Butorphanol provides moderate sedation in dogs and in compromised cats and is appropriate for treatment of short-duration, mild to moderate pain.**
- **Of all of the opioids, butorphanol is least likely to cause excitement in cats and horses.**
- **Moderately expensive.**

Fentanyl

Receptor Binding: Agonist at both mu and kappa receptors.

DEA Class: 2.

Products: Available as an injectable solution and transdermal patches.

FDA Approval: None.

Routes of Administration: IV (bolus or infusion), IM, SQ, epidurally, and transdermally.

Dose: 1 to 5 microg/kg bolus (up to 20 microg/kg). Most commonly used as an infusion. For dosages, see Chapter 7.

Onset of Action: < 1 to 2 minutes.

Duration of Action: 20 to 30 minutes from a single IV bolus; 72 hours transdermal patch: for infusion duration, see Chapter 7.

Clinical Use: As a bolus just before induction to decrease induction drug dose and 'smooth' induction. Also as infusions, transdermally, or as a bolus to boost analgesia just before something really painful is done.

KEY POINTS

- Fentanyl is a very potent opioid that is effective for treatment of moderate to severe pain.
- Most commonly used at induction (bolus) and during maintenance (IV boluses or infusions); and as a transdermal patch for post-operative pain.
- Occasionally used as a premedication when brief, profound analgesia is required (e.g., in cesarean sections, see case examples in Chapter 9).
- Moderately, but not prohibitively, expensive in most countries.

Hydromorphone

Receptor Binding: Agonist at both mu and kappa receptors.
DEA Class: 2.
FDA Approval: None.
Route of Administration: IV (bolus or infusion), IM, SQ, or epidurally.
Dose: Dogs 0.1 to 0.2 mg/kg; Cats 0.1 mg/kg.
Onset of Action: 1 to 5 minutes IV; 10 to 20 minutes IM.
Duration of Action: 2 to 4 hours depending primarily on intensity of pain and patient sensitivity to pain but influenced somewhat by the route of administration.
Drug Specific Information: Hydromorphone is the opioid most often associated with opioid-induced hyperthermia in cats but this may be due to the fact that hydromorphone is one of the most commonly used opioids in cats. Since this adverse effect seems to be more common in certain geographic areas than others, the hyperthermia could also be due to genetic factors in specific populations of cats that make them more sensitive to this effect.
Clinical Use: Same as morphine.

KEY POINTS

- Hydromorphone is inexpensive and provides profound analgesia.
- Effects and adverse effects are very similar to those provided by morphine.
- Hydromophone-induced hyperthermia in cats may be more common in certain populations of cats.

Methadone

Receptor Binding: Methadone is a mu and kappa agonist.
DEA Class: 2.
FDA Approval: None.
Routes of Administration: IV (bolus or infusion), IM, SQ, or epidurally.
Dose: Dog 0.2 to 0.3 mg/kg IV; 0.3 to 0.6 mg/kg (up to 1.0 mg/kg) IM or SQ; Cat 0.1 to 0.3 mg/kg IV; up 0.5 mg/kg IM or SQ; 0.6 mg/kg OTM; Infusion and epidural dosages are in Chapter 7.
Onset of Action: 1 to 5 min IV; 10 to 20 min IM; 15+ SQ.
Duration of Action: 2 to 4 hours depending primarily on intensity of pain and patient sensitivity to pain but influenced somewhat by the route of administration.
Drug Specific Information: Vomiting is very uncommon with methadone, thus it may

be a good choice for patients in which vomiting is contraindicated (e.g., patients with esophageal foreign bodies or increased intracranial pressure, or those with upper airway dysfunction in which regurgitation and aspiration is a concern). Methadone antagonizes the N-methyl-D-aspartate (NMDA) receptors to some degree and may aid in prevention or treatment of pain of central sensitization (or "wind-up pain"). The magnitude of this effect from methadone is unknown (see Chapter 7 for more information).

Clinical Use: Same as morphine.

KEY POINTS
- Methadone provides profound analgesia.
- Effects and adverse effects are very similar to those provided by morphine.
- Methadone may cause enhanced analgesia through NMDA-receptor blockade.
- It is the least likely of the mu agonist opioids to cause vomiting.
- Expensive in the US but very inexpensive in many other countries.

Morphine
Receptor Binding: Morphine is a mu and kappa receptor agonist.
DEA Class: 2.
Products: Available as an injectable solution; preservative-free injectable solution (used for epidural injection, see Chapter 7) and oral tablets (sometimes used for treatment of chronic pain).
FDA Approval: None.
Routes of Administration: IV (bolus or infusion), IM, SQ, IV, epidurally (regular morphine or preservative-free morphine), or intra-articularly (i.e., in the joint space).
Dose: Administer 0.25 to 1.0 mg/kg for dogs; 0.1 to 0.3 mg/kg for cats. For both species, use low-end of the dose for IV administration and in compromised, neonatal or geriatric patients. Epidural and infusion dosages are in Chapter 7.
Onset of Action: 5 minutes IV; 10 to 20 minutes IM; 15+ minutes SQ.
Duration of Action: 2 to 4 hours depending primarily on intensity of pain and patient sensitivity to pain but influenced somewhat by the route of administration.
Drug Specific Effects: Histamine release may occur if administered rapidly IV but slow administration and constant rate infusions do not cause this effect.
Clinical Use: It is the most commonly used opioid for premedication, intraoperative and postoperative boluses and infusions, and injection into the epidural space.

KEY POINTS
- Morphine provides moderate to profound analgesia.
- Morphine is the 'Gold standard' to which other opioids are compared so comments like 'more (or less) potent than morphine' are common. This is not because it is 'better' than other opioids but because it has been available the longest.
- Very inexpensive in the US.

Nalbuphine

Receptor Binding: Nalbuphine is an antagonist at the mu receptor and agonist at the kappa receptor.

DEA Class: Not controlled.

FDA Approval: None.

Routes of Administration: IV (bolus), IM or SQ.

Dose: 0.2 to 0.4 mg/kg.

Onset of Action: Similar to butorphanol.

Duration of Action: Similar to butorphanol (45 to 90 minutes).

Clinical Use: Nalbuphine is not widely used. It can be used in place of butorphanol but is not a good sedative.

KEY POINTS

- **Nalbuphine is very similar to butorphanol but provides minimal to no sedation.**
- **It provides mild analgesia of short duration.**
- **Moderately expensive.**

IMPORTANT POINT:

The effects of all opioids are reversible.

Table 4-2
Opioid Premedication for Dogs and Cats.

Opioid	Analgesia	Onset/ Duration	Comments and Adverse Effects	Dose in **mg/kg** unless otherwise indicated
Morphine	Profound analgesia; Full mu and kappa opioid receptor agonists; all are DEA Class II opioids	1 to 5 mins IV or 10 to 20 mins IM / 2 to 4 hours	Adverse effects are minimal; nonpainful animals may vomit following IM injection; May cause histamine release if administered fast IV; May cause excitement in cats - use with a tranquilizer, inexpensive.	Dog: 0.25 to 1.0 IM or slowly IV Cat: 0.1 to 0.3 IM or slowly IV Typical starting dose: Dog 0.5 (0.25 for geriatric & compromised patients) IM, cat 0.2 IM
Hydromorphone		Similar to morphine	Similar to morphine but no histamine release. May cause hyperthermia in cats, especially at doses >0.1 mg/kg; inexpensive.	Dog: 0.1 to 0.2 IM or IV Cat: 0.1 IM or IV Typical starting dose: Dog & cat 0.1 IM
Methadone		Similar to morphine	Similar to morphine but no histamine release and little to no vomiting; is also an N-methyl-D-aspartate antagonist but efficacy is not known; expensive.	Dog & Cat: 0.2-0.4 IV; 0.2-0.6 (up to 1.0 in dogs) IM; Cat 0.6 oral transmucosal Typical starting dose: Dog & cat 0.4 IM
Fentanyl	More potent than the drugs listed above; mu and kappa agonist; DEA Class II	< 1 to 2 min / 20 to 30 minutes IV Transdermal patch: CAT: 6-12 hrs/3-4 days DOG: 12-24/3 days	Less likely to cause adverse effects than other full opioid agonists; Duration of action is short so most commonly used as bolus for brief painful stimulus, as an infusion or in a transdermal patch; moderately expensive.	Dog & cat: 1 to 5 micrograms/kg IV. Can administer up to 20 microg/kg; information on infusions and transdermal patch in Chapter 7.

83

Table 4-2 continued

Butorphanol	Mild to Moderate analgesia; kappa agonist, mu antagonist; DEA Class IV opioid	3 to 5 mins IV or 5 to 15 mins IM /20 to 60 (dog) to 90 (cat) minutes	<u>EXTREMELY SHORT DURATION OF ACTION:</u> Decent sedative in both dogs and cats, especially if combined with a tranquilizer; same adverse effects as other opioids but effects are generally mild; Unlikely to cause excitement in either cats or horses so commonly used in these species; moderately expensive.	Dog & Cat: 0.2 to 0.4 IM or IV Typical starting dose: Dog & cat 0.4 for surgery, 0.2 for sedation without surgery
Nalbuphine	Same as butorphanol; Not DEA controlled	Similar to butorphanol	Similar to butorphanol but not very sedating. One of the best uses of butorphanol is for sedation.	Dog & Cat: 0.2 to 0.4 IM or IV
Buprenorphine	Mild to Moderate analgesia; partial mu agonist; DEA Class III opioid	10 to 30 mins / 4 to 8 hours, depending on pain intensity & dose	Long duration of action but slow onset of action and minimal to no sedation; same adverse effects as other opioids but effects are generally mild or nonexistent; moderately expensive. Commonly used transmucosally to administer postop at home or for chronic pain in cats. Can also be used by this route in dogs but volume is large unless dog is really small.	Dog & Cat: 0.01 to 0.03 IM, IV. May need to double the dose for transmucosal delivery. Typical starting dose: Dog & cat 0.03 Simbadol® is an FDA-approved buprenorphine for cats only that provides analgesia for 24-hrs. The dose is 0.24 SQ, 0.12-0.18 should be considered for sick, geriatric and pediatric cats.

Premedication: Tranquilizers/Sedatives
(In alphabetical order; Table 4-3)

Acepromazine Maleate

General Information: Acepromazine, classified as a phenothiazine tranquilizer, is one of the most commonly used sedatives in veterinary medicine. 'Ace' provides mild to moderate, fairly long-term (several hours) sedation without analgesia. The effects are not reversible.

Mechanism of Action: Primarily an antagonist at dopaminergic receptors.

Metabolism/Clearance: Primarily hepatic.

Reversal Drugs: The effects are not reversible, must be metabolized.

Routes of Administration: IV, IM and SQ.

Species Used: All mammals.

Dose: Dog 0.01 to 0.05 mg/kg; Cat 0.03 to 0.05mg/kg by all routes.

Onset of Action: 15 to 30 minutes.

Duration of Action: 2 to 8 hours with residual effects possible (but rare) for up to 48 hours.

FDA Approval: Dogs, cats and horses.

DEA Class: Not controlled.

Effects: Mild to moderate, long duration (hours) sedation.

Adverse Effects: Minimal. Because of vasodilation, may contribute to lowered blood pressure and body temperature but this is generally not a problem in healthy patients receiving clinically appropriate dosages.

Species Specific Effects/Adverse Effects: None in small animals.

Clinical Use: Acepromazine is commonly used for premedication, long duration light to moderate sedation, and to smooth out rough recoveries (although its slow onset makes early administration [i.e., as a premedication] or combination with faster acting drugs necessary when used for the latter purpose). It is not generally used in compromised, geriatric, anemic, hemorrhaging or hypotensive patients, nor in patients with hepatic disease, for the reasons described below.

Precautions

• Because of the decrease in circulating red blood cells (see 'margination' below), acepromazine should be avoided or used with caution in patients that are anemic, hemorrhaging or have platelet dysfunction.

• Hypotension secondary to vasodilation can occur but is primarily dose dependent and is more likely in patients that are already vasodilated or hypotensive. Thus, acepromazine should be avoided in patients that fit either of these categories.

• Acepromazine should be avoided or administered at very low doses in patients with hepatic dysfunction and in geriatric patients since patients from either of these groups may have difficulty metabolizing the drug, resulting in a more pronounced effect and/or a prolonged duration of action.

Absolute Contraindications: None.

KEY POINTS

- Acepromazine is inexpensive, provides no analgesia, is not reversible, and requires hepatic metabolism.
- It can cause the PCV to decrease up to 50% within 30 minutes post administration. This occurs due to a vasodilation (primarily in the spleen) and 'margination' of the red cells along the vessel walls. The PCV will return to normal within several hours.
- It can be useful in patients with some cardiac diseases because of its mild anti-arrhythmic effects. Mild vasodilation can also be useful in some cardiac patients by reducing cardiac afterload, which means that the heart does not have to work as hard to eject blood into the vessels. In this instance, a very low dose (0.01mg/kg) should be used to avoid hypotension.
- It has mild anti-emetic properties.
- DOES NOT CAUSE SEIZURES - this is an old myth that has been proven false.
- May cause Boxer dogs to collapse, but there is little evidence and this may be a myth.
- There is a specific gene mutation (MDR-1) that makes Collies sensitive to the adverse effects of drugs like ivermectin and may cause an exaggerated response to some drugs, one of them being acepromazine.

Alpha-2 Agonists

Class Information: This class of drugs provides both sedation AND analgesia in all species.

Mechanism of Action: Binds to alpha-2 receptors in the central nervous system to provide sedation and analgesia. Provides differing degrees of analgesia depending on the alpha-2: alpha-1 receptor binding ratio. A higher ratio = more profound analgesia.

Metabolism/Clearance: Metabolized by the liver but the effects are also reversible with alpha-2 antagonists.

Reversal Drugs: All alpha-2 agonists can be reversed with all alpha-2 antagonists, which are atipamezole, yohimbine and tolazoline. However, only atipamezole is specifically designed for reversal of medetomidine and dexmedetomidine so it provides a more complete reversal. It is also safer than the other reversal drugs because it competitively binds to the alpha-receptors, which displaces the alpha-2 agonist. It has no (or very minimal) effect on its own.

Routes of Administration: IV (as boluses or infusions), IM, SQ and epidurally (although not commonly used by this route in small animals).

Species: All.

FDA Approval: See specific alpha-2 agonists

DEA Control: No drugs in this class are DEA controlled.

Effects: Provides dose-dependent sedation with mild to moderate analgesia.

Side/Adverse Effects: Vasoconstriction which can cause hypertension and increase cardiac work (because it is harder for the heart to eject blood into small vessels than into big vessels). The hypertension causes reflex bradycardia. The vasoconstriction is most prominent in peripheral vessels like the skin and mucous membranes, thus, the mucous membranes often look pale and the pulse oximeter may not work very well on the lip or the tongue for the first 5 to 15 minutes (depending on the dose) after alpha-2 administration. Use other monitors - blood pressure, capillary refill time, etc. Remember that the blood did not leave the patient - just left the mucous membranes. The blood moves centrally and the organs are perfused. The bradycardia is a NORMAL reflex to the high blood pressure caused by the vasoconstriction. It is NOT an adverse effect and doesn't need to be treated since the blood pressure is HIGH. Only treat bradycardia if blood pressure is LOW. This can happen following alpha-2 agonist administration in patients on inhalant anesthetic drugs because the vasoconstriction may dissipate (or be overcome by the vasodilatory effects of the inhalants) but the heart rate may not increase in anesthetized patients. Alpha-2 agonists can cause vomiting, especially xylazine. Alpha-2 agonists cause decreased insulin release and patients will become transiently hyperglycemic, which is unlikely to cause a clinical impact. They also cause increased urine production and patients often need to urinate soon after waking from sedation. Some patients have transient muscle twitching that has been confused with mild seizures but is NOT seizures.

Species Specific Effects/Adverse Effects: The effects are the same in all species but the alpha-2 agonists have a wider dosage range between species than any of the other anesthesia-related drugs. In large animal species, small ruminants are particularly sensitive and require the lowest dosages, pigs are the least sensitive and require the highest dosages. Among common small animal patients, dogs are the most sensitive, cats a little less sensitive and small pocket pets (rabbits, rodents, etc.) are the least sensitive. See specific drugs for dosing information.

Clinical Use: Commonly used as a preanesthetic and for procedural sedation (i.e., sedation for 'procedures' that don't require general anesthesia - like taking radiographs, suturing small lacerations, etc.) in all species. Can be combined with analgesic drugs and injectable anesthetic drugs (like ketamine) for a commonly used anesthetic protocol. Also frequently used to treat dysphoria and pain in patients experiencing dysphoria in the recovery phase of anesthesia.

Hints for Clinical Use

• The most predictable and profound sedation will occur in patients that are calm and that receive an opioid in addition to the alpha-2 agonist. Sedative/tranquilizers work by decreasing the release of excitatory neurotransmitters. When the excitatory neurotransmitters are already circulating (in aggressive, excited or extremely fearful patients), the sedative/tranquilizers will not work as well.

• Try to keep the patient calm and quiet before administering the alpha-2 agonist. If the patient is excited, keep the patient in a quiet, darkened environment after the administration of the alpha-2 agonist.

• Use a high dose in excited patients, a low dose is unlikely to work and having to stick the patient again with a needle to administer a second dose can make the patient even more excited.

• Adding an opioid will increase the predictability of the sedation, even if the procedure that the patient is being sedated for is not painful. Choose the opioid based on pain level and/or duration of procedure (e.g., hydromorphone or morphine can be used for painful procedures or procedures that last > 1 hour; butorphanol can be used for nonpainful or minimally painful, short procedures).

IMPORTANT POINT:

Don't treat the bradycardia! It is a normal reflex to the increased blood pressure. Check the blood pressure and treat the bradycardia ONLY if the patient is hypotensive. If the blood pressure is normal, leave the heart rate alone. If treatment is necessary, you can reverse the effects of the alpha-2 agonist or use an anticholinergic - the 'rule' that anticholinergics should not be used in patients that received alpha-2 agonists only applies if the heart rate is low AND the blood pressure is high. **If both the heart rate AND the blood pressure are LOW, anticholinergic administration is acceptable**.

• Don't reverse all patients. It is not necessary to reverse most of the patients - let them sleep! Reversal takes away the analgesia as well as the sedation and adds to the overall cost of the drugs. Definitely reverse if you are concerned about any adverse effects or if you need to send the patient home right away. There is more information on reversal in the section on drugs used during recovery from anesthesia at the end of this chapter.

TIP:

Use this drug class in cats! It is efficient and easy to use since you can administer it IM. Dexdomitor® (dexmedetomidine) is FDA approved for use in cats.

Precautions

• Vasoconstriction increases cardiac work, which is detrimental in patients with cardiac disease.
• Alpha-2 agonists can worsen bradycardic arrhythmias, like second-degree AV block.
• Vomiting can occur especially after IM or SQ administration. The vomiting is often beneficial since it empties the stomach but vomiting can be detrimental in some patients, like those with esophageal foreign bodies; head trauma or brain lesions (vomiting increases intracranial pressure); patients with specific upper airway dysfunction causing the epiglottis not to completely cover the laryngeal opening (which could lead to aspiration pneumonia); and patients with some ocular diseases (vomiting causes increased intraocular pressure).
• Some people feel that the alpha-2 agonists are contraindicated in diabetic patients because of the transient hyperglycemia where others feel that this is not clinically important since it is of such short duration. Transient hyperglycemia is safer than transient hypoglycemia. We commonly use alpha-2 agonists in diabetic patients.

Absolute Contraindications: Do not administer to patients with most types of cardiac disease.

KEY POINTS

• Alpha-2 agonists provide dose-dependent sedation. The sedation dose is highly variable among species.

• All alpha-2 agonists provide moderate analgesia but, because of more specific alpha-2 receptor binding, medetomidine and dexmedetomidine provide better analgesia than xylazine.

• The alpha-2 mediated vasoconstriction increases cardiac work so the drugs should not be used in patients with most, but not all, types of heart disease.

• Bradycardia is a normal physiologic response to the increase in blood pressure secondary to the vasoconstriction. Don't treat the bradycardia - check blood pressure and leave the heart rate alone if the pressure is good.

• Alpha-2 agonists may cause vomiting, which is not a problem in most patients. Vomiting can be prevented by pre-administration of maropitant (Cerenia®).

• The effects of alpha-2 agonists are reversible with atipamezole (the most commonly used antagonist in small animals).

• However, not all patients need to be reversed - consider letting most of them wake up without reversal.

• Remember that reversing the sedation also reverses the analgesia so provide other means of pain relief. See information on 'partial reversal' in the recovery section of this chapter.

Specific Alpha-2 Agonists

(in alphabetical order)

Dexmedetomidine

Alpha-2: Alpha-1 Receptor Binding: 1620:1.

FDA Approval: Approved as a general and preoperative sedative/analgesic in dogs and a general sedative/analgesic in cats.

Species: Any but primarily used in small mammals (ruminants, dogs, cats, rabbits, ferrets, rodents, etc.); can be used in birds, reptiles, chelonians, etc...; sometimes used in horses as an intraoperative CRI.

Dose: There is a label dose that should be consulted for preanesthesia and sedation in the dog and cat. Clinically, the following dosages are commonly used for premedi-cation or light to medium sedation: Dogs; 0.004 to 0.015 mg/kg; Cats: 0.008 to 0.03 mg/kg. For both species, use the low end of the dose for IV administration and a higher dose for IM administration. Also use the low end of the dose (IV or IM) for calm or geriatric patients and for patients that only require light sedation.

Onset of Action: 1 to 5 minutes IV; 5 to 15 minutes IM; 10+ SQ.

Duration of Action: 30 minutes to 3 hours depending on individual sensitivity to the drug class, dose of the drug and route of administration.

Clinical Use: Commonly used as a preanesthetic and for procedural sedation (taking radiographs, suturing small lacerations, etc.) in all species. Can be combined with analgesic drugs and injectable anesthetic drugs (like ketamine) for a commonly used anesthetic protocol. Also frequently used to calm patients in the recovery phase of anesthesia.

Medetomidine

Dexmedetomidine is 'purified' medetomidine. Medetomidine is the racemic mixture (i.e., it has both dextrorotary and levorotary isomers) while dexmedetomidine is just the dextrorotary isomer (hence the name 'Dexdomitor'). Thus all information for medetomidine is the same as that listed for dexmedetomidine, except the dose.
Dose: There is a label dose that should be consulted for sedation in the dog. Clinically, the following dosages are commonly used for premedication or light to moderate sedation: Dogs; 0.008 to 0.03 mg/kg; Cats: 0.015 to 0.06 mg/kg. For both species, use the low end of the dose for IV administration and a higher dose for IM administration. Also use the low end of the dose (IV or IM) for calm or geriatric patients and for patients that only require light sedation.

KEY POINTS and DRUG SPECIFIC INFORMATION
- **Dexmedetomidine and medetomidine cause identical physiologic and analgesic effects.**

Xylazine

Alpha-2: Alpha-1 Binding: 160:1.
FDA Approval: Sedation in cats, horses, deer, and elk.
Species: Any, primarily horses and agricultural animals (e.g., cows, goats, sheep, etc.) but still used some in small animals.
Routes of Administration: IM, IV and SQ.
Dose: There is a label dose that should be consulted for sedation in both the dog and cat. Clinically, the following dosages are commonly used for premedication or light to moderate sedation in both species: 0.2 to 0.5 mg/kg. Up to 1.0 mg/kg can be used IM in especially fractious animals.
Onset of Action: 1 to 5 minutes IV; 5 to 15 minutes IM; 10+ SQ.
Duration of Action: Analgesia lasts 15 to 30 minutes; sedation lasts 1 to 2 hours depending on individual sensitivity to the drug class, dose of the drug and route of administration.
Clinical Use: Same as dexmedetomidine but higher incidence of adverse effects in small animals has led to limited use when compared to medetomidine and dexmedetomidine.

KEY POINTS and DRUG SPECIFIC INFORMATION
- **Xylazine is more likely to cause arrhythmias in dogs and cats than medetomidine or dexmedetomidine, and provides less analgesia than other alpha-2 agonists.**
- **Xylaxine is used as an emetic (induces vomiting) in cats.**
- **Other key points are the same as those for alpha-2 agonists in general.**

Benzodiazepines

Class Information: Diazepam and midazolam are the two benzodiazepines used for anesthesia. These drugs are not potent sedatives but may produce calming when combined with an opioid in neonatal, geriatric or compromised patients. If used alone in healthy, young patients, a paradoxical excitement often occurs and can be quiet dramatic. Both have a very wide safety margin, and cause virtually no cardio-vascular or respiratory changes. Generally used at induction as a muscle relaxant (especially when used with ketamine, which can cause muscle rigidity) and to decrease the dose of the induction drug (See protocols in Chapter 9). Diazepam and midazolam have no analgesic effects.

Mechanism of Action: Binds to the gamma-amino-butyric-acid (GABA) receptor in the central nervous system and causes an increase in the release of inhibitory neurotransmitters.

Metabolism/Clearance: Metabolized by the liver but effects are reversible with a benzodiazepine antagonist.

Reversal Drug: Flumazenil.

Routes of Administration: IV (both drugs), IM (midazolam only).

Species: All.

Dosage: 0.1-0.4 mg/kg for both drugs when used for premedication or part of anesthetic induction (higher dosages are used to treat seizuring patients).

DEA Control: Both are DEA Class 4.

FDA Approval: None are approved for use in veterinary medicine.

Effects: Calming (not true sedation) and muscle relaxation.

Side/Adverse Effects: Can cause paradoxical excitement in healthy patients.

Clinical Use: As a premedication, especially in really sick, really young, or really old patients. More commonly used as part of induction.

Species Specific Effects/Adverse Effects: None.

Precautions: Do not use as a premedication in excited or aggressive patients as the excitement or aggression may become worse. Can, however, use as part of induction.

Absolute Contraindications: None.

KEY POINTS

- The benzodiazepines are not potent sedatives and are most commonly used as part of induction rather than premedication.
- Administration with an opioid generally causes mild sedation in geriatric, neonatal and sick patients.
- If used as a premedication in healthy patients, combine with an opioid and/or a sedative (e.g., an alpha-2 agonist).
- The effects of the benzodiazepines are reversible with the antagonist flumazenil. Most practices don't have flumazenil because the effects of benzodiazepines very rarely need to be reversed.

Specific Benzodiazepines
(in alphabetical order)

Diazepam
Onset of Action: 2 to 3 minutes.
Duration of Action: 1 to 4 hours.

KEY POINTS And DRUG SPECIFIC INFORMATION
- Administer IV ONLY! Can be painful when administered IM and is not well absorbed by this route so effects are very unpredictable.
- Can cause hypotension if administered rapidly IV, probably because of the propylene glycol, which is the carrier of the drug.
- Do not store diazepam in any sort of plastic container because the drug adheres to plastic. This may even be a problem in patients on diazepam infusions administered through plastic IV lines, but the clinical impact appears to be minimal to nonexistent.
- Diazepam precipitates with many other drugs so cannot always be combined in the same syringe with other anesthetic drugs. Can be combined with ketamine without precipitating.

Midazolam
Onset of Action: < 1 to 2 minutes IV; 5-10 minutes IM
Duration of Action: 15 to 80 minutes IV or IM.

KEY POINTS And DRUG SPECIFIC INFORMATION
- Midazolam can be administered IM so is more likely than diazepam to be used as a premedication. IM administration is extremely useful in very small patients (e.g., rabbits, rodents, etc.).
- Midazolam can be mixed with most other drugs without precipitating.
- Midazolam is more potent, has a faster onset time and shorter duration compared to diazepam, but this is rarely (if ever) clinically impactful when using benzodiazepine drugs for anesthetic premedication or induction.

Table 4-3
Sedative/Tranquillizers Used in Dogs and Cats.

Drug	Onset/ Duration	Comments	Dose in mg/kg unless otherwise indicated
Acepromazine	15 to 30 mins / 2 to 8 hours (or longer if metabolism is impaired)	May cause hypotension at higher doses or in patients already prone to hypotension; generally don't exceed 3 mg/dog even if large dog; Metabolized by hepatic enzymes; not reversible; no analgesia. DOES NOT CAUSE SEIZURES - that is an old myth.	Dog: 0.01 to 0.03 (up to 0.05) IM or IV Cat: 0.03 to 0.05 IM or IV Typical starting dose: Dog 0.02, cat 0.03
Dexmedeto-midine (alpha-2 agonist)	1 to 5 min IV or 5 to 15 mins IM / 30 mins to 3 hours (dose dependent)	Analgesia & sedation; effects are reversible (atipa-mezole); causes vasoconstriction which causes hypertension, increased cardiac work, decreased cardiac output and reflex bradycardia.	Dog: 0.004 to 0.015 IM or IV (low end of dose for premed or IV dosing) Cat: 0.008 to 0.03 IM or IV (low end of dose for premed or IV dosing) Typical starting dose for light sedation: Dog 0.005 to 0.008, cat 0.007 to 0.010
Medetomidine (alpha-2 agonist)	1 to 5 min IV or 5 to 15 mins IM / 30 mins to 3 hours (dose dependent)	Analgesia & sedation; effects are reversible (atipa-mezole); causes vasoconstriction which causes hypertension, increased cardiac work, decreased cardiac output and reflex bradycardia.	Dog: 0.008 to 0.03 IM or IV (low end of dose for premed or IV dosing) Cat: 0.015 to 0.04 (MAYBE to 0.06) IM or IV (low end of dose for premed or IV dosing) Typical starting dose: 2x dexmed dose
Diazepam (benzodiazepine)	2 to 3 mins IV / 1 to 4 hours	IV administration - but not IM - for predictable effects; minimal sedation & no analgesia; effects are reversible (flumazenil); can cause paradoxical excitation and or aggression; DEA Class IV.	Dog & cat: 0.1-0.4 IV. Typical starting dose 0.2.
Midazolam (benzodiazepine)	1 to 2 mins IV or 5 to 10 mins IM / 15 to 80 minutes IV or IM	Good absorption with IM administration; minimal sedation & no analgesia; effects are reversible (flumazenil); can cause paradoxical excitation and or aggression; DEA Class IV.	Dog & cat: 0.1-0.4 or IV. Typical starting dose 0.2.

Other Drugs that may be used as Premedications
Ketamine, Telazol and Alfaxalone
Ketamine and Telazol® are potent anesthetic drugs that can be administered IV or IM to produce anesthesia. They are most often used as induction drugs and are discussed in further detail later in this chapter. However, they may be administered in low dosages as part of the premedication in aggressive or extremely frightened patients. With the low end of the dose ranges listed later in this chapter, deep sedation or very light anesthesia may be achieved. An example is the combination of ketamine, an alpha-2 agonist and an opioid. Administration of this combination (generally administered IM) can be used to induce a patient to anesthesia for a surgical procedure, to deeply sedate a patient (called 'chemical restraint') for diagnostic or other non-surgical procedures, or as premedication prior to induction and general anesthesia **(Table 4-4)**.

Alfaxalone is also an induction drug that is discussed in more detail later in this chapter. It can be administered IM for light sedation (NOT INDUCTION) in geriatric or sick cats at 0.5 to 1.0 mg/kg. The degree of sedation is more consistent if the alfaxalone is combined with an opioid. The advantage of alfaxalone in this scenario is that it causes less cardiovascular impact when compared to alpha-2 agonists and is cleared more quickly than acepromazine. However, in healthy cats this is unlikely to provide adequate sedation and dexmedetomidine or acepromazine is generally preferred. Alfaxalone can also be administered IM in small dogs but the volume is large even in small patients and prohibitively large in medium sized dogs or bigger. Alfaxalone is a common choice for sedating or even anesthetizing small mammals, reptiles, etc... The fact that it can be administered IM is very beneficial in these patients in which venous access is difficult or even impossible.

Support Drugs: Anticholinergics
The only support drugs that are routinely administered preoperatively are the anticholinergics, atropine and glycopyrrolate. Other support drugs may be necessary in selected patients. Support drugs, including the anticholinergics are discussed in Chapter 6.

Nonsteroidal Anti-Inflammatory Drugs (NSAIDs)
Class Information: This is a very effective class of drugs because they treat pain by decreasing the source of pain (inflammation). NSAIDs are fairly safe (think of how many doses are administered [LOTS!] vs how many adverse effects are reported. There are FDA-approved NSAIDs for both the dog and the cat and the class includes both traditional NSAIDs and the prostaglandin inhibitor, grapiprant (Galliprant®). NSAIDs are often administered prior to anesthesia because they are more effective when administered before pain starts (called 'preemptive analgesia'). NSAIDs may be administered postoperatively because they are more

likely to cause adverse effects if the patient becomes hypotensive - which can occur during anesthesia. Regardless of the timing of the first dose, NSAIDs are often used to control postoperative pain. There is more information on NSAIDs in Chapter 7.

Maropitant (Cerenia®)

This drug approved to control vomiting but also has a role in pain management, especially the management of visceral pain when used as part of a multimodal analgesic protocol. It is often administered as part of the premedications to control vomiting associated with the patient's disease and/or vomiting from drugs like the potent opioids. In addition to the maropitant-induced analgesia, the decrease in vomiting adds to the patient's overall comfort. Patients that receive maropitant also return to normal eating after surgery more quickly than patients that don't receive maropitant. Maropitant can be administered IV or SQ (1 mg/kg) in dogs and cats and is most effective if administered at least 60 minutes prior to administering premedicants that might cause vomiting. SQ injections sting. Oral maropitant is also effective (2 mg/kg dog; 1 to 2 mg /kg off-label cat) but would need to be administered at least several hours prior to administering drugs that might cause vomiting. The owner could potentially administer the oral maropitant the night or morning before the anesthesia.

How to: Choose Premedications

Premedications almost always include an opioid, even if the procedure isn't painful, since opioids are safe, effective, reversible drugs. Opioids improve the efficacy of sedatives/tranquilizers. Opioid choice should be based on both the intensity of pain and the expected duration of the procedure. Alpha-2 agonists are potent, rapidly acting sedatives that are used as premedications in heart-healthy patients. This class of drugs is especially good for very active, aggressive or fearful patients since this group of patients may need moderate to even profound sedation. Acepromazine is slow to act and provides only mild to moderate sedation but is long lasting and is also very inexpensive. This drug is especially good for patients that are already calm and those that need only light sedation. Aggressive patients may benefit from the addition of ketamine or Telazol® to the premedication protocol. Use an anticholinergic if the heart rate is likely to decrease (remember, the decrease with alpha-2 agonists is normal and should not be treated!). Remember to meet your patient before you choose your premedicationss so that you can choose the right drug - and the right dose!

Table 4-4
Other Drugs that may that may be Used as Premedications.

Drug	Duration	Advantages	Disadvantages	Dose (dog and cat) mg/kg unless otherwise indicated
Atropine (Anticholinergic)	90 mins	Crosses blood-brain-barrier; fast onset	Profound tachycardia	0.02–0.04 IM
Glycopyrrolate (Anticholinergic)	120 mins	Less tachycardia than atropine	Tachycardia, doesn't cross BBB	0.005 to 0.02 IM
Maropitant (Cerenia®) (Anti-emetic)	24 hours	Decreases or eliminates nausea and vomiting preoperatively and postoperatively; provides some analgesia	Really none except needs to be administered 30 TO 60 minutes prior to premedications that might cause vomiting or will decrease/eliminate postoperative, nausea/vomiting. May sting on SQ injection, less sting if refrigerated, none if administered IV.	1 IV or SQ in dogs and cats; oral maropitant would also be effective but should be administered several hours prior to administering drugs that cause nausea/vomiting at a dose of 2 dog and 1 to 2 cat.
Non-steroidal anti-inflammatory drugs	Variable, generally 24 hours.	Anti-inflammatory. Most effective if administered preoperatively but postoperative administration is also effective.	Adverse effects include GI upset or ulceration and hepatic or renal dysfunction.	More information in Chapter 7.

Drugs used in the Induction Phase of Anesthesia

Induction drugs are administered to produce unconsciousness in the patient. Induction should occur rapidly and smoothly and drugs should be dosed 'to effect', meaning that the patient should receive only enough drug to provide the appropriate effect - which would be a level of unconsciousness that would allow intubation of the patient or allow completion of a minor, brief procedure. The adverse effects of induction drugs are almost always dose-dependent, thus the dose should be decreased as much as possible, and this is generally achieved by using premedications. Induction drugs include propofol, ketamine, Telazol®, etomidate and alfaxalone. Inhalant anesthetic drugs are sometimes used for induction but this is not recommended for routine cases. Drugs that may be administered with the induction drugs to enhance their effects include opioids, sedative/tranquilizers and muscle relaxants. None of the induction drugs are reversible. Three of the drugs are DEA controlled: ketamine and Telazol® are Class III drugs and alfaxalone is a Class IV drug (See Table 4-1).

Specific Induction Drugs

In alphabetical order; All dosages are for dogs and cats unless otherwise specified (Table 4-5).

Alfaxalone (Alfaxan®)

Classification: Neurosteroid induction drug.
DEA Class: IV.
FDA Approval: Dogs and cats.
Species: Any, but primarily dogs, cats and species of similar size or smaller. Large volume and cost limits use in large animals.
Route of Administration: IV; IM in some circumstances but not for routine use in dogs and cats. Commonly used IM in small mammals like rodents, rabbits, etc… since venous access is limited.
Dose: 2 to 3 mg/kg dogs; 5 mg/kg cats. Titrate to effect as a lower dose may allow intubation, especially following adequate premedication.
Onset of Action: 30 to 60 seconds.
Duration of Action: 5 to 10 minutes (maybe up to 20 minutes).
Clinical Use: Similar to propofol. For routine induction in dogs and cats; especially appropriate for use in compromised dogs and cats since the drug can be easily titrated to effect and cleared from the body by multiple routes. Should be administered following premedication to decrease the alfaxalone dose. Can be used at low dose IM for light sedation in geriatric or sick cats.
Metabolism/Clearance: Primarily hepatic.
Effects: Very rapid induction to anesthesia so it is easy to titrate to effect.
Adverse Effects: Dose-dependent cardiovascular and respiratory depression. Can contribute to hypotension, especially in critical patients. May cause slightly less

respiratory depression than propofol but this is not consistent and depends on the dose of each drug.

Precautions: Dose carefully to minimize the dose-dependent cardiovascular and respiratory depression. It can cause excitement and paddling in recovery. Use with sedatives/tranquilizers and analgesic drugs.

Absolute Contraindications: None.

KEY POINTS
- **Alfaxalone may cause less respiratory depression than propofol but this is not consistent and probably only significant if a high dose of alfaxalone is compared to a high dose of propofol.**
- **Because of the alfaxalone-induced respiratory depression, preoxygenation is recommended in compromised patients.**
- **Large boluses administered rapidly are most likely to result in respiratory depression, hypotension, and reduction in myocardial contractility so administer fairly slowly (but quickly enough that it actually induces sleep).**
- **Alfaxalone can cause hyperexcitability in recovery, especially if a benzodiazepine is the only other drug administered (this precaution is listed on the label of the drug).**
- **Alfaxalone can be used IM in small patients (rabbits, rodents, etc...). Reportedly effective IM in cats but causes moderate to profound hyperexcitability and ataxia in healthy, young cats if dose is large enough for induction. Because of these effects it is not recommended as an IM induction drug in healthy cats. However, lower dosages IM (0.5 to 1.0 mg/kg) can provide light sedation in compromised cats.**
- **In the US, alfaxalone is a DEA class IV drug.**

Barbiturates
Classification: Barbiturates used in anesthesia are classified as 'ultra short' acting. An example is thiopental, whose effects and dosing are described here.

DEA Class: 3.

FDA Approval: Not currently available in the US for any species but available in other countries.

Species: Any.

Route of Administration: IV ONLY. Extra-vascular injections are very painful and cause tissue necrosis.

Dose: Thiopental: 6 to 15 mg/kg with premedication; up to 20 mg/kg without premedication.

Onset of Action: 30 to 60 seconds.

Duration of Action: 5 to 15 minutes.

Metabolism/Clearance: Primarily hepatic.

Effects: Fairly rapid induction with profound muscle relaxation.

Adverse Effects: Dose-dependent moderate-to-profound cardiovascular and respiratory depression.

Species Specific Effects/Adverse Effects: None - but there is a breed effect.

Greyhounds metabolize barbiturates more slowly than other breeds of dogs, which can lead to a prolonged recovery, especially if more than one dose is administered.

Precautions: Profound effects on the cardiovascular and respiratory system makes this drug class less than ideal for compromised patients. Dependence on hepatic metabolism can lead to prolonged recovery in patients with hepatic dysfunction if multiple or large doses are needed for induction.

Absolute contraindications: None.

KEY POINTS

• Thiopental is not currently available in the US but is available in other countries.

• Thiopental decreases cerebral oxygen consumption and intracranial pressure, decreases incidence of seizures in actively seizuring patients and in patients in which seizures might be induced (patients undergoing myelograms with certain contrast agents that induce seizures).

Etomidate

Classification: Etomidate is a non-barbiturate induction drug.

FDA Approval: No veterinary approval.

Species: Almost exclusively used in dogs and cats. Expense and lack of need limits use in large animals.

Route of Administration: IV.

Dose: 1 to 3 mg/kg.

Onset of Action: 30 to 60 seconds.

Duration of Action: 5 to 15 minutes.

Clinical Use: Almost exclusively used for patients with severe cardiac disease.

Metabolism/Clearance: Primarily hepatic.

Effects: Anesthesia with no cardiovascular effects.

Adverse Effects: When used without adequate sedation, etomidate can cause muscle rigidity, paddling, muscle twitching and vocalization.

Species Specific Effects/Adverse Effects: None.

Precautions: Etomidate suppresses adrenocortical function so it may not be appropriate for patients that need an adrenocortical response for survival, like septic patients.

Absolute Contraindications: None.

KEY POINTS

• There are virtually no cardiovascular effects with etomidate. It is Ideal for induction in patients with severe cardiac disease.

• Use with sedation and a benzodiazepine or patient may paddle, vocalize, and go through periods of muscle rigidity.

• It suppresses adrenocortical function for up to 3 hours following administration. The clinical significance of this is unknown.

• Etomidate decreases cerebral oxygen consumption and intracranial pressure. It may also decrease the incidence of seizures in seizuring patients.

Ketamine

Classification: Ketamine is a dissociative anesthetic and N-methyl-D-aspartate (NMDA) receptor antagonist.

FDA Approval: Ketamine is aproved for anesthesia or restraint in cats and restraint in subhuman primates by intravenous injection.

Species: Any.

Route of Administration: It can be administered IV or IM. Ketamine stings when administered IM, and the large volumes that would be necessary to provide anesthesia in large patients limits IM dosing to small patients (cats, small dogs, pocket pets, and reptiles).

Dose: Dose 1 to 5 mg/kg IV or 5 to 10 mg/kg IM.

Onset of Action: 1 to 2 minutes.

Duration of Action: 10 to 30 minutes, depending on dose and route of administration.

Clinical Use: Appropriate as a routine induction drug in dogs and cats. Administer following premedication or concurrently with a tranquilizer and/or a muscle relaxant or muscle rigidity can occur.

Metabolism/Clearance: It is metabolized in the liver and metabolites are excreted by the kidney. In cats, the active metabolite (norketamine) and unchanged ketamine are excreted by the kidney. In cats, the active metabolite (norketamine) and unchanged ketamine are excreted by the kidney.

Effects: Anesthesia marked by lack of muscle relaxation but also minimal to no cardiovascular and respiratory depression. In fact, heart rate, blood pressure and cardiac work generally increase slightly because of sympathetic nervous system stimulation.

Adverse Effects: Muscle rigidity occurs if it is used without a muscle relaxant. Unlikely, but may contribute to seizures in patients already prone to seizuring but does not cause seizures and may actually be neuroprotective. Can cause hypersalivation. May contribute to emergence delirium in patients with inadequate sedation or patients receiving an excessively high dose of ketamine. Unlikely, but may contribute to sympathetic nervous system induced arrhythmias or tachycardia. None of these effects occur when ketamine is administered as a CRI because the CRI dose is very low.

Species Specific Effects/Adverse Effects: None.

Precautions

• **Ketamine is metabolized by the liver (dogs and cats) AND excreted by the kidney (cats) so elimination may be delayed in patients with hepatic and/or renal disease.**

• **Ketamine may exacerbate some tachyarrhythmias and is used cautiously in patients that are already tachycardic (e.g., patients with cardiac disease or diseases that impact heart rate, like hyperthyroidism).**

• **Ketamine may increase intracranial pressure (ICP) by increasing cerebral blood flow and is generally not used in patients that could have increased ICP, like those with a space occupying lesion in the brain.**

Absolute Contraindications: None, although should be used with caution or not at all in patients with increased ICP or tachyarrhythmias. Patients with hepatic or renal insufficiency should receive as low a dose as possible.

KEY POINTS
- Use in combination with sedation and an opioid IM in cats for profound sedation or light-medium plane of anesthesia.
- IMPORTANT POINT: Patients eyes will remain open after the use of ketamine so eyes should be well lubricated with artificial tears to help prevent drying of the eye.
- There may be an increase in heart rate following IV injection.
- There is minimal to no cardiovascular or respiratory depression.
- Ketamine is metabolized by the liver and partially cleared unchanged by the kidneys (in cats) so use caution in cats with renal disease and in both dogs and cats with hepatic disease.
- Ketamine plays an important role in pain management. See Chapter 7 (CRI's).

Propofol
Classification: Non-barbiturate.
FDA Approval: Dogs and cats.
Products: Propofol is available with and without preservative. Propofol with preservative (Propoflo28®) has a much longer shelf life once the bottle is opened (28 days) compared to propofol without preservative (6 hours). The preservative is NOT toxic to cats in clinically used propofol dosages (Taylor et al 2012).
Species: Any, but the large volumes needed and the expense of the drug limit or even preclude its use in large animals.
Route of Administration: IV.
Dose: 3 to 6 mg/kg with premedication; up to 8 mg/kg without premedication.
Onset of Action: 30 to 60 seconds.
Duration of Action: 5 to 10 minutes.
Clinical Use: For routine induction in dogs and cats; especially appropriate for use in compromised dogs and cats since the drug can be easily titrated to effect and cleared from the body by multiple routes. Should be administered following premedication to decrease the propofol dose.
Metabolism/Clearance: Various routes, not dependent on hepatic metabolism or renal clearance for elimination.
Effects: Very rapid induction to anesthesia so easy to titrate to effect.
Adverse Effects: Dose-dependent cardiovascular and respiratory depression. Can contribute to hypotension, especially in critical patients.
Species Specific Effects/Adverse Effects: Repeat dosages in cats may cause a small increase in Heinz bodies (abnormal structures in red blood cells) but this is clinically insignificant and propofol can be used repeatedly in cats (Matthews et al. 2004).
Precautions: Because the base for the drug is a lipid (which is why it is white), it can support bacterial growth. The preservative in Propoflo28® prevents bacterial growth and the open bottle can be used for up to 28 days. For both formulations

of propofol, titrate carefully to minimize the dose-dependent cardiovascular and respiratory depression.

Absolute contraindications: None.

KEY POINTS

- Fast onset and short duration make it easier to titrate to effect without overdosing so it is considered 'safer' for compromised patients, which tend to have greater physiologic depression from high drug dosages than healthy patients have.
- Because of the propofol-induced respiratory depression, preoxygenation is recommended in compromised patients.
- Administration of a benzodiazepine (midazolam or diazepam at 0.2 mg/kg IV) in conjunction with, or 30 seconds to 1 minute prior to, propofol administration will drastically decrease propofol dose, and thus decrease dose-dependent adverse effects.
- Propofol is appropriate for patients with renal and/or hepatic dysfunction because it is metabolized and cleared by multiple routes.
- Large boluses administered rapidly are most likely to result in respiratory depression, hypotension, and reduction in myocardial contractility so administer fairly slowly (but quickly enough that it actually induces sleep).
- Decreases cerebral oxygen consumption and intracranial pressure and may decrease incidence of seizures in seizuring patients.
- Propofol and Propoflo28® can be used safely in both dogs and cats.

Telazol® (Zoletil®)

Classification: Telazol is a dissociative anesthetic + benzodiazepine (combination of tiletamine and zolazepam). It antagonizes NMDA-receptors like ketamine.

FDA Approval: For IM administration in dogs and cats for restraint and short-duration anesthesia and for IV administration in dogs for induction to anesthesia.

Species: Primarily dogs, cats and exotic species. Poor recoveries limits its use in horses.

Route of Administration: IV or IM.

Dose: Dose 2 to 5 mg/kg IV or 5 to 10 mg/kg IM. Very low doses are used if Telazol® is reconstituted with an alpha-2 agonist and opioid (see maintenance section in this chapter). See information on use of Telazol® as a sedative/tranquilizer earlier in this Chapter.

Onset of Action: 1 to 2 minutes following IV administration, 5 to 10 minutes following IM administration.

Duration of Action: 10 to 60 minutes (dose dependent).

Clinical Use: Can be used as a routine induction drug and can be used for maintenance (see next section in this chapter). Very potent, dose carefully. Be sure to use with a sedative/tranquilizer to decrease the chance of excitement in recovery (especially in dogs). Commonly used in exotic species in which venous access is difficult (because they are really small or can't be restrained) because a small volume can be administered IM to produce anesthesia. Excellent choice for IM administration in really excited or aggressive patients.

Metabolism/Clearance: Probably the same as ketamine. Not as well researched.

Effects: Rapid induction to anesthesia. Muscle relaxation because of the benzodiazepine. VERY POTENT.

Adverse Effects: Same as ketamine except there is no muscle rigidity. Recoveries can be prolonged and marked by excitement and dysphoria, especially in dogs (see below).

Species Specific Effects/Adverse Effects: More likely to cause excitement in recovery in dogs than cats because dogs metabolize the zolazepam first, leaving the tiletamine, which is a dissociative like ketamine and likely to cause rough recoveries.

Precautions: Same as ketamine.

Absolute Contraindications: None.

KEY POINTS

- Clinical use is, for the most part, similar to the use of ketamine.
- Telazol® is a combination of 50% benzodiazepine and 50% dissociative anesthetic.
- VERY POTENT.
- Very effective choice for IM injection in aggressive dogs and cats.
- Commonly administered by IM injection for large exotic species in which restraint for IV induction would be difficult (e.g., large carnivores).
- The recovery from IM inductions will be very long if no sedative is used to decrease the Telazol® dose.
- Dogs metabolize zolazepam first and before tiletamine and recovery from tiletamine alone may cause a rough recovery. This can be avoided with concurrent administration of sedatives.
- The role of Telazol® in analgesia is unknown, it may have the same role as ketamine (See Chapter 7).

Mask/Inhalant Induction

This is a poor choice for induction in almost any patient and should definitely not be used as the routine method of induction because of the following reasons:

- Inhalant induction in patients that receive no other drugs contributes to anesthesia-related mortality (Brodbelt 2009). This is because inhalants are drugs and have serious dose dependent adverse effects. They require a high dose (high percentage setting on vaporizer) to achieve induction and cause dose-dependent hypotension and respiratory depression.
- The induction time is increased compared to IV agents. **Increased time = increased dose.**
- Mask or inhalant induction also requires a prolonged period with an unprotected airway (no endotracheal tube) with an increased risk of airway compromise or obstruction. Because of this, inhalant induction is contraindicated in brachycephalic patients and other patients with upper airway dysfunction (e.g., laryngeal paralysis). It is also contraindicated in any patient that is likely to vomit since the airway will be unprotected for a prolonged time, increasing the time that vomiting/

aspiration could occur.
- The excitatory phase of anesthesia (See Table 1-1) is exaggerated and prolonged with this type of induction, which increases the dose necessary to achieve induction. **Increased dose = increased adverse effects.**
- Once the patient is induced, a higher concentration of inhalant is required for the maintenance phase when compared to the dose of inhalants required to maintain anesthesia in patients that also had premedications or injectable induction drugs. **Increased dose = increased adverse effects.**
- Risk of arrhythmias increases due to excitement and the high dose of inhalants.
- This method of induction exposes staff unnecessarily to anesthetic agents, which can cause health problems with chronic exposure.

Inhalant induction MAY be acceptable if the patient is already very sedate (but not just obtunded - will still need opioids or benzodiazepines to decrease the dose of inhalant required for maintenance) or if deep sedation is required rather than a surgical plane of anesthesia. However, the staff will still be exposed to the inhalant so, for staff safety, this technique even in very sedate patients should have only limited (or no) use.

Drugs Administered Concurrently with Induction Drugs
Opioids
Occasionally the opioids are administered just prior to induction drugs in patients with IV catheters. This provides a more rapid onset of action and eliminates the need to wait for drugs administered IM to take effect. This technique might be used just for convenience to speed up the anesthetic process or because the patient needs to be anesthetized as soon as possible, as with many patients anesthetized for emergency surgery.

Sedative/Tranquilizers
Especially the alpha-2 agonists. These drugs are often combined with the induction drug and administered simultaneously (e.g., ketamine + alpha-2 agonist or a benzo-diazepine).

Muscle Relaxants
The benzodiazepines are the most commonly used muscle relaxants in small animals and they may be administered just before the induction drug (commonly done with propofol) or with the induction drug (commonly done with ketamine). This will provide muscle relaxation and also allow a decrease in the dose of the induction drug. Dose diazepam or midazolam at 0.2 mg/kg IV. Midazolam can be administered IM but uptake is too slow to use this route in the induction period. Administer slowly over 5 to 10 seconds. Administer the induction drug within 30 seconds of administration of the benzodiazepine. Mild dysphoria may occur if too much time elapses between benzodiazepine and induction drug delivery. Another

option is to administer 10 to 25% of the propofol or alfaxalone dose prior to the benzodiazepine, then administer the benzodiazepine and continue with propofol or alfaxalone to effect. When administered with ketamine, the benzodiazepines are dosed by volume. Reminder: DEA Class 4 drugs, no analgesia, effects are reversible with flumazenil.

How to: Choose an Induction Drug

The dose of the induction drug is more important than the drug itself in almost all patients. For all induction drugs, premedication should be used to decrease the dose required to produce sleep.

• Propofol and alfaxalone are easiest to titrate 'to effect' because of their rapid onset of action, thus these drugs are often chosen for critical patients. Both drugs cause dose-dependent cardiovascular and respiratory depression so dose carefully.

• Ketamine provides anesthesia of 10 to 30 minutes duration so short procedures can be completed without inhalants in some circumstances (e.g., cat castration). Ketamine can be administered IM, which is an advantage in patients in whom venipuncture is difficult. Ketamine is not ideal in patients with cerebral injuries or masses.

• Telazol® is very similar to ketamine but more potent so a small volume can be injected to achieve the same results. The duration of action is longer than with ketamine. Remember to sedate dogs or they can have a very bad recovery.

• Etomidate can be used for patients with severe cardiovascular disease but the availability of this drug is limited in most practices. An opioid can be used, followed by a benzodiazepine, followed by a low-dose of propofol, alfaxalone or ketamine for most patients with mild to moderate cardiovascular disease.

• Inhalant induction should be used only when no other method of induction can be utilized - or not be used at all in most practices. For feral cats (which is where most clinics think inhalant induction is necessary), use the ketamine or Telazol® protocols. The cat can be restrained with gloves or a 'cat bag' or a towel for the quick injection.

Table 4-5
Anesthetic Induction Drugs Used in Dogs and Cats.

Drug	Onset / Duration	Comments	Dose (dog & cat) mg/kg unless otherwise indicated
Propofol	30 to 60 secs / 5 to 10 mins	Fast onset, short duration so easy to titrate to effect. Cleared by multiple mechanisms so appropriate for patients with organ dysfunction. Moderate DOSE DEPENDENT respiratory & cardiovascular depression	3 to 6 IV; Can decrease the dose if administered concurrently with or immediately preceded by 0.2 benzodiazepine IV.
Alfaxalone	30 to 60 secs/5 to 10 mins (up to 20 mins IM)	Very similar to propofol in both good and adverse effects. Can be administered IM, used by this route primarily in 'pocket pets', reptiles and other small 'exotic' patients & sometimes cats for light sedation. DEA Class IV	2 to 3 IV in dogs, up to 5 in cats; Same benzodiazepine comment as for propofol. IM sedation in cats 1.
Ketamine	1 to 2 mins IV / 10 to 30 minutes IV or IM (dose dependent)	Use with a benzodiazepine or alpha-2 agonist; Can be combined with sedatives and used IM in cats - IM volume is generally too large for medium–big dogs; Ketamine may increase intracranial pressure and is generally not used in patients that are seizuring. Minimal to no cardiovascular and respiratory depression. Hepatic (dog,cat) and renal (cat) clearance so use low-dose in patients with hepatic or renal disease. DEA Class III.	1 to 5 IV; 5 to 10 IM (cats or really small dogs - volume is too big for big dogs). Can combine in same syringe with benzodiazepine for IV administration
Telazol	1 to 2 mins IV; 5 to 10 mins IM / 10 to 60 minutes IV or IM (dose dependent)	POTENT. Advantage: small volumes for injection; Disadvantage: easier to overdose because of potency. Slow recovery from IM inductions. Adverse effects similar to those of ketamine. Dogs metabolize zolazepam first and tiletamine recoveries are very rough. USE SEDATIVES. Can reconstitute Telazol powder with dexmedetomidine	2 to 5 IV; 5 to 10 IM. Dose lower if Telazol is reconstituted with alpha-2 agonist and opioid.

| Etomidate | 30 to 60 secs / 5 to 15 mins | Virtually no cardiovascular effects - ideal for induction in patients with severe cardiac disease. Use with sedation or patient may paddle, vocalize and go through periods of muscle rigidity. | 1 to 3 IV |
| **Inhalants (isoflurane, sevoflurane and desflurane)** | | NOT APPROPRIATE FOR ROUTINE INDUCTION. High dosage required for induction can cause profound cardiovascular and respiratory depression. This method of administration also exposes the anesthetist to anesthetic gas, which may cause health problems. See chapter text for more information. | |

Drugs used in the Maintenance Phase of Anesthesia

Introduction

Anesthetic maintenance can be achieved by either inhalant or injectable drugs. The primary - and very important - advantage of inhalant anesthetics is that they are terminated by exhalation of the drugs, with minimal metabolism required **(Table 4-6)**. Thus, even patients that may have difficulty metabolizing drugs can recover fairly quickly from inhalants. The inhalants can be easily dosed 'to effect' and allow a more rapid and precise control over anesthetic depth. The disadvantages are that inhalant anesthetics can take longer to increase anesthetic depth (when compared to IV injectable anesthesia) and administration of inhalant anesthetics requires expensive (when compared to the needle and syringe needed for injectable anesthesia) and bulky equipment.

The main advantages of injectable anesthetics are that they are fairly inexpensive and easy to administer, with no special equipment required. However, a means to supply oxygen should be available for patients regardless of how they are anesthetized since general anesthesia tends to cause some degree of respiratory depression. Anesthesia can be more quickly induced with IV injectable drugs than with inhalant drugs but change in anesthetic depth and recovery from anesthesia are slower and less precise as the body must metabolize and/or clear the drugs in order to terminate anesthetic effects.

Regardless of the type of anesthesia chosen, the drugs should be dosed to effect as much as possible (this is most difficult with drugs administered IM) and monitoring, support, and analgesia must all be addressed (See Chapters 5-7). All dosages in this chapter are for both dogs and cats unless otherwise specified.

Inhalant Anesthetics

Class Information

Isoflurane and sevoflurane are the most commonly used inhalant anesthetics. Desflurane is used occasionally but requires a special heated vaporizer. Halothane is still used in some countries but is not available in the US.

All inhalants cause **dose-dependent** cardiovascular and respiratory depression. Adequate analgesic and sedative premedications in combination with intraoperative analgesia such as opioid infusions and/or local and regional analgesic techniques (see Chapter 7) will reduce the dose of inhalant needed for maintenance of a surgical plane of anesthesia.

▌IMPORTANT TIP
▌lower dose = less incidence of adverse effects.

Table 4-6
Drugs Used for Maintenance of Anesthesia in Dogs and Cats.

DRUG	Comments	Dose (dog & cat)
Inhalant Drugs		
Isoflurane	Most commonly used, least expensive	Vaporizer usually 1 to 3%
Sevoflurane	Next most commonly used, rapid induction/recovery & rapid change of anesthetic depth, moderately expensive	Vaporizer usually 2 to 4%
Desflurane	Least commonly used because heated vaporizer needed for use, very rapid induction/recovery & change of anesthetic depth	Vaporizer usually 6 to 10%
Injectable Drugs		
Ketamine	Short-medium duration, commonly combined with a sedative and an opioid and used as maintenance drug for short procedures especially in cats, inexpensive	See protocols in chapter text
Telazol	Medium-long duration, moderately expensive, see comments under induction	See protocols in chapter text
Propofol or alfaxalone infusions	Can titrate to effect for as long as needed. Useful in situations where inhalant anesthetics are unavailable or surgery is in the airway so inhalants can't be delivered. Propofol moderately expensive, alfaxalone expensive	See protocols in chapter text

Inhalants must be delivered using an agent-specific precision vaporizer (see Chapter 3), otherwise, the inhalant concentration delivered to the patient can be very dangerous. Inhalants can be used in all species. None are DEA controlled.

As mentioned, the inhalants require minimal metabolism since the anesthetic effects are primarily eliminated when the gas is exhaled. This does mean that respiratory rate and depth impact recovery time, however, duration of anesthesia and body temperature will have a much greater impact on recovery time. Premedication with sedatives is often erroneously blamed for long duration anesthesia. However, premedicants allow a decrease in maintenance drug dosages and patients that are maintained at lower inhalant dosages actually recover more quickly. It is true that patients that are calm and pain-free from adequate sedation and analgesia may sleep longer. There is a difference between prolonged anesthesia and physiologic sleep. See more information in the recovery section of this chapter.

> **IMPORTANT TIP**
> Long duration of anesthesia = prolonged recovery; hypothermia = prolonged recovery.

> **IMPORTANT TIP**
> Inhalants do not provide analgesia, they just make the patient unconscious so the brain doesn't process the pain - but the pain pathway is still activated and the adverse effects of pain (See Chapter 7) will occur. Don't forget analgesia!

Isoflurane
The most commonly used inhalant anesthetic because it is the least expensive. The typical maintenance range is 1 to 3%. It is FDA approved for dogs and horses.

Sevoflurane
Less soluble in blood than isoflurane so it causes a quicker induction, quicker change of anesthetic depth and quicker recovery than isoflurane. This can make the use of sevoflurane safer for critical patients because it can be more easily titrated 'to effect'. So the gas isn't safer, but the way it can be used might make it safer in some patients. The typical maintenance range is 2 to 4%. Sevoflurane is moderately expensive and FDA approved for dogs.

Desflurane
Less soluble in blood than isoflurane or sevoflurane so it causes a quicker induction, quicker change of anesthetic depth and quicker recovery than isoflurane or sevoflurane. The typical maintenance range is 6 to 10% (may be slightly higher in cats). Desflurane is moderately expensive but the heated vaporizer is more expensive than the vaporizers used for isoflurane and sevoflurane. It has a very pungent odor and can cause breath holding if delivered by mask. It is not FDA approved in veterinary species.

Injectable Anesthetics
The drugs in this section have been described in detail earlier in this chapter. Injectable drugs can be delivered by either the IM or IV routes for maintenance of anesthesia. For compromised patients, IV administration is safer because the drugs can be more easily administered to effect. For medium to large patients, IV administration is more appropriate because the volume of drugs needed to produce anesthesia can be large and injections of large volumes of drugs IM can be painful. However, IM drug delivery is often ideal in very small patients in which venous access is limited because of size or temperament of the patient.

Ketamine Combinations

Ketamine is commonly combined with an opioid and an alpha-2 agonist or a benzo-diazepine and administered IM or IV for 10 to 30 minutes of anesthesia, which may be enough for very short procedures. Ketamine may contribute to pain relief (see Chapter 7) but ketamine alone does not provide surgical analgesia so don't forget analgesia!

Ketamine + benzodiazepine: A typical protocol is to administer ketamine and midazolam or diazepam mixed in the same syringe in a 1:1 ratio by volume with a total dose of 1 ml/10 kg IV in a patient without sedatives or 1 ml/20 kg IV in a sedated patient (which is preferable). Example: A sedated 20 kg patient would receive ½ ml diazepam + ½ ml ketamine. This will provide about 10 to 20 minutes of anesthesia. The addition of opioids or local anesthetic blocks will provide analgesia and improve the predictability of the anesthesia.

Ketamine + opioid + alpha-2 agonist (e.g., dexmedetomidine): Ketamine combined with opioids and alpha-2 agonists are commonly used, especially in cats, for anesthesia of 20 to 30 minutes duration. A common combination is:
0.1 to 0.2 mls PER 4.5 KG of each of the following drugs:
* medetomidine or dexmedetomidine,
* buprenorphine, butorphanol (10 mg/ml) or hydromorphone [morphine will work but use 0.03 to 0.05 mls of 15 mg/ml morphine per 4.5 kg),
* ketamine

Combine the drugs in the same syringe and administer IM or IV (use the low end of the dose for IV administration and/or for patients needing deep sedation but not anesthesia). Adjust the dosage for the size of the cat (e.g., increase the mls for cats over 4.5 kg, decrease if under 4.5 kg). Onset of anesthesia occurs in 5 to 10 minutes after IM injection, 1 to 2 minutes after IV injection. Inhalant anesthesia may be needed if the injectable protocol does not provide adequate anesthesia, or you can 'top off' with ¼ to ½ of the original dose of the combination. This protocol can be used in dogs but the volume gets fairly big so it is most appropriate for fairly small dogs if delivered IM.

Telazol®

Telazol® alone (2 to 5 mg/kg IV; 5-10 mg/kg IM) will provide anesthesia of 10 to 30 minutes, depending on the dose. Administration without concurrent use of a sedative requires a fairly high dose to produce anesthesia. The high dose can significantly prolong recovery time and lead to poor (or 'rough') recoveries, especially in dogs since they metabolize the zolazepam first and the remaining tiletamine can contribute to excitement. Opioids or local anesthetic blocks will provide analgesia and improve the predictability of the anesthesia. See dosages and concerns regarding Telazol® earlier in this chapter.

Telazol® Combinations

TKX (Telazol®, ketamine, xylazine) is an older combination that is effective, but provides minimal analgesia. A combination that provides better analgesia is Telazol®, dexmedetomidine (or medetomidine) and butorphanol (More information and expanded dosing charts are available in Ko et al. 2010). This combination is made by reconstituting Telazol® powder with 2.5 ml of 10 mg/ml butorphanol and 2.5 ml dexmedetomidine (or medetomidine). The combination can be administered IV or IM in dogs and cats. The chart below includes dosages in **mls** of the combination for IM administration in dogs and cats. Decrease the dosages by 10 to 25% for IV administration:

0.005 ml/kg = light sedation
0.01 ml/kg = moderate sedation
0.02 ml/kg = profound sedation
0.03-0.04 ml/kg = surgical anesthesia.

NOTE: There is only moderate analgesia with this protocol so use multimodal analgesia!

Propofol Infusions

Propofol can be used as an IV infusion (or repeated boluses) to maintain anesthesia in patients that are not appropriate for the longer lasting ketamine or Telazol® protocols. Dose at 0.4 to 0.8 mg/kg/minute following sedation and induction with a standard dose of propofol. You can also repeat propofol boluses of 1 to 2 mg/kg as needed if an infusion is not convenient or possible. Anesthesia is very difficult to maintain with propofol alone but a sedative used as a premedication or in combination with the propofol will improve the efficacy of this protocol. Benzodiazepines (usually IV) are commonly used if the technique is being used in critical patients, alpha-2 agonists (IV or IM) are commonly used for healthy patients. The patient should be on oxygen during anesthesia with propofol. Propofol does not provide pain relief so don't forget analgesia!

Alfaxalone Infusions

Alfaxalone can be used as an IV infusion (or repeated boluses) to maintain anesthesia in patients that are not appropriate for the longer lasting ketamine or Telazol® protocols. Anesthesia is very difficult to maintain with alfaxalone alone but a sedative used as a premedication or in combination with the alfaxalone will improve the efficacy of this protocol and may decrease the likelihood of excitement in recovery. Benzodiazepines (usually IV) are commonly used if the technique is being used in critical patients, alpha-2 agonists (IV or IM) are commonly used for healthy patients. The patient should be on oxygen during anesthesia with alfaxalone. Alfaxalone does not provide pain relief so don't forget analgesia!

Dose from the label:
• Premedicated dogs: 6 to 7 mg/kg/hour (0.10 to 0.12 mg/kg/minute) or boluses of

1.0 to 1.2 mg/kg for 10 minutes of maintenance anesthesia.
• Unpremedicated dogs: 8 to 9 mg/kg/hour (0.13 to 0.15 mg/kg/minute) or boluses of 1.3 to 1.5 mg/kg for 10 minutes of maintenance anesthesia.
• Premedicated cats: 7 to 8 mg/kg/hour (0.11 to 0.13 mg/kg/minute) or boluses of 1.1 to 1.3 mg/kg for 10 minutes of maintenance anesthesia.
• Unpremedicated cats: 10 to 11 mg/kg/hour (0.16 to 0.18 mg/kg/minute) or boluses of 1.6 to 1.8 mg/kg for 10 minutes of maintenance anesthesia.

How to: Choose a Maintenance Drug

The decision should be based on: 1) duration of the procedure, 2) health of the patient, and 3) location of the patient. Patients anesthetized for longer than 30 minutes should be maintained on inhalant anesthetics or recovery can be long since administration of drugs that need to be metabolized will have an impact on recovery, especially if repeat administration is necessary for longer-duration anesthesia. Patients that have impaired metabolism should be anesthetized with inhalant anesthetics (for the same reason as above). Injectable anesthetics are appropriate for short procedures in healthy patients. Injectable anesthetics are also appropriate when anesthesia must be done at a remote location where inhalant anesthetic equipment is not available. Infusions (or repeat IV boluses) of propofol or alfaxalone may be chosen for patients that only require a very brief procedure, patients that may not be able to metabolize ketamine or Telazol®, or patients that cannot be intubated (e.g., patients having surgery of the upper airway or trachea).

Drugs used in the Recovery Phase of Anesthesia

Recovery is often the most dangerous phase of anesthesia and there is a higher mortality rate during this phase (Brodbelt 2009). Patient status generally falls into one of 3 categories during recovery: 1) Normal recovery, no treatment needed, 2) Dysphoric or painful recovery, analgesia and/or sedation needed, or 3) Excessively long recovery, attentive monitoring and support required (See Chapters 5, 6 and 10) and reversal drugs are potentially needed (Table 4-7).

Pain and Dysphoria

Pain and dysphoria can be very hard to differentiate - but this really isn't all that necessary. If a patient is having a bad recovery, IT SHOULD BE TREATED. Excitement and/or pain are not appropriate in recovery and pain itself can cause dysphoria. Of course, a very short period of excitement right at the time of extubation may occur but if it does not stop within 30-60 seconds or if it is extreme for any amount of time, treatment is necessary. The following drugs are appropriate for treatment.

Table 4-7
Drugs Used in the Recovery Phase of Anesthesia in Dogs and Cats.

Drug	Comments when used for recovery	Dose (mg/kg) All species if not indicated
Analgesics (opioids)	Pain in recovery is common - opioids are an excellent choice for treatment of postoperative pain since they are potent and have rapid onset.	
ANY!	TREAT PAIN! Even if your analgesic protocol is excellent, patients may experience pain in recovery. Ideally, repeat the opioid that was used for premedication. Remember that buprenorphine has a fairly long time to onset so it may not be ideal for really painful patients.	Full or half of premedication dose, depending on apparent intensity of pain and time since previous dose.
Sedative	Some patients need longer term sedation or at least calming. Be sure to address pain first!	
Acepromazine	Effective for providing long-duration calming but not fast-acting and no analgesia so best to combine with an opioid and/or an alpha-2 agonist.	Dog: 0.01 to 0.02 IV or IM Cat: 0.02 to 0.03 IV or IM
Sedative/analgesics	Pain is difficult to differentiate from dysphoria in recovery. Sedative/analgesics treat both pain AND dysphoria so you don't have to try to differentiate.	
Dexmedetomidine (alpha-2 agonist)	Analgesia and sedation = excellent choice for dysphoric recoveries since both excitement and pain are treated. Generally administer IV for fast onset but IM acceptable if IV access difficult - which is more common in cats.	Dog: 0.001 to 0.005 IV if possible, IM okay just slower onset Cat: 0.003 to 0.01 IM or IV *For both species, low end of dose range IV. Typical starting dose: Dog 0.002 to 0.003, cat 0.005 to 0.007
Medetomidine (alpha-2 agonist)	Same as for dexmedetomidine	Dog: 0.002 to 0.01 IV if possible Cat: 0.005 to 0.015 IM or IV *For both species, low end of dose

Reversal drugs	If the patient is recovering very slowly, consider reversing drugs that cause sedation, but remember that long duration of surgery and hypothermia are the biggest contributors to prolonged recovery. Don't forget to address pain if analgesic drugs are reversed.	
Atipamezole	Alpha-2 agonist reversal. Best choice for small animals because it causes minimal to no adverse effects in these species. Tolazoline & yohimbine are more commonly used in large animals - primarily because of cost. Generally administered IM but IV okay - just be ready for fast return to consciousness!	Dose at a volume equal to or lesser than the volume of medetomidine or dexmedetomidine administered; ¼ to ½ of the alpha-2 agonist volume is usually effective. Or 0.1 to 0.4 mg/kg if another alpha-2 agonist was used.
Naloxone	Opioid reversal. Will reverse ALL opioid effects of any opioid administered (although the effects of buprenorphine can be difficult to reverse due to tight buprenorphine binding to opioid receptors). Treat pain before reversing!!!	Dose at 0.01 to 0.02 IV, IM, SQ. Best for IV is to dilute with saline (any volume) and administer over 1 to 2 minutes 'to effect'.
Buprenorphine	Opioid reversal, partial reversal at mu receptors. Will not reverse all of the analgesia. Should be used for mild effects - not emergencies or profound sedation. Slow onset - so butorphanol is often better for reversal.	0.01 to 0.02 IV for more rapid effect, IM okay.
Butorphanol	Opioid reversal, full reversal at mu receptors. Will not reverse all of the analgesia. Should be used for mild effects - not for emergencies or profound sedation.	0.2 IV for more rapid effect, IM okay.
Flumazenil	Benzodiazepine reversal. This drug class rarely needs reversal so most practices don't carry flumazenil.	0.01 to 0.04 usually IV or IM but may be used by other routes.

Opioids

Opioids are potent analgesic drugs and should be considered first since pain is a common cause of excitement in recovery. Even if the analgesic protocol is very good, break-through pain often occurs immediately postoperatively. When deciding whether or not to administer an opioid and/or which opioid to choose, consider: 1) the potency of the opioid that was administered during premedication and/or intra-operatively; 2) the dose of opioid administered during premedication and/or intra-operatively; and 3) the amount of time that has elapsed since that opioid was administered compared to the expected duration of action of that opioid. For rough recoveries, consider administering ½ to full dose of the same opioid that was administered as a premedication. Ideally, a potent opioid like morphine, hydromorphone or methadone is used. Because IV administration provides the most rapid onset, this delivery route should be used if the patient appears moderately to severely painful. IM administration is appropriate for patients experiencing mild pain or those in which IV administration will be difficult. Consider application of a fentanyl patch or administration of the long-acting buprenorphine (Simbadol®). The longer acting drugs will not only provide analgesia in recovery but also into discharge.

Alpha-2 Agonists

Alpha-2 agonists are an excellent addition to the opioid, or substitution for the opioid if the rough recovery is more likely due to anesthesia-induced excitement or dysphoria rather than pain. Fortunately, alpha-2 agonists provide both sedation AND analgesia, making them a good choice if the cause of the bad recovery is uncertain. A low or 'microdose' of an alpha-2 agonist will provide 10 to 20 minutes of sedation and analgesia. Recommended dosages are 1 to 5 microg/kg dexmedetomidine or 2 to 10 microg/kg medetomidine. Remember that cats require a higher dose than dogs so use the high end of the range in cats. Administer IV if possible, for faster action, but IM is acceptable. Some clinicians are concerned that sedation + analgesia could 'mask something' that is going wrong. We agree - you are masking something - PAIN! Fortunately, we have MANY parameters other than pain to monitor to see if 'something is going wrong'. For instance, check the capillary refill time (CRT) and examine the surgical site for signs of complications.

Acepromazine

Acepromazine is appropriate if 1) you are sure that the patient is not experiencing pain or you have administered analgesic drugs and 2) the patient is not frantic. The first point is important because it is possible to sedate a patient to the point that it will not exhibit pain, even if it is in pain, and this is inhumane and not good medicine. So give opioids first! The second point is important because acepromazine takes 10 to 20 minutes to take effect so a dysphoric patient will be dysphoric for a long time before the acepromazine is effective. One way around this is to administer the microdose of the alpha-2 agonist (fast onset, moderate sedation) AND the acepromazine (long duration, mild sedation). Use the low end of the dose, usually 0.01 mg/kg for dogs and 0.03 mg/kg for cats IV or IM.

Constant Rate Infusions

Continue any analgesic infusions that were being administered intraoperatively or start infusions if necessary. See Chapter 7 for more information.

Excessive Anesthetic Depth or Prolonged Time in Recovery

Patients can be excessively sedated and need to have drug effects reversed. If you think this is necessary, be sure that the patient isn't just sleeping because it is comfortable. Appropriate use of analgesic drugs pre- and intra-operatively will actually promote sleep, which is normal and important for healing. To determine whether the patient is experiencing sleep or anesthesia, see if you can wake the patient. If you can wake it, it is sleeping and does not need to be reversed. If you can't wake it, be sure that there is not another cause of prolonged recovery like a very long anesthesia time (long surgeries are the number one cause of long recoveries), hypothermia or hypoglycemia. Finally, if you decide to reverse the patient, be sure to address analgesia. If you reverse an analgesic drug without providing another source of analgesia, the patient can become extremely dysphoric from pain.

There is actually no need to reverse most patients, but reversal is appropriate in: 1) patients that are having a very prolonged recovery, 2) patients that cannot be observed during recovery and need to be completely conscious (like those that need to be recovered in an area remote from the surgery area for some reason), and 3) patients that will be discharged right away.

Drugs whose effects can be reversed include the opioids, alpha-2 agonists and the benzodiazepines. No other anesthetic drugs are reversible.

Opioid Reversal

The effects of full agonist opioids (e.g., morphine, hydromorphone, methadone, fentanyl) can be partially reversed using opioids that antagonize mu-receptor mediated effects (i.e., butorphanol) or opioids that compete for mu-receptor binding and cause only a mild effect at those receptors (i.e., buprenorphine). The advantage of using these drugs for reversal is that the patient will have less pronounced opioid effects and thus will most likely regain consciousness (although may still be somewhat sedated) but will also retain some analgesia. If the butorphanol or buprenorphine doesn't work within 10 to 15 minutes, naloxone can be administered if necessary. The low end of the normal clinical doses (0.2 mg/kg butorphanol; 0.01 mg/kg buprenorphine) should be administered IV if possible (for a faster response). If the patient is in an emergency situation (so deep that it is close to death) do not use this technique, use naloxone. Naloxone will reverse all of the opioid effects - sedation, dysphoria and analgesia - of any opioid administered (although the effects of buprenorphine can be difficult to reverse since the drug binds very tightly to the opioid receptors and is difficult to displace). Be sure to administer something for the pain!!! The dose is 0.01 to 0.04 mg/kg IV, IM or SQ.

The best way to administer the drug is to dilute the patient's naloxone dose with saline and administer the drug over 1 to 2 minutes 'to effect'. The desired effect is generally a patient that is more awake but still calm and maybe somewhat 'sleepy'.

Alpha-2 Agonist Reversal
Any alpha-2 agonist can be revered with any alpha-2 antagonist (atipamezole, yohimbine or tolazoline). However, atipamezole is most specific for the alpha-2 receptor and provides the most predictable reversal with minimal to no adverse effects (the other two drugs can cause excitement, vasodilation and other minor adverse effects). Atipamezole (trade name Antisedan®) is the most commonly used alpha-2 antagonist in small animals. The dose is a volume equal to or lesser than the volume of medetomidine or dexmedetomidine administered. Or it can be dosed at 0.1 to 0.4 mg/kg if an alpha-2 agonist other than medetomidine or dexmedeto-midine was used (because then the 'same volume' dose might not be the correct dose). A dose of ¼ to ½ of the alpha-2 agonist volume is usually effective since some of the alpha-2 agonist will be metabolized by the time you reverse - meaning the effects will already have begun to dissipate. The lower dose may also result in a 'partial reversal', meaning that some minor sedation and analgesia may remain. However, it is <u>impossible to predict how much analgesia will remain</u> so other analgesic drugs should be administered prior to reversal of the alpha-2 agonist. Atipamezole is most commonly administered IM but SLOW IV is acceptable - just be ready because the patient will wake up very quickly! Yohimbine and tolazoline are more commonly used in large animals (See Chapter 11).

Benzodiazepine Reversal
Although the effects of benzodiazepines are so mild that they rarely need to be reversed, they can be reversed with flumazenil at 0.01 to 0.04 mg/kg administered IV or IM.

Drugs for Postoperative Pain after Discharge
Anti-inflammatory Drugs
The non-steroidal anti-inflammatory (NSAID) drug class is one of the most effective analgesic classes because these drugs control not only pain, but the source of pain (i.e., inflammation). Since post-operative pain is primarily inflammatory pain, NSAIDs should be considered in all patients. However, patients with conditions that would preclude NSAID use (e.g., renal insufficiency, hepatic disease and clotting dysfunction) should receive drugs from other analgesic classes (See Chapter 7). The NSAID class includes both traditional NSAIDs (eg, carprofen, meloxicam, deracoxib, firocoxib, robenacoxib) and the prostaglandin inhibitor grapiprant (Galliprant®). Grapiprant has a wide safety margin and may be appropriate for some patients that should not receive traditional NSAIDs, although administration for acute pain is off-label.

Opioids

Buprenorphine can be sent home for OTM administration. The dose may be 0.01 to 0.02 mg/kg BID-TID but absorption from this route is not as good as we once thought it was and dosages of 0.03-0.05 mg/kg administered as often as QID should be considered, especially if the pain is severe. This is especially useful and cost effective in cats and very small dogs. The FDA-approved 24-hour duration buprenorphine (Simbadol®) is also an excellent choice in cats. The ability to administer drugs once daily is more convenient for the veterinarian and less annoying for the cat. Butorphanol tablets are occasionally sent home as analgesics but the efficacy is questionable and this use of butorphanol is not recommended. For moderate to severe pain of intermediate duration (e.g., many orthopedic injuries/surgeries), consider application of transdermal fentanyl patches, which will provide analgesia for 3 (or more in cats) days. More potent oral opioids are an option (e.g., codeine, morphine, etc...) but these are DEA Class II controlled drugs and should only be sent home with trusted clients. Tramadol is DEA Class IV and one of the most commonly dispensed drugs for postoperative pain in veterinary medicine, yet its efficacy is highly variable and IT SHOULD NOT BE DISPENSED AS THE SOLE ANALGESIC FOR POSTOPERATIVE PAIN. Tramadol may be more appropriate for multimodal analgesia in mild to moderate chronic pain than in acute post-surgical pain (which can be fairly severe).

Other Drugs

There are a few other options for postoperative analgesia (e.g., gabapentin) and these are discussed in Chapter 7.

How to: Choose an Analgesic Drug to Discharge with the Patient

One of the best ways to make a patient comfortable postoperatively is to be aggressive with preoperative and intraoperative analgesia! This alleviates the chance for central sensitization of the pain pathway and makes any postoperative pain less intense and more manageable with standard analgesic drugs. Preoperatively or in recovery, unless NSAIDs are contraindicated in the patient, START WITH AN NSAID! Opioids, tramadol or gabapentin, can be combined with the NSAID. Simbadol® will provide analgesia for 24 hours and NOCITA® will provide analgesia for 72 hours, so technically both of these drugs are part of discharge analgesia, even though they are administered while the patient is in the hospital.

References/Reading

Brodbelt D. Perioperative mortality in small animal anaesthesia Vet J 2009; 182:152-161.

Ko JC, Berman AG. Anesthesia in shelter medicine. Top Companion Anim Med. 2010;25(2):92-7.

Maney JK, Shepard MK, Braun C, Cremer J, Hofmeister EH. A comparison of cardiopulmonary and anesthetic effects of an induction dose of alfaxalone or propofol in dogs.Vet Anaesth Analg. 2013;40(3):237-44.

Matthews NS, Brown RM, Barling KS, Lovering SL, Herrig BW. Repetitive propofol administration in dogs and cats. J Am Anim Hosp Assoc. 2004 Jul-Aug; 40(4):255-60.

Taylor PM, Chengelis CP, Miller WR, Parker GA, Gleason TR, Cozzi E. Evaluation of propofol containing 2% benzyl alcohol preservative in cats. J Feline Med Surg. 2012 Aug: 14(8):516-26.

Chapter 5
Monitoring the Anesthetized Patient

Shona Meyer, BS, LVT, VTS (Anesthesia/Analgesia)

Introduction

The most effective way to deal with anesthetic complications and emergencies is to prevent them by using appropriate 1) preparation/stabilization of the patient, 2) selection of type and dosage of anesthetic drugs, 3) preparation of anesthesia equipment, 4) monitoring of physiologic systems, and 5) pre-, post- and intra-operative support of the patient. This will make the anesthetic episode safer and decrease the likelihood of anesthetic complications. In fact, in a study on risk factors for anesthesia-related mortality, many factors increased the risk of death but only one - monitoring - statistically decreased the risk of death (Brodbelt 2009). Monitors should be used for EVERY anesthetized patient and should never be "optional".

Monitoring Equipment

There are many monitors available. However, all monitors have advantages and disadvantages and it is important to know the uses and the limitations of each monitor. Monitoring equipment can give deceptive readings, so it is critical that the person monitoring anesthesia watch the patient, and evaluate the results against the clinical picture and not rely solely on the anesthesia monitoring equipment. Actually LOOKING AT and TOUCHING the patient is most important - which makes the best monitor the anesthetist, not a machine! Monitoring should include data both from the anesthetist AND from the machines.

TIP
If the monitor provides values that you do not think are correct, FIRST CHECK THE PATIENT, NOT THE MONITOR. Then ask yourself, 'Is the measurement repeatable, does the measurement fit the clinical presentation?' If the answer is yes, fix the patient. If no, fix the equipment.

What to Monitor

Anesthesia causes depression of all organ systems but changes in the central nervous, cardiovascular and respiratory systems are those that are most immediately life-threatening. Thus, most monitoring focuses on these systems. Also, by supporting these systems and insuring appropriate anesthetic depth, blood pressure and blood oxygen content, support for all of the other organ systems is provided. Additional monitoring includes body temperature in all patients and selected parameters like packed cell volume/total protein, serum glucose concentration and urine output in specific patients.

For all monitored parameters, trends of changes are generally more important than the changes themselves. For instance, a heart rate of 60 in a medium-sized dog is not likely to be a cause for concern, but a heart rate of 60 that was 80 just 5 minutes ago is definitely a cause for concern. Therefore, it is very important that monitored parameters are recorded on AN ANESTHETIC RECORD (Figure 5-1 A&B) so that the physiological trends can be referenced, and identified before an emergency occurs.

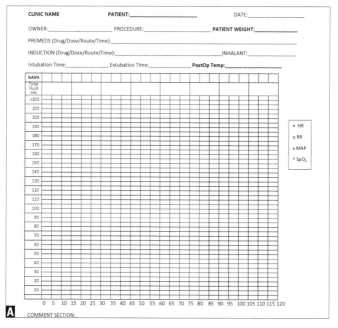

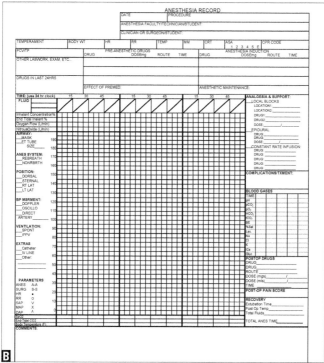

Figure 5-1. A simple anesthetic record **(A)** and a more complex anesthetic record **(B)**. Both are appropriate for use in any practice.

Monitoring the Central Nervous System (CNS) = Monitoring Anesthetic Depth

Anesthetic drugs must cause depression of the CNS to cause unconsciousness, but excessive CNS depression can cause depression of all the other systems and can cause death.

Basic (but Essential) Monitoring:

Response to Stimulus

The stimulus can be a surgical incision, toe pinch **(Figure 5-2)**, or other method, which may cause an increased heart or respiration rate, flinching or even movement. A slight response (a minor increase in heart or respiration rate) can be normal and indicate a light but appropriate plane of anesthesia, but a pronounced and/or persistent response (major increase in heart or respiration rate, or movement) may indicate that the plane of anesthesia is too light or that the patient is experiencing pain. If the patient is too lightly anesthetized, the vaporizer setting should be increased or an additional bolus of injectable drug should be administered. If pain is the issue, analgesics (rather than anesthetics) are the best choice to decrease the patient's response. On the other end of the anesthetic depth spectrum, no response at all can be detrimental because it might indicate an excessive depth of anesthesia. If the patient is extremely deep, dramatically decrease the vaporizer setting (or turn the vaporizer off if the patient is in danger), empty the rebreathing bag (it is full of a high concentration of anesthetic gas) and continually assess for emergencies until an appropriate plane of anesthesia is reached. If the patient is only slightly deep or you can't determine exactly what the depth is, decrease the vaporizer only slightly (by ½-1 percent) and reassess the patient in 5 minutes.

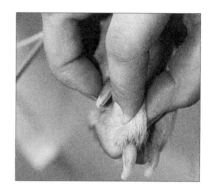

Figure 5-2. Although not as stimulating as making a surgical incision, patient response to strongly squeezing a digit ('toe pinch') indicates that the patient is at a very light plane of anesthesia.

Eye Reflexes

The palpebral, or 'blink', reflex **(Figure 5-3)** is tested by gently tapping at the lateral or medial canthus of the eye (these are the outside or 'lateral', and inside, or 'medial', corners of the eyelid) or gently stroking the eyelashes. Either action should create a partial or complete closure of the eyelids ('blink'). The palpebral reflex should be slow and weak or just absent at a plane of anesthesia satisfactory for surgical stimulus. The reflex can become desensitized if tested too frequently in rapid succession, meaning that the patient stops 'blinking' even at a light plane of anesthesia. This 'desensitization' only lasts a few minutes and then the reflex returns.

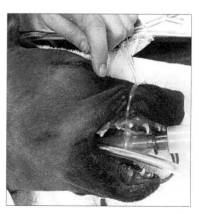

Figure 5-3. The palpebral, or 'blink', reflex is tested by gently tapping at the lateral or medial canthus of the eye or gently stroking the eyelashes and observing a partial or complete closure of the eyelids. At a surgical plane of anesthesia, the blink reflex should be very slight or have disappeared.

Muscle Tone ('Jaw Tone')

Skeletal muscles become more relaxed and offer little resistance to movement as anesthetic depth increases. The degree of muscle relaxation is assessed primarily by testing jaw tone, which is evaluated by moving the mandible up and down with light pressure **(Figure 5-4)**. Strong resistance to movement means that the patient is very lightly anesthetized, whereas slight muscle tone is present in light planes of anesthesia and becomes more flaccid as the depth of anesthesia increases. The amount of tone in the jaw is subjective between people assessing the tone and is also greatly impacted by the size of the patient (i.e., small dogs and cats = easy to move the jaw; big dogs = harder). As with the other assessment parameters, a change in jaw tone is more indicative of anesthetic depth than jaw tone at any one time. Some drugs promote muscle relaxation (benzodiazepines, alpha-2 agonists) and some increase muscle tone (ketamine, Telazol®) so the drugs themselves can have an impact on this parameter.

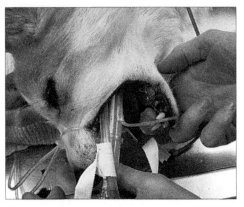

Figure 5-4. Jaw tone is used to assess skeletal muscle relaxation since the muscles become more relaxed and offer little resistance to movement as anesthetic depth increases. Jaw tone is evaluated by moving the mandible up and down.

Eye Position

This is somewhat useful in the dog and cow but not very useful in other species. In an awake patient the eye is in the central position (the pupil is directly in the center of the ring made by the eyelids) and the pupils may be slightly dilated. As the patient moves into a light to moderate depth of anesthesia, the eye rotates to the middle and down (towards the sternum) so that the white sclera is all or mostly all that can be seen between the eyelids **(Figure 5-5)**. As the patient moves to a deeper plane of anesthesia, the eye rotates back to central but the pupil is often more profoundly dilated. For many patients, the rotated eye with the sclera showing indicates a surgical plane of anesthesia, but for some patients the centrally located eye is more predictive of appropriate anesthetic depth. Gravity has some effect on eye position when the patient is placed in dorsal recumbency so patient position should be considered when using this parameter for monitoring.

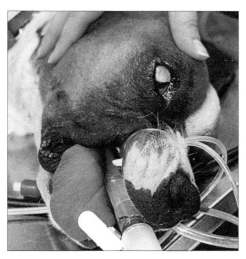

Figure 5-5. Eye position changes as anesthetic depth changes. In a light to moderate depth of anesthesia, the eye rotates to the middle and down so that the white sclera is all or mostly all that can be seen between the eyelids, as in this photo.

Pupil Constriction/Dilation

The pupil in an awake patient will constrict and dilate in response to light. In the anesthetized patient, the pupil size may change (although not consistently) as the patient moves through different anesthesia stages and phases. As the patient moves into stage II (excitement phase) or a deeper plane of anesthesia the pupil becomes slightly dilated. The pupil returns to normal once the patient reaches stage III (surgical plane of anesthesia). As anesthesia moves into deeper planes the pupil becomes more and more dilated. Remember that pupil size is often dictated by the drugs administered rather than anesthetic depth (atropine causes pupillary dilation, opioids can cause dilation or constriction depending on the species).

Lacrimation (production of tears)

Lacrimation during anesthesia might indicate a light plane of anesthesia, but this is much more useful in horses than in other species.

CNS Advanced Monitoring

Assessment of anesthetic depth using advanced monitoring techniques is becoming more common in human medicine but is currently rarely used in veterinary medicine except for research. The main technique for assessment of anesthetic depth is based on evaluation of brain activity using the electroencephalogram (EEG) or bispectral index system (BIS). Species differences in brain activity changes in response to anesthesia may continue to limit this technique in veterinary medicine. **Figure 5-6** shows BIS electrodes under the skin on the head of a cat.

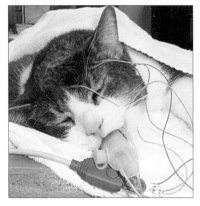

Figure 5-6. Bispectral index **(BIS)** electrodes under the skin on the head of a cat. BIS and electroencephalogram **(EEG)** measure brain activity and can be used to assess anesthetic depth. These protocols are used almost exclusively for research in veterinary medicine.

Summary

Anesthesia-induced changes in the central nervous system can cause major complications, including death. The best way to avoid complications is to identify deleterious trends by monitoring the patient and recording physiologic parameters on an anesthetic record. Monitoring of the central nervous system = monitoring of anesthetic depth, which should include constant assessment of physiologic parameters like heart rate, respiratory rate and blood pressure along with physical changes like response to stimulus and presence of palpebral reflex. Finally, consideration of the dose of anesthetic administered should be a critical part of central nervous system monitoring.

Monitoring the Cardiovascular System

The cardiovascular system is comprised of the heart, the blood vessels (arteries and veins) and the blood & plasma that is pumped by the heart through the vessels. The ultimate goal of the cardiovascular system is to work with the respiratory system to deliver oxygen to the working cells. On the cardiovascular side of oxygen delivery, a decrease in delivery is caused by a decrease in tissue perfusion which can be caused by anything that decreases output from the heart (e.g., decreased contractility, arrhythmias, very slow or very fast heart rate, etc.), decreases the amount of circulating red blood cells (e.g., anemia, hemorrhage, excessive fluid administration, etc.) or drastically changes the diameter ('tone') of the blood vessels (e.g., sepsis, shock, vasoconstrictor/vasodilator drugs, etc.).

Basic (but Essential) Monitoring
Heart Rate (Table 5-1)

• The rate at which the heart pumps blood contributes to blood pressure. Blood pressure can be determined by the formula:
  • Blood Pressure = Systemic Vascular Resistance x Cardiac Output
    • Systemic vascular resistance is blood vessel (primarily arterial) tone.
    • Cardiac output is the amount of blood ejected by the heart over time.

- Cardiac output = Heart Rate x Stroke Volume
  - Stroke volume is the amount of blood ejected by the heart with each beat.
    - Thus, changes in heart rate can cause hypotension or hypertension.
- Changes in heart rate can also be an indicator of other changes that need to be investigated, like anesthetic depth, presence of pain, blood pressure abnormalities, electrolyte imbalance, hydration or circulating volume status, etc.
- Putting this information all together: changes in heart rate can CAUSE problems and/or can INDICATE problems.

Table 5-1
Normal Heart/Pulse Rates

Patient	Heart/Pulse Rate in beats per minute (bpm) in dogs and cats		
Dogs	Small	Medium	Large
	80 to 120	60 to 80	40 to 60
Cats	120 to 180	NOTE: some references list 150 to 200bpm as normal but in most healthy adult cats this rate is generally only 'normal' when cats are scared - like during a physical exam - and not really the normal resting heart rate.	

How to: Monitor the Heart Rate
The best way is to put your fingers on a pulse or listen to the heart using a stethoscope or esophageal stethoscope. Count for 15 seconds and multiply the number of beats by 4 to get an accurate rate in beats/minute.

TIP
Do not rely on the ECG to count the heart rate as the machine often miscounts, especially if the patient has arrhythmias or if the complexes are abnormal sizes. See more information in the ECG section of this chapter.

TIP
Esophageal Stethoscopes (Figure 5-7) are INEXPENSIVE, efficient tools that allow the anesthetist to hear both the heart beat and respiratory sounds. They are especially useful when the anesthetized patient is completely covered by drapes and can't be accessed with a standard stethoscope. The probe is placed in the esophagus to the level of the heart and connected either to traditional ear pieces (like the ear pieces used in standard stethoscopes or to a speaker (like the one used by Dopplers).

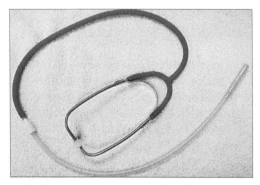

Figure 5-7. Esophageal stethoscope: An inexpensive, efficient tool that allows the anesthetist to hear both the heart beat and respiratory sounds.

> **TIP**
> **Attach a long piece of tape to the oral end of the probe (the end that is in the mouth) so that the stethoscope can still be pulled out, even if the probe advances down the esophagus past the patient's pharynx.**

Pulse Rate

The number of pulses counted over time is technically called the pulse rate rather than the heart rate but the pulse rate and heart rate should be the same. In the initial physical exam for all patients, and especially in patients with cardiovascular disease or diseases that cause major cardiovascular changes, the pulses should be palpated at the same time the heart is being ausculted. The pulse rate should synchronize with the ausculted heart rate and a pulse should be present with every normal beat on the ECG.

To feel the pulse, place your fingers lightly but firmly over a peripheral artery. Too much pressure will occlude the artery but too little pressure will make the artery difficult to feel. The femoral, dorsal pedal, plantar metatarsal, palmar metacarpal (or palmar common digital), brachial, coccygeal, and lingual arteries are the most commonly palpated arteries in small animals **(Figure 5-8)**. As with ausculting the heart rate, count for at least 10 to 15 seconds to get an accurate count.

Common Heart Rate Abnormalities

Bradycardia (heart rate slower than normal for that patient's species, breed, body size and age) and tachycardia (heart rate faster than normal for that patient's species, breed, body size and age) commonly occur during anesthesia. Specific types of bradycardia and tachycardia are presented in the ECG section of this chapter. The cause of these arrhythmias should be investigated and treated, if necessary.

Impact of Abnormalities on Heart Rate

Extreme bradycardia or tachycardia can be life threatening. Extreme bradycardia

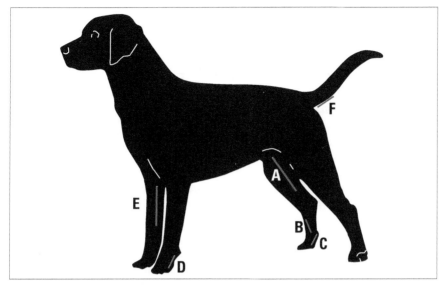

Figure 5-8. Commonly palpated arteries in small animals. The femoral *(A)*, inside the rear leg behind the stifle, dorsal pedal *(B)*, inside of the rear leg just below the hock, plantar metatarsal *(C)*, just above the main foot pad on the back of the hind paws, palmar metacarpal *(D)*, also called palmar common digital, just above the main foot pad on the back of the fore paws, brachial *(E)*, along the inside of the forearm, coccygeal *(F)*, on the underside of the tail and lingual (not shown) on the underside of the tongue.

can occur just before the heart stops completely (asystole) and extreme tachycardia can lead to life-threatening arrhythmias (like ventricular tachycardia). Also, since heart rate is a component of blood pressure, drastic changes in heart rate may cause hypotension, and RARELY hypertension in the anesthetized patient.

If the heart rate is slow AND blood pressure is low, administer drugs to increase the heart rate (e.g., anticholinergics like atropine or glycopyrrolate). However, in most patients with a healthy cardiovascular system, changes in blood pressure are controlled more by stroke volume and systemic vascular resistance than by heart rate, so the blood pressure can be normal even if the heart rate is low. Therefore, if the heart rate is low but blood pressure is normal, DO NOT 'TREAT' THE HEART RATE. As long as the blood pressure is normal, leave the heart rate alone. Physiologically, **blood pressure is more important than heart rate** and normal physiologic reflexes will cause changes in heart rate, stroke volume and systemic vascular resistance in order to keep blood pressure normal.

Although increased heart rate will generally increase blood pressure, profound tachycardia can actually contribute to hypotension. If the heart rate is too high, the chambers of the heart (right and left atria; right and left ventricles) do not have time to adequately fill with blood, thus stroke volume decreases and this is likely to cause a reduction in blood pressure. Profound tachycardia can also have a negative impact on the heart muscle (myocardium). The myocardium receives its blood flow (perfusion) when the muscle is not contracting (diastole) but cannot be perfused during contraction (systole) since contraction of the muscle collapses the myocardial blood vessels. If the heart is in systole most of the time (as with tachycardia), the myocardium may not receive enough blood, which will decrease the oxygen delivery to the myocardial fibers, which can lead to arrhythmias, decreased contractility and even cardiac arrest.

IMPORTANT POINT
It is VERY important to monitor overall cardiovascular function, not just heart rate since the blood pressure may be perfectly normal even though the rate is a little slower or a little faster than you are comfortable with. The body's natural reflexes will cause changes in heart rate in an attempt to keep blood pressure within a normal range.

IMPORTANT POINT
Some drugs such as alpha- 2 agonists (xylazine, medetomidine, dexmedetomidine) will cause systemic vasoconstriction (constricted blood vessels) which causes HYPERTENSION. The normal physiologic reflex to this increase in blood pressure is a decrease in the heart rate in order to decrease the work of the heart muscle. This bradycardia DOES NOT require treatment as long as the blood pressure is normal.

IMPORTANT POINT
Pediatric patients (<3 months) have less contractile tissue in the myocardium than adults, and therefore are not able to increase stroke volume as readily as adults and are more dependent on an adequate heart rate to maintain cardiac output.

Mucous Membrane Color
The color of the mucous membranes is influenced by blood volume (the amount or volume of blood in the body), oxygen saturation of hemoglobin (i.e., the measurement obtained by the pulse oximeter), vessel tone (dilated or constricted), and some systemic diseases. Blood volume and vessel tone are controlled by the cardiovascular system while oxygen saturation is controlled by the respiratory system.

Normal Mucous Membrane Color
The normal color is pink to slightly pale pink, cats often slightly paler than dogs; (Figure 5-9).

How to: Assess Mucous Membrane Color
Evaluate mucous membrane color in the oral cavity or conjunctiva (mucous membranes of the eyelids). If the head is covered with a surgical drape, color can be evaluated in the walls of the vagina or at the opening of the prepuce.

Common Mucous Membrane Color Abnormalities

Pale/White may be caused by anemia (decreased volume of red blood cells), vasoconstriction (due to drugs like the alpha-2 agonists, hypothermia etc.), or decreased perfusion secondary to any cause of decreased cardiovascular function (decreased myocardial contractility, severe arrhythmias, etc.).

Blue/Purple is called 'cyanosis' and is due to decreased oxygen delivery to the tissues. This can be due to low oxygen saturation of the hemoglobin or severely low cardiac output.

Bright or 'Brick' Red may be caused by profound vasodilation and/or venous congestion ('pooling' of blood in the vessels due to poor circulation). This often occurs during sepsis, toxemia and late phases of shock. Carbon monoxide poisoning can also cause very red mucous membranes.

Yellow is called icterus and is due to liver failure or liver disease (the color is due to increased bilirubin in the blood). A slight yellow color can be normal in fasted horses.

Capillary Refill Time (CRT)

The CRT is the time that it takes blood to refill the capillaries after it has been 'forced' from the capillaries by pressure.

KEY POINT

This is a very useful tool for basic assessment of perfusion. Although not a perfect test - and certainly not equivalent to measuring blood pressure, the CRT is more specific than mucous membrane color for assessment of perfusion.

How to: Assess CRT

Apply firm digital (using your 'digit' or finger) pressure to a capillary tissue bed (typically at a mucous membrane like the oral cavity). This forces the blood from the capillaries in the tissue under your finger. When the pressure is removed, the tissue will be 'blanched' (pale) because there is no blood in that area of tissue. Color should return to the area as perfusion of the site returns to normal (i.e., as blood returns to the capillaries). The time it takes the color to return to normal is called the capillary refill time (CRT) **(Figure 5-9 A, B, C)**.

Normal CRT

Normal CRT should be *equal to or less than 2 seconds*.

Common CRT Abnormalities:

• A prolonged CRT is caused by poor tissue perfusion (or 'hypoperfusion'). Hypoperfusion can be caused by severe vasoconstriction (which can impede blood flow) and any cause of hypotension (for instance, decreased cardiac contractility, excessive vasodilation and hypovolemia). It is important to distinguish global

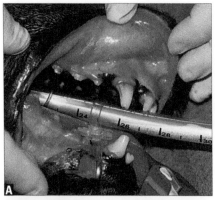
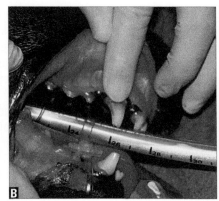
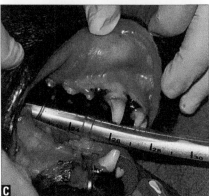

Figure 5-9. Assessing the Capillary Refill Time (CRT). Notice the normal pink color of the mucous membranes just above the canine tooth **(A)**. Apply firm pressure to the mucous membrane with your finger **(B)**. This 'pushes' blood from tissue under your finger. When the pressure is removed, the tissue will be 'blanched' because there is no blood in that area **(C)**. The time that it takes the blood to return to the blanched area is the CRT which is normally 2 seconds.

(whole body) hypoperfusion from localized hypoperfusion since occasionally local blood flow can be compromised even if global blood flow is adequate. An example of this is an excessively tight endotracheal tube tie which has occluded blood flow to the mucous membranes of the jaw in the area in front of the tie, creating a prolonged CRT just in that area.

• An almost instantaneous CRT could indicate hypertension or a 'hyperdynamic' cardiovascular state, as occurs in early phases of shock.

Assessment of Pulse Quality or 'Pulse Pressure'

Pulse pressure represents the difference between systolic and diastolic blood pressure. Pulse pressure is useful since vessel tone is also palpated during the evaluation of pulse pressure. A vessel that has good tone most likely represents better blood pressure than a vessel that is very flaccid and can be collapsed easily. A 'strong' or 'weak' pulse should be noted - especially if the pulse was strong at the last assessment and has changed to weak. Pulse pressure should be assessed in all patients, but there are some disadvantages to this tool:

Pulse quality assessment is:
• Subjective with no real definition of what the anesthetist should feel.
• Difficult to assess in obese patients since the artery can be hard to palpate due to the fat in the tissues.
• Difficult to assess in very small patients due to the small size of the artery.
• Potentially misleading since very different blood pressures can result in the same pulse pressure. For instance,
    • a systolic pressure of 120 mmHg with a diastolic pressure of 80 mmHg results in a pulse pressure of 40 mmHg,
    • but a systolic pressure of 80 mmHg and a diastolic pressure of 40 mmHg could also result in a pulse pressure of 40 mmHg.
    • However, the mean arterial pressure **(MAP)** between these patients would be very different - which means the vessel tone would also be very different and the artery in the patient with 120/80 blood pressure should be much easier to feel than the artery in the patient with 80/40 blood pressure.

How to: Assess Pulse Quality
With your fingers on an artery, attempt to determine the strength of the pulse (strong or weak) and vessel tone (easily collapsible or maintains shape). Also compare trends in pulse quality at different locations. Vessels commonly palpated in small animals are depicted in Figure 5-8.

Normal Pulse Quality
It is hard to define normal since this is a subjective assessment, but a 'strong' pulse should be felt, especially on palpation of the femoral artery. The shape of the vessel (a cylindrical shape) should also be palpable if pressure is good.

Common Pulse Quality Abnormalities
• Poor pulse quality is caused by decreased perfusion requiring immediate general patient assessment and may be grounds for immediate patient treatment - especially if the pulse quality is deteriorating. Causes include general hypotension, hypovolemia, vasoconstriction, and decreased cardiac contractility.
• A 'bounding' pulse (strong systolic pulse but a vessel that nearly collapses during diastolic pulse) may represent excessive vasodilation which may occur, for example, during shock. A bounding pulse is also described in patients with some cardiac conditions, such as patent ductus arteriosus.

Packed Cell Volume (PCV) and Total Protein (TP)
The fluids pumped by the heart through the vessels (blood and plasma) are part of the cardiovascular system. Packed cell volume (PCV), sometimes called hematocrit or 'crit', is a measure of the percentage of circulating red blood cells compared to

the total volume of circulating fluid, which is why PCV is reported as a percent. Red blood cells contain hemoglobin, and hemoglobin carries oxygen. Thus, an adequate number of red blood cells is critically important for oxygen delivery.

Total protein (TP) is a measure of the amount of protein in the plasma. Total protein is comprised primarily of albumin and globulins. Other components of total protein include clotting factors, enzymes and hormones.
• Albumin provides 'oncotic pressure' which is an intravascular 'force' that 'pulls' inward and keeps fluids (such as those normally in the body and the IV crystalloid fluids that we administer during anesthesia) in the vasculature. Low albumin can cause fluid to leak from the vessels, which can lead to edema.
• The amount of albumin can affect the degree of activity of many drugs, including many anesthetics and analgesics. Many drugs are strongly bound to albumin (meaning that a very large percent of the drug dose is attached to albumin). The 'free fraction' of drugs is the percentage of the dose that is not bound to albumin and this is the active percentage. If the albumin is low, so there is less protein for the drug to bind to, the free fraction increases and a normally appropriate dosage of a drug may cause an exaggerated response, or even an overdose.
• Globulins are a component of the immune system and are not as important to this discussion.

NOTE
Total protein is sometimes called 'total solids' but this is not technically correct. Total solids include protein PLUS other components like glucose and cholesterol. However, these terms are commonly used interchangeably.

TIP
PCV and TP should be repeatedly measured in any patient that is anemic, hypoproteinemic, receiving a large volume of IV fluids or hemorrhaging during surgery.

How to: Measure PCV and TP:
Fill a microhematocrit tube with whole blood and seal the end of the tube with special wax. (**Figure 5-10 A**). Spin the tube in a specified centrifuge for 5 minutes at 12,000 rpm. Read the column of blood in the tube using a micro-capillary reader (**Figure 5-10 B**). For TP, break the microhematocrit tube so that the portion with the clear fluid (which is the protein portion) breaks free from the blood portion. Drip some of the fluid onto a refractometer chamber (**Figure 5-11**) and read the result in g/dL.

IMPORTANT POINT
The refractometer may make erroneous measurements if the plasma contains a large amount of other solids (like high lipid concentration) so serum chemistry should be evaluated in diseased patients.

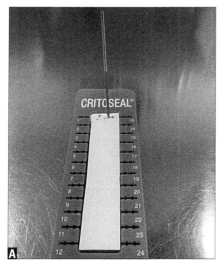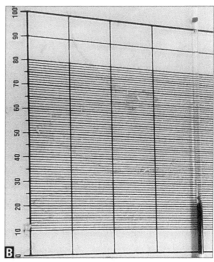

Figure 5-10. Measuring the packed cell volume (PCV). Fill a capillary tube with blood, seal one end of the tube with wax **(A)** and centrifuge the tube to separate the blood cells from the serum. Place the top of the wax 'seal' on the line at the bottom of the capillary tube reader card **(B)**. Keeping the top of the wax seal on the line at the bottom of the card reader, move the tube along the the card until the top of the serum column lines up with the 100 line (this is 100%) at the top of the card. Read the PCV at the junction of the blood and serum. In this example the PCV is 21%.

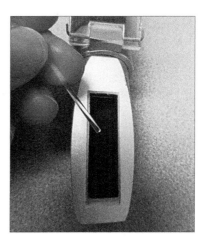

Figure 5-11. Measuring the total protein using a refractometer. Break the microhematocrit tube so that the part with the serum portion breaks free from the blood portion. 'Drip' the fluid onto the refractometer surface. Look through the refractometer. The total protein is measured in g/dL at the junction of the light and dark fields (not shown in this photo).

Normal Values

The normal ranges will differ slightly between laboratories, species, breeds and even age groups (neonatal vs adult patients). The reference values reported below are from the WSU clinical pathology lab for dogs and cats >1 year of age (Table 5-2).

Table 5-2
Normal Values for PCV and Total Protein in Adult Dogs and Cats

PARAMETER SPECIES	Dog	Cat
PCV (%)	36 to 56	30 to 46
TP (g/dL)	5.5 to 7.5	6.2 to 8.5

Common Abnormalities in PCV/TP

Anemia (low red blood cell count), polycythemia (high red blood cell count), hypoproteinemia (low protein) and/or hyperproteinemia (high protein).

Anemia can be caused by any disease or condition that causes blood loss, failure to produce new red blood cells, and/or decreased iron availability (e.g., hemorrhage, chronic kidney disease, gastro-intestinal ulcers, cancer, chronic inflammation) and can be caused transiently by excessive IV fluid administration (called 'dilutional' anemia). Excessively low PCV (< 18 to 25% in acute anemia and < 15 to 18% in chronic anemia) requires a blood transfusion.

Polycythemia can be caused by dehydration and by diseases that cause chronic hypoxemia, like some heart defects. This condition is almost always due to dehydration in anesthetized patients without those heart defects, so increased IV fluid administration is required.

Hypoproteinemia can be caused by any disease that causes protein loss (e.g., kidney disease, gastro-intestinal protein losing diseases, large wounds that 'ooze' protein); decreased protein production (hepatic disease); hemorrhage; and excessive IV fluid administration (called 'dilutional' hypoproteinemia). If protein is excessively low, a blood or plasma transfusion may be required.

Hyperproteinemia generally indicates that the patient is dehydrated and requires IV fluid therapy. In some chronic diseases, globulins can be elevated and cause hyperproteinemia. This can be identified on a serum chemistry panel.

TIP
We generally use total protein measurement as an estimate of albumin, but if you really need to know how much of the total protein is albumin and how much is globulin, you have to run a serum chemistry panel.

Impact of Abnormalities:

Anemia - decreased tissue oxygen delivery.

Polycythemia - if severe, can also cause decreased tissue oxygen delivery because the 'thick' blood does not flow well (it 'sludges' in the vessels) thus, does not provide normal perfusion of the organs.

Hypoproteinemia causes numerous adverse effects including:
• Loss of fluid from the blood vessels due to decreased oncotic pressure. This can lead to edema.
• Excessive blood loss due to decreased clotting factors.
• Relative drug overdose due to decreased protein binding of drugs.

Cardiovascular System Advanced Monitoring

Electrocardiograph (ECG)

The contraction of the heart muscle is generated by electrical impulses that pass through the myocardium. These electrical impulses can be recorded by placing electrical connections (the ECG clips and leads) on the surface (skin) of the animal to produce an electrocardiogram or ECG. Anesthetic drugs and changes that occur during anesthesia (e.g., hypoxemia, hypercarbia, electrolyte imbalance) can cause arrhythmias, thus ECG monitoring is important in anesthetized patients.

Normal Electrical Conduction Pathway

Electrical activity starts at the sinus node (the pacemaker of the heart, located at the right atrium) moves through the atria to the atrioventricular (AV) node (located at the junction of the atria and ventricles) and then on to various structures in the ventricles **(Figure 5-12)**.

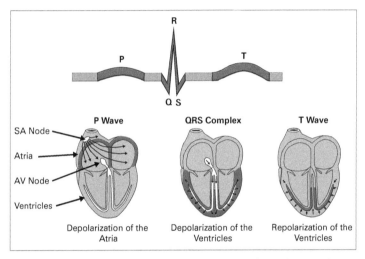

Figure 5-12. Diagram of heart with the normal electrical conduction pathway and a normal ECG.

Normal ECG Complex

A normal ECG complex will have a P, QRS and T wave. In a healthy heart with a normal contraction in response to the electrical impulse, the P wave represents the atrium contracting, the QRS wave represents the ventricles contracting, and the T wave represents the ventricles relaxing.

Advantage

Electrocardiography is easy to use and provides critical information about the electrical activity of the heart.

139

Disadvantage

The presence of normal electrical activity on the ECG does not mean that cardiac output is normal. The heart can have normal electrical activity with little or no mechanical response (muscle contraction). Thus, BLOOD PRESSURE should be monitored along with the ECG. The worst case scenario is called 'pulseless electrical activity' in which there is no contraction in response to the electrical activity, this rapidly leads to death.

How to: Set Up the ECG

Three leads are most commonly used in anesthetized patients. Up to 12 leads can be used for diagnostic purposes but are usually not necessary for assessing changes that might occur during anesthesia.

Place the leads **(Figure 5-13)** with the right arm electrode or 'clip' (**RA** usually white) in the axillary region (i.e., behind the elbow) of the right forelimb of the patient; and the left arm electrode (**LA** usually black) in the axillary region of the left forelimb; and the left leg electrode (**LL** usually red) in the lower flank or stifle region of the left hindlimb. This creates a 'triangular pattern' around the patient's heart. The electrical activity between the right arm and left leg leads produces the ECG tracing and the left arm lead is an electrical ground in Lead II.

TIP

To help remember where to put the ECG clips, use the saying: White on right (white clip on right forelimb); smoke (black clip on left forelimb) over fire (red clip on left hindlimb). The smoke would be 'over' the fire if the animal stood on its hindlimbs.

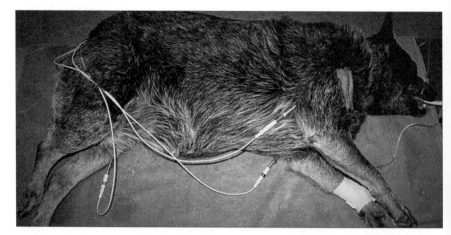

Figure 5-13. Correct placement of the ECG leads. Place the leads with the right arm electrode or 'clip' ([RA] usually white) in the axillary region of the right forelimb; and the left arm electrode ([LA] usually black) in the axillary region of the left forelimb; and the left leg electrode ([LL] usually red) in the lower flank or stifle region of the left foreleg.

TIP
Place gel on the ECG clips before attaching to the patient or squirt the clips with alcohol once they are attached to the skin. Dry clips do not conduct electricity very well. The leads may need to be re-moistened periodically throughout a long procedure.

Impact of Arrhythmias
- Arrhythmias can cause hypotension (through decreased cardiac output) and should be identified and treated (if necessary).
- Arrhythmias can be fatal.

Common Abnormalities (Common Arrhythmias)
The most common arrhythmias occurring in patients under anesthesia are sinus tachycardia, sinus bradycardia and ventricular premature contractions. Ventricular tachycardia, ventricular escape beats and second-degree AV block can also occur in anesthetized patients.

Treatment of these arrhythmias is described in Chapter 10. The patient may present to anesthesia with all types of arrhythmias, but we will only discuss arrhythmias that commonly occur as a result of anesthetic drugs or physiologic changes that occur during anesthesia.

Sinus Tachycardia and Sinus Bradycardia
(Figure 5-14)

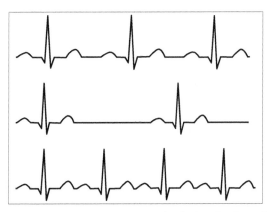

Figure 5-14. ECG tracing depicting normal heart rate (top), sinus bradycardia (middle) and sinus tachycardia (bottom). Regardless of the rate, the ECG tracing has a normal configuration, indicating that the electrical impulse originated at the sinus node and followed the normal electrical pathway through the heart.

- Sinus tachycardia and sinus bradycardia are the most commonly encountered changes in heart rate.

- They are termed 'sinus' because the electrical activity originates at the sinoatrial (or 'sinus') node, which is the normal initiation point for the electrical activity.
- Thus the ECG has a normal configuration but the rate is fast (tachycardia) or slow (bradycardia).
- These rhythms are generally due to an underlying cause (see Chapter 10) and don't require treatment unless the rate causes a decrease in blood pressure.

IMPORTANT POINT
If the heart rate is changed but the ECG is normal, these changes are termed sinus bradycardia and sinus tachycardia. The rate is slow or fast but the heart beat is still normal and produced by an electrical impulse from the sinoatrial (SA) node, which is also called the sinus node (See Figure 5-12).

Sinus Arrhythmia
(Figure 5-15)
Also called 'normal sinus rhythm' because it is a commonly occurring normal alteration in the ECG pattern. The rhythm is initiated at the sinus node and the heart rate increases when the patient inhales and slows when the patient exhales.

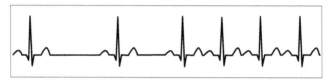

Figure 5-15. ECG tracing depicting sinus rhythm or 'sinus arrhythmia'. This is a normal rhythm, especially in large dogs. The heart rate increases when the patient inhales and decreases when the patient exhales.

Ventricular Premature Contractions (VPCs)
(Figure 5-16)

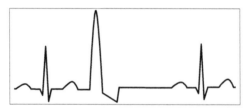

Figure 5-16. ECG tracing depicting ventricular premature contraction (VPC). VPCs occur when the electrical impulse originates in the ventricles instead of the sinus node. Note that the VPC (second complex from the left) occurs early (before the next normal beat would have occurred). The complex has no P wave, but does have a very large and abnormally configured QRS complex and a large inverted T wave. There is a long pause before the next normal beat. The overall heart rate is usually normal.

- VPCs occur when the electrical impulse originates in the ventricles instead of the sinus node.

- These are intermittent early beats (meaning that they occur before the next normal, sinus node generated beat) and the associated complexes are taller, wider and abnormal in appearance (some references use the term 'bizarre' appearance) in comparison to a normal ECG complex. The complex can be upright OR inverted ('upside down')
- They do not have a P wave associated with the QRS complex and the T wave is also large, wide, abnormally configured and usually pointed in the opposite direction of the QRS complex.
- The VPC is usually a single beat typically followed by a compensatory pause - meaning that the next beat will not occur at its normal time, instead there will be a length of time before the next beat occurs - and the heart rate is usually normal.
- VPCs can be caused by many factors, including underlying cardiac disease, age (so they are more common in geriatric patients), hypotension, hypoxemia, hypercarbia, electrolyte imbalance, excessively deep plane of anesthesia, excessively light plane of anesthesia and pain.
- A few VPCs are generally not concerning and don't require treatment, especially if the heart rate and blood pressure are normal. VPCs become concerning, and require treatment, if they occur frequently enough to cause hypotension.
- The underlying cause of the arrhythmia should be investigated since treatment of the cause may be necessary.

Ventricular Tachycardia
(Figure 5-17)

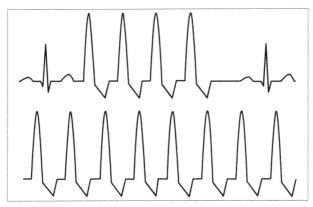

Figure 5-17. ECG tracing depicting ventricular tachycardia. Note that the complexes look like rapidly occurring VPCs. They can be intermittent (top tracing) or continuous (bottom tracing).

- With ventricular tachycardia, the heart rate is fast and there are multiple ventricular beats which may be interspersed with normal beats or may occur with no normal beats at all.
- The ECG tracing reveals a fast rhythm (faster than normal HR) that is composed of all (or mostly) complexes that look like VPCs.

- This is an important arrhythmia to diagnose because it is likely to cause hypotension and can quickly convert to a life threatening arrhythmia such as ventricular fibrillation.
- Ventricular tachycardia can be caused by many factors, including underlying cardiac disease, hypotension, hypoxemia, hypercarbia, electrolyte imbalance, excessively deep plane of anesthesia, excessively light plane of anesthesia and pain.
- Both the arrhythmia and the underlying cause will require treatment.

Ventricular Escape Beats
(Figure 5-18)

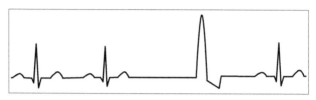

Figure 5-18. ECG tracing depicting ventricular escape beat. The complex looks like a VPC but the beat occurs late (after the next normal beat would have occurred). The heart rate is usually slow.

- Escape beats occur when an electrical pulse originates in the ventricles in response to profound bradycardia.
- These are intermittent late beats (meaning that they occur after a normal beat should have occurred but didn't) and the associated ECG complexes often look like a VPC.
- Escape beats are an attempt by the heart to increase cardiac output (and blood pressure) in the presence of severe bradycardia.
- Anything that causes profound bradycardia can result in ventricular escape beats.
- It is very important to distinguish VPC's (early beat, HR normal) from escape beats (late beat, HR slow) because the treatments are very different. The arrhythmia itself isn't important but the underlying severe bradycardia is likely to contribute to hypotension and will probably require treatment.

2nd Degree AV Block
(Figure 5-19)

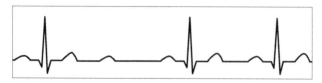

Figure 5-19. ECG tracing depicting 2nd degree AV block. The second P wave from the left does not have an accompanying QRS complex or T wave.

- This arrhythmia is identified on the ECG as an atrial contraction (P wave) without a subsequent ventricular contraction (QRS T).
- The arrhythmia can occur with cardiovascular disease but most often occurs with anything that increases vagal tone (e.g., patients that are very athletic, surgeries of the eye or GI tract) and following administration of alpha-2 agonists.
- The arrhythmia only becomes important if the lack of ventricular contractions causes hypotension - then treatment may be required.
- The arrhythmia occurs commonly and is generally not concerning in horses.

Troubleshooting the ECG Monitor:
Abnormally Shaped ECG Complexes
- First check the patient to determine whether the abnormalities on the ECG tracing are truly an arrhythmia. Feel the pulse, listen to the heart, look at the pulse wave on the pulse oximeter tracing or arterial blood pressure tracing and listen for changes in the sound of the Doppler. If the abnormal tracing is indeed caused by an arrhythmia, proceed to diagnose it as described above.
- Second check for ECG artifacts. An artifact will not be associated with a pulse, the ECG complex will probably not look like a normal complex, the artifact will not interrupt the rhythm - meaning that every P, QRS and T wave will occur at the expected point on the ECG tracing and the interval between R waves (the R-R interval) will not change. An artifact rhythm is usually irregular and the rate of the artifact is variable.

Extra Spike
If a single 'spike' occurs that does not look like any component of a normal ECG complex, does not cause a change in the normal components of the ECG complex and does not cause a pulse deficit:
- Insure that the patient does not have a pacemaker - pacemakers cause a 'spike' just before the normal ECG complex.
- Start turning off electrical appliances (e.g., water blankets, clippers, etc.) since electrical appliances, especially as they are turned on/off, can cause a spike on the ECG tracing.

Rapid, Continuous Peaks or Spikes
If the baseline is wide and looks like continuous, rapid 'spikes' **(Figure 5-20)**, this is probably electrical Interference, but BE SURE to check the patient since it could

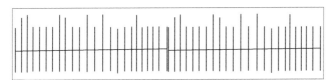

Figure 5-20. ECG tracing with rapid continuous spikes. These are most commonly due to electrical interference. They do not look like a normal ECG tracing and would not be associated with a pulse.

be a rapid ventricular arrhythmia. This interference is most commonly due to a disrupted baseline because of improper grounding. To correct:
- Check for poor contact of the electrodes with the skin,
- Clean the electrode clips, reapply conducting gel and alcohol,
- Ensure that the leads are not contacting metal (like the metal table),
- Remove electrical devices from the table,
- Change the outlet that the monitor is plugged into.

Square Wave
Artifacts that look like a large 'square' wave are most likely caused by the machine calibrating. There are no square arrhythmias.

Wandering Baseline (also called 'waving' or 'undulating' baseline)
If you can see P, QRS, and T complexes but the baseline isn't steady - it 'undulates' up and down **(Figure 5-21)** - it is called a wandering or 'undulating' baseline and is probably due to patient movement.
- If the patient is still conscious (like during a preanesthesia physical exam), try to hold it still for a few minutes.
- If the patient is in recovery, make sure it is not shivering.
- If the patient is anesthetized, make sure that the electrodes for the ECG leads aren't right on the thorax - the movement of breathing can be enough to cause a wandering baseline.

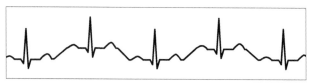

Figure 5-21. ECG tracing showing a wandering baseline (also called 'waving' or 'undulating' baseline). This is most likely due to patient movement.

No ECG Complexes or 'Flatline'
If there are no ECG complexes on the screen assume the worst and quickly check the patient for a heartbeat! If the problem is indeed the patient, go directly to the CPR section in Chapter 10. If there is a heartbeat focus on the machine.
- Check to be sure that all the electrodes are still attached and making good contact with the patient's skin (a lead that has come off is the most common cause of this trouble).
- Make sure that the leads are plugged into the cable and the cable is plugged into the machine.
- Change leads (for example, go to Lead 1 or Lead 3 if you are in Lead 2).
- Increase the amplification of the complexes. This is commonly required in small dogs and cats. If the patient is okay and none of this works, it is probably time to replace the leads and/or the cable.

ECG Incorrectly Counting the Heart Rate
The ECG will not count the heart rate correctly if:
* the patient's rate is too slow;
* the complexes are too small for the machine to count (commonly occurs in cats);
* the rate is random (sometimes slow, sometimes fast);
* the patient has a second degree AV block or other arrhythmia;
* there is a wandering baseline;
* there is electrical interference;
* two peaks in the P-QRS-T complex are the same size (this is common in ECG tracings with very low amplitudes like those often obtained in patients of very small body size like cats). Since the machine is programmed to count the highest peaks it counts both peaks ('double counts') if they are equal (or close to equal) amplitude.

* Fix inaccurate counting by:
  * changing the lead that the machine is reading, e.g., change from Lead II to Lead III (should fix 'double counting');
  * changing amplification of the complexes (should fix complexes that are too small);
  * changing the location of the leads (should fix wandering baseline and maybe double counting and complexes that are too small);
  * wet the contacts at the skin with alcohol or gel;
  * turn off unnecessary electrical appliances;
  * or best choice, just count the rate yourself and don't rely on the machine for rate.

Arterial Blood Pressure
Adequate blood pressure is required for adequate oxygen delivery to the tissues (assuming that the blood is carrying oxygen). Oxygen is a substrate, or 'fuel', that is required for normal cell function. Lack of oxygen = cell damage. Cell damage = tissue damage = organ damage.

IMPORTANT POINT
MOST ANESTHETIC DRUGS CAN CONTRIBUTE TO HYPOTENSION, which can cause decreased oxygen delivery to the cells. Thus, blood pressure should be measured in EVERY anesthetized patient.

CRITICAL POINT!
Blood pressure cannot be determined by heart rate since changes in blood pressure are often due to changes in stroke volume or vessel tone, and not necessarily changes in heart rate. SO BLOOD PRESSURE MUST BE MEASURED.

How to: Monitor Arterial Blood Pressure:

There are three choices:

1) Noninvasive blood pressure (NIBP) measurement using a Doppler **(Figure 5-22)**;
2) Noninvasive blood pressure (NIBP) measurement using oscillometric blood pressure units **(Figure 5-23)**;
3) Invasive blood pressure measurement using a catheter in a peripheral artery. The latter is common in horses but uncommon, and generally unnecessary, in most small animal practices.

Measured parameters include systolic arterial blood pressure **(SAP)**; mean arterial blood pressure **(MAP)** and diastolic arterial blood pressure **(DAP)** (Table 5-3).

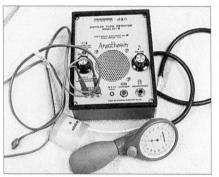

Figure 5-22. Doppler setup for noninvasive blood pressure measurement. The Doppler unit with the probe ('crystal') to place over the artery to amplify sound, the blood pressure cuff, and the bulb used to inflate the blood pressure cuff. Inflation of the cuff stops sound from the Doppler by restricting arterial blood flow. Note the manometer (or 'pressure gauge') that will indicate systolic arterial pressure **(SAP)** as the pressure on the cuff is released and blood flow through the arteries returns.

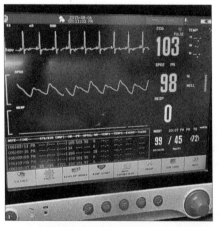

Figure 5-23. The screen of an oscillometric noninvasive blood pressure monitor. In the display in the lower right corner, the systolic arterial blood pressure **(SAP)** is 99 mmHg, the diastolic arterial blood pressure **(DAP)** is 45 mmHg and the mean arterial blood pressure **(MAP)** is 72 mmHg. This is normal blood pressure for an anesthetized dog or cat.

Table 5-3
Normal Ranges for Arterial Blood Pressue in Anesthetized Animals

Systolic	80 to 120 mmHg
Mean*	60 to 100 mmHg
Diastolic	40 to 80 mmHg

IMPORTANT POINT

Invasive monitoring (arterial catheterization) is the most accurate way to monitor blood pressure and is important for horses anesthetized with inhalant drugs (because horses in this situation are highly prone to hypotension) and in research animals (where exact blood pressure readings are important). Invasive blood pressure monitoring is generally not practical in most small animal practices, but may be important for critical small animal patients.

IMPORTANT POINT

Noninvasive blood pressure monitors do not provide an exact measurement of blood pressure but they do provide an approximate blood pressure value and they provide blood pressure trends. Trends are generally more important than the blood pressure at any one point in time and are more likely to be used to make treatment decisions.

How to: Set up the Noninvasive Blood Pressure Monitor:

• For both the Oscillometric and Doppler monitors, an inflatable blood pressure cuff is used to occlude the artery.

• The *width* of the blood pressure cuff should be 40 to 60% of the diameter of the tail or the limb on which the cuff will be placed **(Figure 5-24)**. The length of the cuff is not important as long as it is long enough for the Velcro to keep the cuff securely closed.

• For the Doppler, the hair should be shaved from the site on which the probe will be placed. The probe (or 'crystal') should be coated with ultrasound gel **(Figure 5-25).** Ultrasound gel does not contain 'salts' that will degrade the silicone on the probe. The probe is then placed over an artery on the limb or tail.

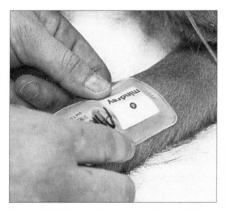

Figure 5-24. The width of the cuff should be 40 to 60% of the circumference of the tail or the limb on which the cuff will be placed. The length of the cuff is not important if it is long enough for the Velcro to keep the cuff securely closed.

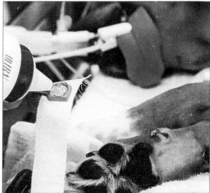

Figure 5-25. The surface of the Doppler probe that will contact the skin should be covered with ultrasound gel and placed over the artery on the limb or tail. The hair must be shaved at the site of probe placement (spot just above the pads in this photo).

149

- The cuff is then placed above the probe - meaning between the probe and the heart **(Figure 5-26)**. If the cuff is 'below' the probe, it will not occlude blood flow at the site of the probe and blood pressure will not be measured.

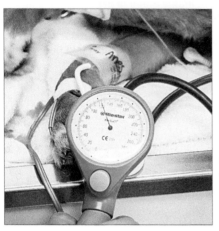

Figure 5-26. The blood pressure cuff is placed above the Doppler probe (between the probe and the heart). The Doppler probe is under the tape behind the pressure manometer and the blood pressure cuff is above the tape. If the cuff is 'below' the probe, it will not occlude blood flow at the site of the probe and blood pressure cannot be measured.

- The blood pressure cuff (oscillometric monitors) or probe (Doppler monitors) should be placed at the same horizontal level as the heart **(Figure 5-27)**. If not at this 'level' the blood pressure reading will not be accurate. This is the same principle as the blood pressure cuff being placed over the upper arm when measuring blood pressure in humans. The upper arm is at the same horizontal 'level' as the heart.

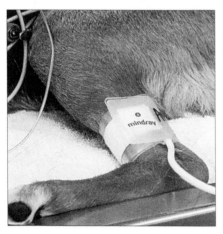

Figure 5-27. For both the oscillometric and Doppler monitors, placement of the blood pressure cuff (oscillometric) or probe (Doppler) must be at the same horizontal level as the heart.

NIBP: Doppler

Works by amplifying the sound of blood flowing through the artery over which the sensor (or 'probe' or 'crystal') is placed. Thus, the sound heard from a Doppler is actually the sound of *blood flow*, not a mechanical noise. The first sound heard when the cuff pressure is being released is systolic arterial blood pressure (SAP).

Advantages of the Doppler
• Other monitors make mechanical noises that can sometimes be caused by inter-ference or other non-patient factors, but this monitor actually amplifies the sound of blood flowing in the patient!
• The equipment is fairly easy to use and can be used in almost any species to amplify the pulsatile blood flow sound, from which the heart rate can be counted.
  • Using Doppler to get blood pressure, however, depends on whether or not a cuff can be placed proximal to the probe.
  • This limits probe placement to distal limbs and the base of the tail for blood pressure measurement.
• Blood pressure determined by the Doppler is not affected by arrhythmias (because the unit is not taking an average pressure over several beats like the oscillometric unit does).
• A blood pressure measurement is more likely to be obtained in really small patients when using the Doppler than when using the oscillometric unit. This is because your ears listening for the blood flow are more sensitive than the oscillometric cuff attempting to detect blood flow.

TIP
Because human ears are more sensitive than a mechanical oscillometric cuff, the Doppler is often more useful than the oscillometric monitor in very small patients like cats and puppies.

Disadvantages of the Doppler
• Blood pressure measurement is manual, not automatic, so the Doppler is a little more work than the oscillometric monitor.
• It measures only SAP, which isn't a problem, just something to remember.
• Hair must be shaved in order to place the probe on the skin (this isn't really a problem but sometimes bothers the owners).
• The probe can be a little tricky to place and especially to tape in place.
• The gel can dry out if the surgery is long, causing the probe to lose contact with the artery.

NIBP Oscillometric Blood Pressure Monitors
These monitors work by detecting the oscillations (caused by turbulence) in blood flow that occur when blood flow returns to an artery that was previously occluded by a pressurized cuff. They measure (or sometimes calculate) systolic, diastolic and mean arterial blood pressure. They can also count heart rate.

Advantages of the Oscillometric Monitor
This monitor is easier to use than a Doppler (place the cuff over an artery and press 'start' on the machine - THAT'S IT!) and provides automatic readings at the time interval set on the monitor (usually every 5 minutes).

Disadvantages of the Oscillometric Monitor
Compared to the Doppler, measurements may be less consistent and/or harder to obtain in small patients, patients with arrhythmias or bradycardia, patients that are moving (or shivering) and extremely hypotensive patients.

Direct (Invasive) Arterial Blood Pressure
Works by directly measuring arterial blood pressure using a catheter inserted into an artery.

Advantages of Direct Arterial Blood Pressure Monitoring
• The most accurate measurement of blood pressure.
• Provides constant, real time blood pressure so that you can respond to problems more quickly.
• SAP, DAP, and MAP are all directly measured and a continuous waveform will be displayed (with the appropriate monitor).

Disadvantages of Direct Arterial Blood Pressure Monitoring
• Arterial catheterization can be difficult and time consuming (arteries are much more difficult to catheterize than veins).
• Many blood pressure monitors do not have the components needed to measure direct arterial blood pressure.

CRITICAL POINT!
*The MAP should be maintained above 60 mmHg in anesthetized patients. A MAP below 50 mmHg is likely to significantly decrease oxygen delivery to the tissues so maintaining the blood pressure above 60 mmHg is more likely to protect the tissues from decreased oxygen delivery.

Common Blood Pressure Abnormalities
The blood pressure may be too low (hypotension), or too high (hypertension). Hypotension is very common in anesthetized patients but hypertension is rare.

Impact of Blood Pressure Abnormalities
Decreased oxygen delivery to the tissues (hypotension); potential damage to some organs (hypertension).

Trouble Shooting Doppler Equipment
Doppler Sound Absent
• Check the patient! If you can palpate a pulse, the problem is almost certainly the equipment.
• The probe may have shifted and is no longer over an artery or has lost contact with the artery.
  • The probe may have poor contact with the skin. In this case, more gel may need to be applied - this happens often in long surgeries since the gel dries out over time.

- Patient movement can disrupt contact between the probe and skin, and the tape or wrap over the probe may need to be adjusted.
- The cuff may still be inflated and occluding the artery.
- The cable may be disconnected from the speaker, the speaker may not be turned on or the speaker battery may be dead.
- You may need a new probe! They wear out - and they often get damaged. Place it on yourself and see if it works.

Doppler Sound is not Diminished by Inflation of the Blood Pressure Cuff
This means that inflation of the cuff is not occluding the artery.
- The cuff is too large or too loose to occlude the artery.
- The cuff or cable may be leaking air and not inflating the cuff.
- The bulb used to pressurize the system may be defective and not inflating the cuff.
- The cuff may be in wrong place (below the probe instead of above it)
- The patient has severe hypertension - the sound should still be abolished if enough pressure is applied to the artery, but it may require a lot more pressure than you expected

False Hypotensive Reading
The Doppler may indicate hypotension that is not plausible for the patient.
- Always check the patient before assuming that the hypotension is false. Palpate the pulse quality and assess the mucous membrane color and CRT. If unsure, turn down the vaporizer and give the patient a bolus of IV fluids.
- Then trouble shoot the equipment.
  - Check cuff size and contact with the patient. A cuff that is too large or too loose will cause false hypotensive readings.
  - Make sure that the Velcro is adequate to keep the cuff snug as it is being inflated. Cuffs and Velcro wear out!
  - Check location of the probe. Placing it higher than the heart will cause false hypotensive readings.
  - Check the probe. It may have slipped or lost contact with the skin, making blood flow difficult to hear.
  - Make sure that the blood flow to the limb is not being restricted. This sometimes occurs with table ties that are too tight.
  - You may be deflating the cuff too rapidly and missing the initial return of flow (i.e., missing the first sound of flow).
  - If the patient is a very small dog or cat the Doppler may not amplify sound enough to hear the first blood flow (SAP), and the first sound you hear may be occurring closer to the MAP.

To trouble shoot, turn down the vaporizer and give the patient a bolus of
fluids. If the pressure comes up, the hypotensive measurement was probably
real. If the blood pressure stays stable, then the patient may be normotensive
and the Doppler is underestimating blood pressure. But you can't just assume
that it is underestimating - you have to challenge the system by trying to
change the blood pressure in order to make a decision.

| NOTE
Manometers may be faulty and/or may need to be recalibrated after heavy use
and/or if the factory tubing has been replaced or shortened. Faulty or uncali-
brated momanometers can give inaccurate measurements.

False Hypertensive Reading
The Doppler may indicate hypertension that is not plausible for the patient.
• Always check the patient before assuming that the hypertension is false.
• Palpate the pulse quality and assess the mucous membrane color and CRT.
• Make sure that the cuff is not too small, too tight or below the level of the heart.

| TIP
To trouble shoot, administer an analgesic drug (hypertension is commonly
due to pain) and/or turn up the vaporizer slightly. If the pressure comes down,
the hypertensive measurement was probably real. If the patient stays stable,
then the patient may be normotensive and the Doppler is overestimating
blood pressure. But you can't just assume that it is overestimating - you have
to challenge the system by trying to change the blood pressure in order to
make a decision.

Trouble Shooting the Oscillometric Blood Pressure Monitor
The Monitor does not Provide any Blood Pressure Results
• Check the patient! If you can palpate a pulse, the problem may be the equipment,
but it is also possible that the patient may really be hypotensive. Check this by
palpating pulse quality and checking mucous membrane color and CRT, and using a
Doppler to listen for blood flow. The human ear is more sensitive than the oscillometric cuff so it is often possible to measure blood pressure with a Doppler even
when the oscillometric unit fails to measure blood pressure.

If the problem is not the patient, trouble shoot the machine:
• Check the cuff, it may be too large or too loose to occlude the artery. Make sure
that the Velcro is adequate to keep the cuff snug as it is being inflated. Cuffs and
Velcro wear out!
• Check the location of the cuff - is it really over an artery?
• Check for leaks in the cuff or cable - if there are leaks, the cuff won't inflate.
• Check the machine - it may be waiting for you to hit the 'start' button or to
program in a time interval for taking the pressure.

- Check the machine to make sure that it is really generating enough air to inflate the cuff (disconnect the cuff from the cable and feel for air coming out of the cable). If not, the machine needs to be serviced.

False Hypotensive Reading

The oscillometric monitor may indicate hypotension that is not plausible for the patient.
- Always check the patient before assuming that the hypotension is false. Palpate the pulse quality and assess the mucous membrane color and CRT. If unsure, turn down the vaporizer and give the patient a bolus of IV fluids.
- Then trouble shoot the equipment.
    - Check cuff size and contact with the patient. A cuff that is too large or too loose will cause false hypotensive readings.
    - Check location of the cuff. Placing it higher than the heart will cause false hypotensive readings.
    - Check all the factors that would affect inflation of the cuff as described in the 'no readings on the oscillometric monitor' section (e.g., leaks in cuff or cable, machine not producing enough air pressure).
    - Make sure that the blood flow to the limb is not being restricted. This sometimes occurs with table ties that are too tight.
    - If the patient is a very small dog or cat the oscillometric unit may not recognize the first blood flow (SAP), and the measurement it provides for SAP may be closer to the MAP.

TIP
To trouble shoot, turn down the vaporizer and give the patient a bolus of fluids. If the pressure comes up, the hypotensive measurement was probably real. If the blood pressure stays stable, then the patient is likely normo-tensive and the oscillometric monitor is underestimating blood pressure. But you can't just assume that it is underestimating - you have to challenge the system by trying to change the blood pressure in order to make a decision.

False Hypertensive Reading

The oscillometric monitor may indicate hypertension that is not plausible for the patient.
- Always check the patient before assuming that the hypertension is false.
- Palpate the pulse quality and assess the mucous membrane color and CRT.
- Make sure that the cuff is not too small, too tight or below level of the heart.

TIP
To trouble shoot, administer an analgesic drug (hypertension is commonly due to pain) and/or turn up the vaporizer slightly. If the pressure comes down, the hypertensive measurement was probably real. If the patient stays stable, then the patient is likely normotensive and the monitor is overestimating blood pressure. But you can't just assume that it is overestimating - you have to challenge the system by trying to change the blood pressure in order to make a decision.

The Blood Pressure Results are Not Consistent

The measurements may be completely erratic - sometimes high, sometimes low. This commonly occurs if:

• The patient is really bradycardic or having arrhythmias (even minor alterations in normal rhythm like sinus bradycardia or tachycardia can cause this problem).

• The patient is being moved so that the cuff position in relation to the heart is changing.

• To troubleshoot:

  • CHECK THE PATIENT FIRST (heart rate, mucous membrane color and capillary refill time)!

  • Watch for the trend of the pressure measurements - it is more useful to monitor a trend of results rather than any one reading.

  • If the patient is stable, hit the start button again and get a new reading.

The Machine does not Accurately Count the Heart Rate

• Check to make sure that the machine is set to read the heart rate from the blood pressure tracing.

• Amplify the signal so that the peaks on the blood pressure tracing are larger.

Trouble Shooting the Direct Arterial Blood Pressure Monitor

Measurements obtained by direct arterial blood pressure monitors are more likely than measurements obtained by noninvasive monitors to truly reflect abnormalities in the patient so, for any abnormality, CHECK THE PATIENT FIRST! Take steps as described in the noninvasive monitor sections to correct any patient abnormalities.

The Monitor does not Provide Blood Pressure Results

• Check the tracing on the monitor, if there are waveforms but no numbers, re-zero the transducer . If there is no waveform, causes include:

  • The catheter is not in the artery.

  • The fluid filled line from the catheter to the transducer is not open.

  • The cable from the transducer to the machine is not connected.

  • The catheter is completely occluded and needs to be flushed with saline or heparinized saline.

  • The transducer wasn't zeroed or is not zeroed correctly. Re-zero.

  • The transducer has malfunctioned and should be replaced.

False Hypotensive Measurement

• Check the tracing, there may be an abnormally small wave form. Causes:

  • The arterial catheter may be partially occluded with a blood clot and should be flushed with saline or heparinized saline. May need to flush more frequently.

  • Blood flow may be partially obstructed because the catheter is placed against an arterial wall. Try flushing first, then try pulling the catheter SLIGHTLY out.

  • The blood flow may be partially occluded if the surgeon is leaning on the patient or the table ties are too tight.

  • Arterial wall constriction from a difficult catheterization can cause a

temporary 'occlusion'. This will dissipate over time.
- The transducer wasn't zeroed correctly. Re-zero.
- The transducer may be placed above the level of the heart.

False Hypertensive Reading
- Check the tracing, there may be an abnormally tall wave form. Causes:
- The transducer may be placed below the level of the heart.
- The transducer wasn't zeroed correctly. Re-zero.

Summary
Anesthesia-induced changes in the cardiovascular system can cause major complications, including death. The best way to avoid complications is to identify deleterious trends by monitoring the patient. Cardiovascular monitoring should include simple techniques like assessment of pulse strength, mucous membrane color and capillary refill time, to more advanced techniques like measurement of arterial blood pressure and evaluation of the ECG.

Monitoring the Respiratory System
The respiratory system is comprised of all of the airway structures from the nares or oral cavity to the alveoli. The ultimate goals of the respiratory system are to work with the cardiovascular system to deliver oxygen to the working cells and to remove carbon dioxide from the blood to prevent acidosis. On the respiratory side of oxygen delivery, a decrease in delivery is caused by anything that prevents oxygen from entering the blood stream. Examples include factors that:
- Decrease oxygen in the lungs:
  - hypoventilation (by far the most common cause),
  - obstructions in the airway or breathing system (e.g., plugged or kinked endotracheal tube, kinked breathing system hoses),
  - decreased inhaled oxygen (e.g., no or low oxygen flow in anesthesia system, excessive nitrous oxide flow),
  - equipment malfunction or error (oxygen line not connected to patient's breathing system, endotracheal tube in the esophagus, etc.),
  - anatomic shunts (e.g., persistent ductus arteriosis [PDA]).
- Decrease the surface area of the lung available for oxygen diffusion:
  - Including, atelectasis (airway collapse), lung tumors or torsions, endobronchial intubation (the ET tube in one bronchi instead of in the trachea so that only one lung receives oxygen), pressure on the diaphragm from abdominal distension or pregnancy and pressure on the rib cage.
- Impair diffusion of oxygen across the alveolar membrane:
  - Pulmonary edema for example.
- Cause equipment malfunction or error (including oxygen not turned on, tank empty or flow too low, malfunctioning one-way valves in breathing system, kinks or occlusion in tubing or endotracheal tubes).

Since the respiratory system is also responsible for eliminating carbon dioxide (CO_2) from the body, factors that cause an abnormal carbon dioxide concentration should be considered and include anything that:
- Changes the rate or depth of ventilation (breathing):
  - Hyperventilation, as may occur with pain, excessively light plane of anesthesia, hypoxemia;
  - Hypoventilation, as may occur with excessive anesthetic depth, drugs that cause respiratory depression, CNS disease, head trauma.
- Alters movement of air through the airways:
  - Upper airway dysfunction (brachycephalic airway disease for example).
  - Lower airway dysfunction (including pneumonia, pressure on the diaphragm, decreased movement of the thoracic wall).
- Cause equipment malfunction or error (including oxygen flow too low in nonbreathing systems, exhausted carbon dioxide absorbent in rebreathing systems, malfunctioning one-way valves in rebreathing systems, kinks or occlusions in breathing system hoses or endotracheal tubes).

CRITICAL POINT!
Ventilation (breathing) and gas exchange (oxygen into the body; carbon dioxide out of the body) are impaired to some degree by almost all of the anesthetic drugs used in pre-medication, induction and maintenance of anesthesia. Hypoventilation (rate too slow or volume of breath too low to provide adequate delivery of oxygen and/or removal of carbon dioxide) is common, and close monitoring of respiratory function during anesthesia is extremely important.

CRITICAL POINT!
Ventilation and gas exchange can also be impacted by malfunctioning anesthesia equipment. Appropriate maintenance and frequent function checks of the equipment are extremely important. The ability to troubleshoot anesthetic equipment when something goes wrong is also important.

Respiratory System Basic (but Essential) Monitoring
Parameters to monitor include respiratory rate, tidal volume (volume of breath), and mucous membrane color.

Respiratory Rate (Table 5-4)
- Respiratory rate is one of the components of breathing, or 'ventilation', needed to maintain normal oxygen and carbon dioxide levels (normal 'gas exchange'). It is the combination of respiratory rate and tidal volume that is important for normal ventilation and gas exchange.
  - Respiratory rate is more obvious than tidal volume so the rate is typically used to evaluate ventilation.

- Respiratory rate x tidal volume (volume of breath, see next section) = minute ventilation (the amount of air moved through the alveoli in a minute).
- Changes in respiratory rate can also be an indicator of other changes that need to be investigated, like anesthetic depth, presence of pain, patient disease, hypoxemia (low oxygen), hypercarbia (high CO_2), equipment malfunction, body temperature, etc.

Table 5-4
Normal Ranges for Respiratory Rate in Breaths/Minute in Anesthetized Patients

Patient	Respiratory rate in breaths per minute (bpm)
Cat or Small Dog	10 to 20
Medium or Large Dog	5 to 10

IMPORTANT POINT
Changes in respiratory rate can CAUSE problems and/or can INDICATE problems.

IMPORTANT POINT
It is the minute ventilation that is responsible for gas exchange. Respiratory rate (RR) and tidal volume (TV) can change dramatically but as long as RR x TV = adequate minute ventilation, then gas exchange will be adequate.

How to: Monitor the Respiratory Rate:
Respiratory rate can be determined by:
- Observing the chest (or 'thoracic') movement (or 'excursions') of the anesthetized patient, which is the simplest way to determine the respiratory rate **(Figure 5-28 A)**.
- Observing movements of the reservoir (or 'rebreathing') bag **(Figure 5-28 B & C)**,
- Ausculting with a stethoscope or an esophageal stethoscope **(Figure 5-28 D & E)**,
- Watching the endotracheal tube 'steam up' with condensation. **(Figure 5-28 F & G)**.
- Some ECG/blood pressure monitors also count respiratory rate, however, the rate should be checked by one of the methods listed above to insure that this number is accurate. The machine counts 'respiratory rate' by counting thoracic movements, therefore any movement (e.g., shivering, strong heart contractions, the leads being bumped by the surgeon, etc.) can cause erroneous readings.

IMPORTANT TIP
Do not rely on the respiratory rate displayed on an ECG machine without double checking using other methods!

Common Respiratory Rate Abnormalities and Causes
Abnormalities are generally due to an underlying cause but may be due to respiratory disease.
- Bradypnea (respiratory rate slower than normal for that patient's species and body size), is most commonly caused by excessive anesthetic depth but can be caused by a variety of diseases;

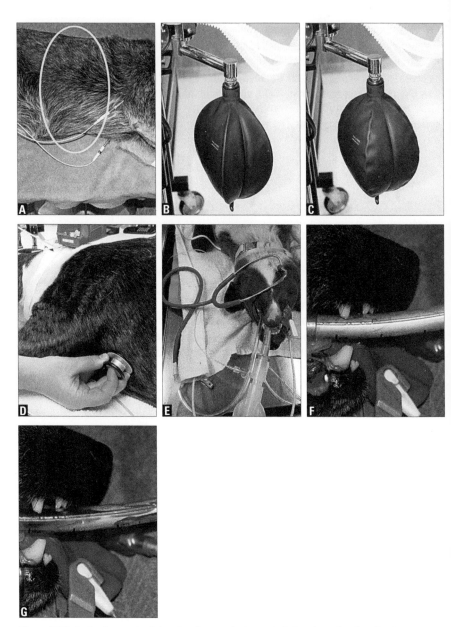

Figure 5-28. A simple way to determine the respiratory rate is by observing the chest movement of the patient. The movement is usually biggest and easiest to see, at the back of the rib cage **(A)**. It can also be determined by observing movement of the reservoir bag. The bag decreases in size when the patient inhales **(B)** and increases in size when the patient exhales **(C)**. Respiratory rate can also be determined by auscultating with a stethoscope **(D)** or an esophageal stethoscope **(E)**. Watching the endotracheal tube 'steam up' with condensation as the patient exhales warm, moist air **(F)** and clear as the patient inhales cold, dry air **(G)** is also useful.

- Tachypnea (respiratory rate faster than normal for that patient's species and body size), is commonly caused by pain, excessively light plane of anesthesia, hypoxemia, hypercarbia, hyperthermia and a variety of diseases;
- Hyperpnea (panting) is caused by the same factors that cause tachypnea and commonly results in decreased tidal volume because the lungs don't have time to fill when the respiratory rate is excessively high;
- Irregular breathing pattern (breath holding, fast rate intermixed with slow rate, etc.) can also occur for a variety of reasons, including all of those listed above;
- Apnea (no breaths) is caused by the same factors that cause bradypnea and can only be tolerated for very short periods of time.

Impact of Abnormalities in Respiratory Rate

There may be no impact if tidal volume changes to compensate for abnormal respiratory rate. Potential impact includes:

- Inadequate oxygen delivery is most commonly caused by bradypnea and apnea but can also be caused by hyperpnea.
  - Defined as hypoxemia (inadequate oxygen in the blood) or hypoxia (inadequate oxygen in the tissues). Hypoxemia is measured by arterial blood gas analysis and is designated PaO_2 (partial pressure of arterial oxygen).
- Inadequate elimination of carbon dioxide (hypercarbia or hypercapnia) with subsequent respiratory acidosis is most commonly caused by bradypnea and apnea but could be caused by hyperpnea.
  - Hypercarbia, excessively high CO_2, measured in the arterial blood and designated $PaCO_2$, or hypercapnia, excessively high CO_2 measured in the exhaled breath or end tidal CO_2 ($ETCO_2$).
- Excessive removal of carbon dioxide (hypocarbia) with subsequent respiratory alkalosis is an important consequence of tachypnea and potentially hyperpnea.
  - Hypocarbia, abnormally low CO_2, measured in the arterial blood and designated ($PaCO_2$) , or hypocapnia, abnormally low CO_2 measured in the exhaled breath or end tidal CO_2 ($ETCO_2$).
- Inadequate uptake of inhalant (which might cause the patient to wake up) may occur with apnea, bradypnea and hyperpnea.
- All of these changes can lead to a variety of adverse effects, including death.

Tidal Volume

Tidal volume, the volume of air inhaled with every breath, is one of the components of breathing, or ventilation, needed to maintain normal oxygen and carbon dioxide levels (normal 'gas exchange'). It is the combination of respiratory rate and tidal volume that is important for normal ventilation and gas exchange.

- **Respiratory rate x tidal volume** = minute ventilation (the amount of air moved through the alveoli in a minute) and it is the combination of these two components that is important for normal ventilation. A decrease in either component will cause hypoventilation. As with respiratory rate, changes in tidal volume can cause abnormal gas exchange.

• As with respiratory rate, changes in tidal volume can also be an indicator of other changes that need to be investigated such as anesthetic depth, presence of pain, patient disease, hypoxemia (low oxygen), hypercarbia (high CO_2), equipment malfunction and body temperature.

IMPORTANT POINT
Changes in tidal volume can CAUSE problems and/or can INDICATE problems.

• Respiratory rate is more commonly monitored because it is easy to assess, but tidal volume is equally important in normal respiratory function.

IMPORTANT POINT
It is important to monitor the overall respiratory function, not just the rate, since rate is only one component of ventilation. Tidal volume may change to compensate for an abnormal respiratory rate or may be ineffective in spite of a high respiratory rate, as often occurs in animals that are panting.

Normal Tidal Volume
10 to 15 ml/kg/breath.

How to: Assess Tidal Volume:
Although not common, tidal volume can be measured using a spirometer **(Figure 5-29)**. More commonly, tidal volume is roughly estimated by watching the movement of the patient's thorax or movements of the rebreathing bag. The thoracic movement (or thoracic 'excursions') during an adequate breath should look about the same as you would expect from a conscious patient. The rebreathing bag should be partly emptied during an adequate breath.

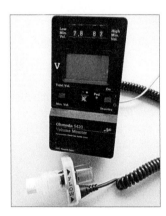

Figure 5-29. A spirometer placed in the exhalant limb of the breathing system, can be used to measure tidal volume.

Example of Assessing Tidal Volume

A 20 kg dog with a 10ml/kg tidal volume is moving 200 mls of air with every breath (20 kg x 10 ml/kg). If there is a 2000 ml reservoir bag (or 'rebreathing' bag) on the machine, the dog should deplete the bag by about 10% (200 mls/2000 mls) with every breath. This is a very rough estimate but it can be useful!

Common Tidal Volume Abnormalities and Causes

• Inadequate tidal volume to support normal oxygenation and elimination of carbon dioxide is usually due to respiratory depression from anesthetic drugs but could be due to anything that:
  • Limits expansion of the thorax (for example, ties/ropes that cross the thorax, legs tied too tightly across the thorax, surgeon leaning on the thorax or fractured ribs);
  • Limits expansion of the lungs (for example, pneumothorax, pyothorax or hemothorax);
  • Limits movement of the diaphragm (for example, ascites, distended abdomen or stomach, obesity or pregnancy;
  • Causes thoracic pain (for example, fractured ribs or contusions), which makes the patient unable to or unwilling to breath normally.
• Excessive tidal volume occasionally occurs, but it is uncommon under anesthesia unless caused by mechanical ventilation.

Impact of Tidal Volume Abnormalities

There may be no impact if the respiratory rate changes to compensate for the abnormal tidal volume. If there is an impact, it will be the same as those listed for abnormalities in the respiratory rate, i.e., abnormally low tidal volume = hypoventilation and abnormally high tidal volume = hyperventilation.

Mucous Membrane Color

The color of the mucous membranes is influenced by blood volume (the amount or volume of blood in the body), oxygen saturation of hemoglobin (i.e., the measurement obtained by the pulse oximeter [SPO_2]), vessel tone (dilated or constricted), and some systemic diseases. From the components on this list, it is primarily the oxygen saturation of hemoglobin that is a component of the respiratory system.

Normal Mucous Membrane Color

The normal color is pink to slightly pale pink (cats are usually slightly paler pink than dogs).

How to: Assess Mucous Membrane Color:

Look at the mucous membrane color in the oral cavity or conjunctiva (mucous membrane of the eyelids). If the head is covered with a surgical drape, color can be evaluated in the walls of the vagina or at the opening of the prepuce.

Common Abnormalities Resulting from Changes in the Respiratory System

Blue/purple is called 'cyanosis' and is due to decreased oxygen delivery to the tissues. This can be due to low oxygen saturation of the hemoglobin or severely low cardiac output. THIS IS A VERY LATE INDICATOR OF INADEQUATE OXYGENATION. A good anesthetist would notice long before the color change that the patient was not ventilating adequately. Other color abnormalities are more commonly due to cardiovascular changes.

Respiratory System Advanced Monitoring

Monitors include: end-tidal carbon dioxide ($ETCO_2$) monitor, pulse oximeter (SpO_2) and the blood gas analyzer.

End Tidal Carbon Dioxide (ET CO_2) Monitor or 'Capnometer'

Other than arterial blood gas, $ETCO_2$ is the best monitor of ventilation.

- CO_2 is <u>more diffusible</u> across the alveolar wall than oxygen, therefore it changes more readily with <u>changing ventilation</u>. Also, there are numerous factors that can change oxygen but <u>altered ventilation</u> is by far the <u>main reason</u> for changes in CO_2. For these reasons, CO_2 is considered to be better than oxygen as an indicator of respiratory function.

- End-tidal CO_2 is the CO_2 measured in the exhaled gas at the end of a normal (or 'tidal') exhalation. The values that the monitor displays are called hypercapnia (if the CO_2 is high) or hypocapnia (if the CO_2 is low).

- The alveolar/arterial membrane is very thin and CO_2 is very diffusible so the exhaled CO_2 concentration should be very close to the arterial CO_2 concentration. However, $ETCO_2$ is generally slightly lower than the arterial CO_2 since not all of the blood that is delivered to the lung arrives at ventilated alveoli to participate in gas exchange, some arrives to perfuse the tissues of the lung and some arrives at alveoli that are not participating in gas exchange. If the CO_2 continues to circulate and is not exhaled, the $ETCO_2$ monitor cannot measure it.

> **IMPORTANT POINT**
> The $ETCO_2$ monitor can only measure CO_2 in the exhaled gas. Thus, CO_2 in the blood may not be the same as CO_2 measured by the $ETCO_2$ monitor, but they are usually fairly similar in patients with normal lungs.

- Most $ETCO_2$ monitors display a capnograph or capnogram (display showing CO_2 graph or 'wave form'). Evaluation of the capnograph can be very valuable for patient assessment.

Normal $ETCO_2$ and $PaCO_2$ Values

For conscious animals 35 to 45 mmHg is normal and is ideal in anesthetized animals.

Up to 55 mmHg is technically defined as mild hypercapnia and down to 30 mmHg is technically defined as mild hypocapnia but both are acceptable in anesthetized patients. $ETCO_2$ or $PaCO_2$ > 60 mmHg will likely cause respiratory acidosis and < 25 mmHg will likely cause respiratory alkalosis. Both conditions should be corrected.

Advantages of CO_2 Monitoring

• The capnometer is a true monitor of ventilation (as compared to the pulse oximeter which is a monitor of oxygenation), is fairly easy to use, and produces results that are usually comparable to CO_2 measured with an invasive arterial blood gas analysis.
• $ETCO_2$ is a continuous monitor, which allows a much shorter response time (when compared to collection and assessment of arterial blood gases) when changes need to be made by the anesthetist to correct abnormal CO_2.
• Presence of a normal $ETCO_2$ value or capnographic wave can be used to confirm tracheal intubation.

TIP
A normal $ETCO_2$ value/ capnograph wave indicates that the ET tube is really in the trachea!

Disadvantages of $ETCO_2$ Monitoring

The monitor is more expensive than and requires a little more work than a pulse oximeter (but a lot less than arterial blood gas collection). The sensor in the airway (main stream monitor) or the tubing from the airway to the sensor (side stream monitor) will build up condensation/moisture over time causing an erroneous reading or an error message. Specific monitors (main stream vs side stream) also have specific advantages/disadvantages.

How to: Measure $ETCO_2$:

There are two types of $ETCO_2$ monitors, main stream and side stream.

Main Stream or 'Nondiverting' Capnometer

The sensor that measures the CO_2 is placed directly in the airway between the end of the endotracheal tube and the breathing system **(Figure 5-30)**.

Advantages of Main Stream Monitoring
The $ETCO_2$ is directly measured in the airway at the site of the sensor, delivering a faster response time and a more accurate result than side stream capnography. Because the gas sample is not aspirated from the airway, the unit does not have to be scavenged.

Disadvantages of Main Stream Monitoring
• The system creates an area where exhaled and inhaled gas can mix ('deadspace'). This means that the patient is inhaling some CO_2 from the last breath it exhaled, decreasing the efficiency of gas exchange.

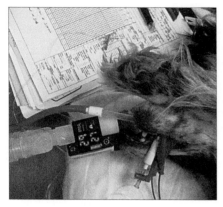

Figure 5-30. A main stream end-tidal carbon dioxide (ETCO$_2$) monitor. The sensor that measures the ETCO$_2$ is directly in the airway between the end of the endotracheal tube and the hoses of the breathing system. The actual reading can be displayed at a remote monitor away from the patient or directly on the monitor in the airway shown here. The advantage of the latter is that it is portable and the disadvantage is that it operates on batteries with no option of conversion to hospital current.

• The carbon dioxide sensor is more likely to be damaged since it has to be handled frequently (connect/disconnect with every patient).
• Mainstream capnometers are generally more expensive than side stream capnometers.

How to: Set Up the Main Stream Capnometer:

Place the sensor in the airway between the endotracheal tube and the breathing system.

Side Stream or 'Diverting' Capnometer

This system 'diverts' or aspirates a sample from the exhaled air at a rate of 50 to 150ml/minute. The sample is aspirated to the sensor which is in the monitor, not in the airway **(Figures 5-31 and 5-32)**.

Advantages of Side Stream Monitoring
• There is less mixing of inhaled and exhaled gas with side stream capnometry (less dead space).
• The carbon dioxide sensor is in the machine so damage to the sensor is unlikely.
• Some units are also designed to measure the concentration of exhaled inhalant gas (isoflurane, sevoflurane, desflurane).

Disadvantages of Side Stream Monitoring
• Scavenging is required since inhalant gas is aspirated into the unit.
• The sample line can get clogged or kinked.
• The accuracy decreases with an increased respiratory rate and/or small tidal volume (so it is not as accurate in really small patients, for example), both of which can make it difficult for the machine to aspirate a consistent airway gas sample.
• The response time is slower than that of mainstream monitors.

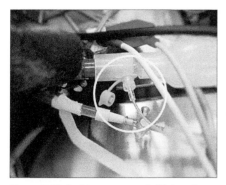

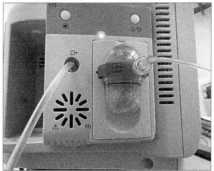

Figure 5-31. A side stream end-tidal carbon dioxide (ETCO$_2$) monitor. There is a small diameter tube attached near the end of the endotracheal tube (yellow circle). It is attached on the other end to the monitor, which is remote from the airway. Exhaled gases are aspirated through the tubing and the ETCO$_2$ is measured at the monitor.

Figure 5-32. The attachment site for the ETCO$_2$ tubing at the anesthesia machine. Note the water trap below the tubing, it is necessary because condensation is aspirated along with exhaled gases. Without the water trap, the condensation could cause occlusion of the tubing.

How to: Set Up a Side Stream Capnometer

Attach one end of the tubing that comes with the monitor to a port on the endotracheal tube **(Figure 5-31)** and the other end to the appropriate site on the monitor **(Figure 5-32)**. Be sure that a scavenger line is attached to a charcoal canister for scavenging of the waste inhalant gas **(Figure 5-33)**.

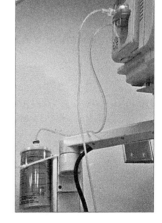

Figure 5-33. The attachment of a small scavenging tube from a sidestream monitor to a charcoal canister, which is necessary because inhalant gas is aspirated from the airway and must be scavenged.

Common CO$_2$ Abnormalities
(Figure 5-34)

• Hypercarbia/hypercapnia: (CO$_2$ too high; > 45 mmHg) is primarily due to hypoventilation, which means any factor that decreases RR or TV. Metabolic changes that cause increased CO$_2$ production, anesthesia equipment malfunction (allowing the patient to rebreath CO_2) and inadequate mechanical ventilation can also contribute to hypercarbia/hypercapnia.

• Hypocarbia/hypocapnia (CO_2 too low; < 35 mmHg) which is primarily due to hyperventilation meaning any factor that increases RR or TV. Excessive mechanical ventilation (anesthetist induced hyperventilation) can also contribute to hypocarbia/hypocapnia.

• These and other abnormalities can be determined by evaluating the capnographic waveform.

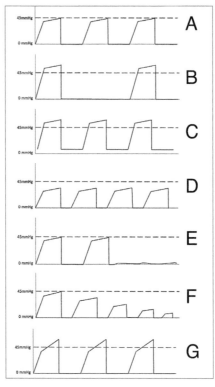

Figure 5-34. Normal/abnormal capnographic waves. The shape of a normal capnographic wave is square or rectangular, the $ETCO_2$ value is in the normal range (35 to 45 mmHg) and the CO_2 value just before inspiration is 0 mmHg (A). In hypoventilation the rate is slow and/or the tidal volume is low so the $ETCO_2$ is above the normal range, but the baseline of the tracing is still zero (B). Retention of CO_2 causes rebreathing of CO_2 by the patient. Low oxygen flow in a non-rebreathing system, exhausted CO_2 absorbent or a faulty expiratory one-way valve are possible causes. The $ETCO_2$ is above normal range and the baseline of the tracing is above zero (C). A below normal $ETCO_2$ can be from hyperventilation or can be artificially low in a small patient with a very fast respiration rate. If artificial, the $ETCO_2$ waves are rounded and more like an oval than a rectangle (D). A sudden loss of the $ETCO_2$ waveform and number can be due to a disconnect of the patient from the breathing system or a sudden loss of blood flow to the lungs (E). Cardiac arrest is the most common cause of loss of blood flow. A rapid, but not sudden, decrease in wave height and $ETCO_2$ number can mean a decreasing blood flow to the lungs. The patient is not in cardiac arrest but is likely headed that way (F). With airway obstruction the wave length looks more like a 'shark fin' than a rectangle (G).

Impact of Abnormalities

Hypercarbia causes respiratory acidosis. Hypocarbia causes respiratory alkalosis. Any change in pH (acidosis or alkalosis) disrupts normal cell function, which is dangerous for the patient and can lead to death.

Trouble Shooting the $ETCO_2$ Monitor

As always check the patient first, check the respiratory rate, tidal volume, mucous membrane color and pulse oximeter values. If available run a blood gas analysis, to compare the $ETCO_2$ and $PaCO_2$.

$ETCO_2$ Values that do not make Sense or are Erratic

Disconnect the monitor from the patient, breathe through the sensor yourself and decide if the resultant values (if any values are displayed) make sense. If the values are normal (35 to 45 mmHg), the patient probably needs ventilation support. If they are abnormal the monitor probably needs servicing. Another way to double check the $ETCO_2$ monitor values is to compare them to a $PaCO_2$ from an arterial blood gas sample.

No $ETCO_2$ Values Displayed

• Check the patient first! If the monitor is not producing any numbers or waveforms, momentarily assume the worst and quickly check the patient since circulatory collapse (cardiac arrest) can cause low/no $ETCO_2$. This occurs because the blood flow is so low that the CO_2 is not moved from the tissue to the lungs where it can be exhaled. Feel for a pulse, listen for a heartbeat, check that the patient is breathing and assess mucous membrane color/CRT.
• Check the equipment:
  • Even if the patient seems okay, the absent reading could still mean something fairly serious so check that the airway is patent (open). Check for occlusions in the ET or breathing system, extubation, esophageal intubation and any other factor that could cause airway compromise.
    • Loss of a patent airway, especially if the airway is occluded can rapidly lead to respiratory arrest followed by cardiac arrest, so act quickly!
  • If the airway is patent, check for a disconnection of the breathing circuit. This is the least serious of the serious conditions but would result in the patient not receiving oxygen or anesthetic gases.
  • Once you are sure that the lack of a CO_2 value isn't due to something life-threatening, check to make sure that:
    • The probe is correctly placed at the end of the endotracheal tube (main stream).
    • The sampling line is connected to both the patient and the monitor (side stream).

- Condensation isn't clouding the sensor (mainstream).
- Condensation has not plugged the sampling line (sidestream).

CRITICAL TIP!
Circulatory collapse (cardiac arrest) can cause low/no $ETCO_2$. This is because blood is not being returned to the lungs so the CO_2 can't be exhaled and measured. If the CO_2 starts to plummet - REACT QUICKLY! In this situation, the change would be rapid.

CRITICAL TIP!
An abrupt loss of the CO_2 value or tracing is one of the best ways to identify disconnection when the patient is covered with drapes and you can't see the breathing system. REACT QUICKLY! In this situation, the change would be immediate.

CRITICAL TIP!
Loss of an $ETCO_2$ value can indicate an endotracheal occlusion. Occluded airways allow pressure to build up in the lungs and this can lead to lung trauma or to cardiovascular collapse. An incomplete occlusion will cause a steep alveolar plateau on the capnograph (See Figure 5-34 *G*) In this situation, the change could be gradual (a slowly growing mucous plug) or abrupt (a kinked ET tube in a patient with hyperflexion of the neck for CSF tap or cervical radiographs, for example).

ADVANCED CRITICAL TIP!
Pulmonary embolism (blood clot or air bubble in the vessels of the lung) can block the flow of blood to the lungs can cause loss of the $ETCO_2$ reading. This is an uncommon cause problem, or uncommonly recognized problem, in veterinary medicine. The change would likely be fairly abrupt.

High $ETCO_2$ Values ('hypercapnia') in a Patient that Appears to be Breathing Normally
- CHECK THE PATIENT FIRST! Insure that the patient is not hypoventilating or hyperthermic (hyperthermia causes increased CO_2 production).
- CHECK THE ANESTHESIA EQUIPMENT! Anesthesia equipment that is malfunctioning may permit rebreathing of exhaled gases. This can occur because of:
  - Exhausted CO_2 absorbent in the rebreathing system.
  - A fresh gas flow that is too low in the nonrebreathing system.
  - Increased dead space due to endotracheal tubes that are too long and stick out beyond the incisors.

Look at the capnograph! Not only can an elevated $ETCO_2$ value diagnose equipment failure, but a capnograph can aid in deciding whether the high $ETCO_2$ is due to increased exhaled CO_2 or retention of CO_2 in the system and rebreathing of CO_2.

In the latter case, the ETCO$_2$ will not return to zero when the patient inhales (See Figure 5-34 *C*).

CRITICAL TIP!
Anesthesia equipment that is malfunctioning may permit rebreathing of exhaled gases, which could lead to dangerously high ETCO$_2$ values!

ADVANCED TIP!
Alveolar collapse (atelectasis) can cause low/no ETCO$_2$. This is because alveolar collapse causes ventilation/perfusion mismatch, which means that some alveoli are ventilated and some are perfused (receive a blood supply) but there may be alveoli that are not both ventilated and perfused. These alveoli do not participate in gas exchange. This may cause low ETCO$_2$ because not all of the blood reaching the lungs arrives at ventilated alveoli and the CO$_2$ is not exhaled for the monitor to measure. In this case, the CO$_2$ in an arterial blood gas would be high.

Low ETCO$_2$ Readings (hypocapnia) when the Patient appears to be Breathing Normally
- Check the patient first! Insure that the patient is not hyperventilating.

- Check the Anesthesia Equipment.
  - A leak (or 'entrainment') of room air into the breathing system will dilute the CO$_2$ and cause artificially low CO$_2$ values. Make sure that there are no leaks anywhere in the system (for example, around the ET tube cuff), holes in any of the breathing system hoses or leaks at any of the connections).
  - ETCO$_2$ monitors do not work efficiently in small patients because of very small tidal volumes and/or very fast respiratory rates. In these instances, the CO$_2$ will not reach a plateau and the machine will underestimate the CO$_2$ concentration.
  - Check the make sure that the probe is correctly placed at the end of the endotracheal tube (main stream) or that the sampling line is connected to both the patient and the monitor (side stream). For main stream, make sure that condensation is not clouding the sensor. For side stream, make sure that condensation has not plugged the sampling line. Also see characteristic capnograph tracings in Figure 5-34 *E* and *F*.

Pulse Oximeter (SpO$_2$)
This is a noninvasive measurement of the percentage of hemoglobin (the oxygen-carrying component of red blood cells) saturated with oxygen in arterial blood. The SpO$_2$ will eventually indicate hypoventilation, but ETCO$_2$ will more quickly indicate hypoventilation, especially in patients breathing supplemental oxygen, like most anesthetized patients. Patients breathing room air (which is 21% oxygen) will desaturate relatively quickly, making the pulse oximeter more useful for identifying hypoventilation. Even though the monitor has this limitation, SpO$_2$ is useful, easy and inexpensive. It should be monitored in every anesthetized patient **(Figure 5-35)**.

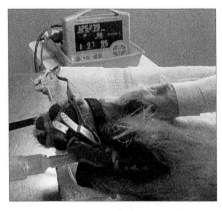

Figure 5-35. Pulse oximeter (SpO$_2$): This is a noninvasive way to measure the percentage of hemoglobin saturated with oxygen in arterial blood. The oxygen-hemoglobin saturation is 97% in this photo.

IMPORTANT POINT
Oxygen is not as good as CO$_2$ as a marker of adequate ventilation, therefore the pulse oximeter is actually a monitor of oxygenation, not ventilation.

TIP
Keep the pulse oximeter in place when taking the patient off of supplemental oxygen and/or when extubating any patient with airway dysfunction. The patient will desaturate if it is not yet ready to be on room air without supplemental oxygen and you can quickly administer oxygen before it develops a respiratory crisis.

Advantages of Pulse Oximetry
EASY to use and inexpensive. Most SPO$_2$ monitors provide a graph ('plethograph' or 'plethogram'). The presence of a waveform on the monitor can be used to count the pulse and the changing amplitude of the waveform can be used to evaluate pulse quality.

IMPORTANT ADVANTAGE OF PULSE OXIMETRY
SpO$_2$ provides some information on both oxygenation and circulation. The patient must be ventilating adequately to bring oxygen into the lungs and the circulation to the lungs must be adequate to pick up the oxygen. Circulation to the probe site must also be adequate or the probe will be unable to detect a pulse.

Disadvantages of Pulse Oximetry
• Can give a false sense of security regarding the adequacy of ventilation in patients breathing 100% oxygen. This is due to the shape of the oxygen-hemoglobin dissociation curve (Figure 5-36). Patients on 100% oxygen can be normally saturated but still not be breathing adequately.
• Can give a false sense of security regarding tissue oxygen delivery in anemic patients. Tissue oxygen delivery is highly dependent on the AMOUNT of hemoglobin (which is dependent on the volume of blood) available to bind to oxygen and

carry that oxygen to the tissues. If the patient is anemic (low blood volume = low hemoglobin concentration), the pulse oximeter will likely read adequate saturation if the patient is on supplemental oxygen, but this does not mean that there is enough saturated hemoglobin to supply oxygen to all of the tissues.

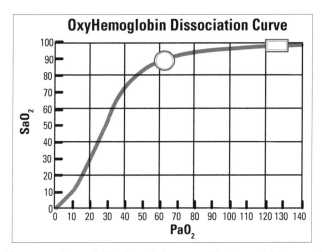

Figure 5-36. The oxygen-hemoglobin dissociation curve. The hemoglobin saturation with oxygen which is designated as SpO_2 (the saturation as measured by the pulse oximeter) or SaO_2 (the saturation as measured by arterial blood gas analysis) cannot be greater than 100% (the numbers on the vertical axis. However, the amount of oxygen in the blood (the numbers on the horizontal axis), which is indicated by PaO_2 and is only available by arterial blood gas analysis, can continue to increase until it reaches about 500 mmHg (normal PaO_2 on room air is 150 mmHg). When the PaO_2 is very high, the SpO_2 and SaO_2 will stay high for a fairly long time (indicated by the values to the right of the rectangle), even if the patient is not breathing. Eventually, the oxygen in the lungs will start to decrease and will cause a decrease in the SpO_2 and SaO_2 (indicated by the circle), but the $ETCO_2$ monitor would have already indicated hypoventilation and high $ETCO_2$. This is why we say that pulse oximetry is not a sensitive measure of ventilation in patients breathing 100% oxygen but is much more sensitive in patients breathing room air. The pulse oximeter is technically called a monitor of 'oxygenation' rather than of ventilation.

CRITICAL POINT!
Pulse oximetry can give a false sense of security regarding the adequacy of ventilation in patients breathing 100% oxygen.

CRITICAL POINT!
Be VERY critical of low saturation in anemic patients. If the saturation drops, start means to increase saturation IMMEDIATELY by breathing for the patient and supplementing with oxygen if not already on oxygen. Because there are fewer molecules of hemoglobin in the blood in anemic patients, it is critically important that all of the molecules are fully saturated with oxygen to increase the likelihood of oxygen delivery to the tissues.

How to: Measure SpO$_2$

The probe should be placed on tissue that is hairless, non-pigmented and fairly thin. The most common site is the tongue but the lips are also very useful. Other sites include the vulva, prepuce and any thin skin like toe webs or the flank. The ear is often too thin, but still worth a try! **(Figure 5-37)**

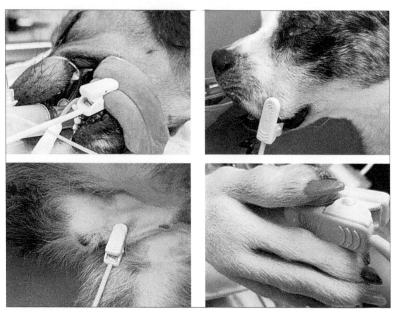

Figure 5-37. Sites for placement of the pulse oximeter probe. In a clockwise direction starting from the upper left hand corner: The tongue usually works the best but if the tongue is not accessible or is extremely cold and vasoconstricted, other sites to try include the lips, toe webs and prepuce. The vulva and fold of the flank (not shown) are also options.

Normal SpO$_2$ Values

The SpO$_2$ range on 100% oxygen should be 95% to 100%. Patients breathing room air should be able to maintain > 90%.

Common SpO$_2$ Abnormalities

A decrease in oxygen saturation (SpO$_2$ < 90%) may occur.

Impact of SpO$_2$ Abnormalities

A decrease in oxygen saturation = decreased oxygen delivery to the tissues. Since oxygen is the fuel that the organs need to function normally, decreased oxygen delivery can lead to a multitude of adverse effects including renal/or hepatic dysfunction, arrhythmias, cerebral dysfunction and death.

Trouble Shooting the Pulse Oximeter

As always, check the patient first. Check the mucous membrane color, respiratory rate, tidal volume, and pulse. If available run a blood gas analysis on an arterial sample and look at the PaO_2 value. THEN check the machine.

SpO_2 Values that do not make Sense or are Erratic

Do not forget that the pulse oximeter probe will need to be replaced periodically! It might be that the probe is faulty. Take it off the patient and put it on your own finger to see if it works. If it works place the SpO_2 probe on a different site on the patient.

No SPO_2 Value or Waveform

• CHECK THE PATIENT! Quickly put your finger on the pulse and check the mucous membrane color and CRT.
• CHECK THE MACHINE! Make sure that:
  • The probe has not become disconnected.
  • The machine is turned on and plugged in.
  • The probe is firmly attached to the patient in a thin, non-pigmented area, preferably one with no hair. A gauze sponge can be placed between the skin and the probe to increase the chance of getting the unit to work, but this is inconsistent.
• If everything else is alright, decide if the patient could be vasoconstricted since the smaller vessel size (most commonly due to hypothermia or administration of vasoconstricting drugs like the alpha-2 agonists) makes it more difficult for the probe to detect a pulse. For hypothermia, warm the patient. For vasoconstriction from alpha-2 agonists, wait for the drug effects to dissipate.

TIP

Don't forget that the pulse oximeter probe WILL NEED to be replaced periodically! It might be that the probe is faulty. Take it off the patient and put it on your own finger to see if it works.

Desaturation (SpO_2 < 90%) in a Patient that Appears to be Breathing Normally

• First, check the patients' pulse/heart rate. If the pulse rate the SpO_2 monitor is providing does not match the patients' actual pulse, the reading is most likely inaccurate. Check the mucous membrane color. A blue color indicates desaturation, but remember that this is a very late sign of desaturation and potentially indicates a very dangerous situation. If the patient does appear to be desaturating, trouble shoot using the information in the previous section on hypoxemia.
• Check the machine!
  • Make sure that the probe is firmly attached to the patient in a thin, non-pigmented area of skin, preferably one with no hair. Make sure that the patient is not hypothermic or experiencing alpha-2 agonist-mediated vasoconstriction.
  • Localized hypoperfusion may be caused by the probe constricting the area where it is placed and will cause a falsely low oxygen reading. Move the probe. This is more likely if the probe has been in one place for an extended period of time

(longer than 60 minutes - or even as short as 30 minutes on really thin skin) since the probe can cause compression of the arteries. This is also common when the tongue is pulled too far out of the mouth and blood flow is occluded by the jaws.
• Check the quality of the pulsatile signal (the size of the pulse wave or the number of 'bars' if the unit does not give a pulse wave), if low or erratic, the reading may be an artifact.

> **TIP**
> Check the patients' pulse/heart rate. If the pulse rate the monitor is providing does not match the patients' actual pulse, the reading is most likely inaccurate.

Arterial Blood Gas Analysis

This is the gold standard for monitoring respiratory function. Arterial oxygen content (PaO_2), saturation (SaO_2), carbon dioxide content ($PaCO_2$) and pH can be measured using arterial blood gas analysis.

Advantages of Blood Gas Analysis

Arterial blood gas analysis is very accurate and precise for diagnosing respiratory function/dysfunction.

Disadvantages of Blood Gas Analysis

Arterial blood gas monitoring requires puncture of an artery and/or insertion of an arterial catheter, both of which can be difficult, especially in small patients. It also requires a special blood gas analyzer, as these are not standard parameters on most blood/serum analyzers.

How to: Collect Arterial Blood for Blood Gas Analysis

See Chapter 8.

Normal Blood Gas Values:

(See table of normal values in Chapter 11).

Common Abnormalities in Blood Gas Analysis

Hypoxemia (low PaO_2 and/or low SaO_2), hypercarbia (high $PaCO_2$) or hypocarbia (low $PaCO_2$) may occur.

Impact of Blood Gas Abnormalities

Hypoxemia may cause decreased oxygen delivery to the tissues, hypercarbia may cause respiratory acidosis and hypocarbia may cause respiratory alkalosis. The two latter conditions cause abnormal pH. All of these conditions can alter many body functions and can lead to death.

Summary

Anesthesia-induced changes in the respiratory system can cause major complications, including death. The best way to avoid complications is to identify deleterious trends by monitoring the patient. Respiratory monitoring should include simple techniques like assessment of respiratory rate, tidal volume and mucous membrane color, and include more advanced techniques like measurement of $ETCO_2$, SpO_2 and maybe even arterial blood gas parameters.

Body Temperature Monitoring
Monitoring Body Temperature

Anesthetic drugs can impact the body's ability to maintain its own temperature by direct impact on the thermoregulatory center in the central nervous system and by causing physical/physiologic changes like vasodilation, which increases the rate of heat loss from the body. In addition, activities that occur during anesthesia (e.g., placing the animal on a cold table, scrubbing the surgical site with excessive amounts of liquid and getting the patient all wet) will add to the drop in body temperature. Shivering is impaired during anesthesia so the body can't respond to falling body temperatures. It is critical that body temperature be monitored and maintained as close to normal as possible **(Table 5-5)**.

Table 5-5
Average Normal Values For Body Temperature

Species	Temperature	
	Degrees Celsius	**Degrees Fahrenheit**
Dog/Cat	38.1 to 39.2 2 (up to 39.4 if nervous)	100.5 to 102.5 (up to 103 if nervous)
Horse	37.0 to 38.3	99.0 to 101.0
Cow	37.0 to 39.3	98.0 to 102.8

Common Abnormalities
Hypothermia

Develops rapidly in patients under anesthesia for many reasons.
• General anesthesia causes direct suppression of the thermoregulatory activity of the hypothalamus.
• Anesthesia-induced vasodilation causes a redistribution of warm blood from the body's core to the skin where heat is released.
• Evaporation of surgical scrub solutions from the body surface, equilibration of core body temperature with ambient temperature through open body cavities, delivery of cold anesthetic gases to the large surface area of the alveoli and a lack of muscle movement also contribute to hypothermia during general anesthesia.

Impact of Hypothermia
- Hypothermia is the main cause of prolonged recoveries from anesthesia. Since recovery is one of the most dangerous periods of anesthesia, the more time spent in recovery, the more likely it is that the patient will have an adverse event.
- Hypothermia causes a variety of complications including, clotting dysfunction, immunosuppression, delayed wound healing, an increased risk of infection, tissue hypoxia, acidosis, abnormal electrical conduction in the heart and myocardial ischemia.
- Hypothermia also causes cerebral effects that decrease the patient's anesthetic needs. Unfortunately, the decreases in anesthetic need are not always recognized and the delivery of anesthesia is rarely changed, resulting in an overdose of anesthetic agents.
- Although shivering in recovery may increase the body temperature, the intensive muscle movements associated with shivering increases oxygen consumption by as much as 200%.
- Hypothermia and shivering contribute to discomfort of the patient.

CRITICAL POINT!
Hypothermia is not benign. It causes a variety of complications including, clotting dysfunction, an increased risk of infection, tissue hypoxia and acidosis, abnormal electrical conduction in the heart and myocardial ischemia. Hypothermia also causes cerebral effects that decrease the patient's anesthetic needs.

Hyperthermia
Causes:
- Metabolic disorders (for example, malignant hyperthermia, which is rare).
- Response to drugs like ketamine and mu agonist opioids [e.g., hydromorphone], especially in cats,
- Over use of patient warming devices.

Impact of Hyperthermia
An elevated body temperature can be life threatening! Hyperthermia can cause abnormalities of numerous organ systems, including seizures, abnormal blood clotting and organ dysfunction or failure.

How to: Monitor: Body Temperature
Some monitors have esophageal temperature probes. These are ideal because they can be inserted and left in place for the entire procedure so that trends in body temperature can be continually assessed. Rectal probes that can be left in place are also useful. Rectal digital thermometers that can be used intermittently are acceptable, as long as the body temperature is checked frequently.

Miscellaneous Monitoring Considerations

This chapter does not provide an exhaustive coverage of monitoring techniques that can be utilized. Patients with specific diseases or complications may require specific monitoring, that might include PCV/TP in anemic or hemorrhaging patients, blood glucose in diabetic patients, electrolytes in patients with a wide variety of diseases and urine output in patients with renal failure.

Reference

Brodbelt D. Perioperative mortality in small animal anesthesia: Vet J. 2009; 182: 152-161

Chapter 6
Support of the
Anesthetized Patient

Shona Meyer, BS, LVT, VTS (Anesthesia/Analgesia)

with contributions from

Mary Albi, LVT

Janel Holden, LVT, VTS (Anesthesia/Analgesia)

Nicole Valdez, LVT, VTS (Anesthesia/Analgesia)

Introduction

The most effective way to deal with anesthetic complications and emergencies is to prevent them! The anesthetist should 1) prepare and/or stabilize the patient, 2) select the appropriate anesthetic/analgesic drugs and the proper dosages of the drugs, 3) prepare the anesthetic equipment, 4) monitor the physiologic systems and 5) provide pre-, post- and intra-operative support of the patient. These steps will make the anesthetic episode safer and will decrease the likelihood of anesthetic complications. Most anesthetic complications occur because steps weren't taken to appropriately prepare, monitor and/or support the patient. Basic support that every patient should receive with the goal of preventing complications will be covered in this chapter. More advanced support for complications (e.g., hypoventilation, hypotension) and emergencies (e.g., apnea, cardiac arrest.) are covered in Chapter 10.

Systemic Impact of Anesthesia

Anesthesia can cause adverse effects in ALL organ systems but adverse effects in the CNS (central nervous system), cardiovascular, and respiratory systems can become acutely life-threatening, especially if depression is profound (e.g., anesthetic overdose) or if the patient is debilitated (e.g., patients with concurrent disease). Thus, we focus our monitoring and support on these three organ systems. Anesthesia-induced changes that may occur in other organ systems (e.g., slowing of hepatic metabolism and decreased renal function) are not generally acutely life-threatening, but they can manifest as complications days to weeks postoperatively. However, supporting the CNS, cardiovascular, and respiratory systems by ensuring appropriate anesthetic depth, blood pressure and blood oxygen content provides support for the other organ systems by promoting adequate oxygen delivery to those systems. Basic support for all patients includes attention to anesthetic depth, provision of analgesia, support of normal respiratory, cardiovascular and thermoregulatory function, and attention to basic husbandry.

Support of the CNS: Attention to Anesthetic Depth and Provision of Analgesia

Anesthetic drugs must cause depression of the CNS in order to produce unconsciousness. The patient must be closely monitored to ensure that excessive anesthetic depth does not occur. Excessive anesthetic depth will cause adverse changes in all of the other organ systems (e.g., hypoventilation, hypotension) and this can create a very dangerous situation, predisposing the patient to anesthesia-related morbidity, or even mortality. Anesthetic drugs, including inhalant drugs, must be dosed 'to effect', meaning administration of the right dose to keep the patient asleep without causing excessive anesthetic depth.

The anesthetist should pay particular attention to administration of the inhalant anesthetics since these drugs can rapidly cause an excessive depth of anesthesia. Normal vaporizer settings during maintenance in healthy patients with appropriate analgesia should be around 1 to 2% for isoflurane and 3 to 4% for sevoflurane. Patients with profound analgesia and/or patients that are old or sick, may need vaporizer settings lower than these guidelines. Always TITRATE THE DOSE TO THE PATIENT'S NEEDS! CHECK the patient and DO NOT BE AFRAID to turn the vaporizer down! If you are nervous, grab a few milliliters of propofol or any other induction drug so that you can rapidly return the patient to an appropriate depth of anesthesia if it gets too light. And remember, patients that have adequate analgesia can be maintained at a lighter plane of anesthesia with less likelihood that they will wake up unexpectedly.

IMPORTANT POINT

One of the most important tips is to administer analgesics whenever possible rather than simply increasing the anesthetic depth when the patient responds to a painful procedure. Increasing the anesthetic depth causes depression of all the organ systems whereas treating pain treats the real problem (pain) without impacting the entire body. This response is physiologically more appropriate when pain is the problem and medically more appropriate since excessive anesthetic depth is avoided. Thus, analgesia administered to a painful patient is not only the ethically, but also the medically, 'right thing to do'. Intraoperative analgesic options (see Chapter 7) include boluses of opioids or alpha-2 agonists, constant rate infusions and local/regional anesthetic blockade.

Myth

Analgesia is not necessary while the patient is under general anesthesia.

Truth

In fact, analgesia in anesthetized patients is extremely important for both improving the safety of anesthesia (because the patient can be maintained at a lower concentration of inhalant anesthetic) and decreasing the degree of postoperative pain (the more aggressive we are at treating intraoperative pain, the more comfortable the patient will be postoperatively). Aggressive treatment of acute pain may also lead to a decreased incidence of chronic pain.

Support of the Cardiovascular System: Blood Pressure Support

The cardiovascular 'system' includes not only the heart but also the blood vessels and the blood/plasma. Anesthesia can negatively impact this system in a variety of ways. For instance, many anesthetic drugs (especially the inhalant anesthetics) can cause abnormal heart rate, impaired cardiac contractility and/or vasodilation, all of which can cause decreased blood pressure with a subsequent decrease in oxygen delivery to the tissues. These adverse effects are magnified in patients with cardiovascular disease and diseases that cause a negative cardiovascular impact (e.g., thyroid disease, shock). Support of the cardiovascular system includes maintenance of adequate blood pressure, normal heart rate and appropriate circulating fluid volume. For normal heart rate and blood pressure values see Chapter 5.

Maintenance of normal blood pressure, which is crucial for oxygen delivery to the tissues, is a critical goal in the anesthetized patient. Blood pressure is determined by the heart rate, myocardial (heart muscle) contractility, circulating fluid volume and blood vessel tone. Thus, we need to consider, and may need to treat, any or all of these components in support of normal blood pressure. Basic support of blood pressure, including maintenance of normal heart rate and volume expansion with intravenous (IV) fluids, is described here. Correction of abnormal blood pressure, including administration of positive inotropic drugs (drugs that increase myocardial contractile strength) and vasopressors (drugs that cause blood vessels to contract) are described in Chapter 10. It is important to realize that some patients will require these drugs as part of normal blood pressure support, especially patients that are geriatric or sick so we suggest that you read Chapter 10 PRIOR to anesthetizing any patient.

IMPORTANT TIP

Positive inotropic drugs and vasopressors can also be used to PREVENT hypotension as part of normal blood pressure support. If you think that a patient might have decreased myocardial contractility (e.g., some geriatric patients or patients with cardiac disease) or that a patient might have excessive vasodilation (e.g., patients in shock), use the drugs described in Chapter 10 as part of prevention and support - don't wait until the blood pressure drops! Start administering the drugs when you start administering the anesthetic drugs since the anesthetic drugs, especially the inhalants, are very likely to add to the hypotension.

Blood Pressure Support: Heart Rate

Heart rate should be supported in order to support blood pressure. Both excessively slow heart rates (bradycardia) and excessively fast heart rates (tachycardia) can cause decreased cardiac output (amount of blood pumped by the heart with each beat) which can cause hypotension. If blood pressure is impacted, the abnormal heart rate should be treated. Basic support information is presented here and more detailed information on causes and treatment of bradycardia and tachycardia is presented in Chapter 10.

Bradycardia

Bradycardia can cause hypotension secondary to decreased cardiac output. Cardiac output = heart rate x stroke volume (the amount of blood ejected by each 'stroke' or beat of the heart). Increased vagal tone from stimulation of the vagus nerve is by far the most common cause of bradycardia. Increased vagal tone can be induced by a variety of perioperative factors **(Table 6-1)**, including some anesthetic drugs (particularly the opioids and alpha-2 agonists), some surgical procedures and some breed predispositions. Anticholinergic drugs (either atropine or glycopyrrolate; **Table 6-2**) should be administered to treat or to prevent the vagally-mediated bradycardia **if the bradycardia causes hypotension**, but are not generally necessary if the blood pressure is normal.

Table 6-1
Common Perioperative Causes of Increased Vagal Tone and Bradycardia

FACTOR INCREASING VAGAL TONE	COMMENTS
Drugs	
Opioids	Opioids cause a direct decrease in heart rate and anticholinergic treatment may be necessary if this leads to hypotension.
Alpha-2 agonists	Alpha-2 agonists cause an INDIRECT decrease in heart rate due to HYPER-TENSION and anticholinergics should NOT be administered if the blood pressure is normal.
Surgeries	
Gastro-intestinal	Traction on the intestine can increase vagal tone.
Ocular	Pressure on the eye can increase vagal tone.
Bladder	Traction on the bladder and pressure from inside the bladder (i.e., full bladder) can increase vagal tone.
Larynx/airway	The vagus nerve has many branches in these areas and stimulation can cause increased vagal tone.
Head/Neck	The vagus nerve may be directly stimulated by surgery in this area.
Patients	
Very athletic dogs	Athletic dogs (racing dogs, some hounds, etc.) that are very fit (actually athletically fit patients of any species) are more likely to have high vagal tone.
Brachycephalic dogs and cats	Brachycephalic patients may have increased vagal tone or may be more likely to have vagal stimulation because they can be hard to intubate and stimulation of the larynx can stimulate the vagus nerve causing bradycardia.

Table 6-2
Anticholinergic Drug Information

Drug	Dosage for Dogs & Cats (mg/kg)	Route of Injection	Time to Onset of Action (minutes)	Duration of Action (hours)
Atropine	0.02-0.04	IV,IM,SQ	1-2 IV 5-15 IM	1-1.5 (up to 3)
Glycopyrrolate	0.005-0.02	IV,IM,SQ	3-4 IV 5-15 IM	2-4 (up to 6)

Anticholinergic Drugs
Nicole Valdez LVT, VTS (Anesthesia/Analgesia)

Specific Drugs: Atropine, Glycopyrrolate
Mechanism of Action
Anticholinergics block acetylcholine (which is a neurotransmitter and gives the class its name 'anticholinergics') at a variety of sites throughout the body, including parasympathetic sites on the vagus nerve.
FDA Approval
Glycopyrrolate is approved in both dogs and cats.
Species
Used for all species, but slowing of GI motility may cause colic in horses and GI complications in ruminants. The clinical impact of this effect in small animals is minimal to nonexistent.
Routes of Administration
IV, IM and SQ.
Dose
Atropine 0.02 to 0.04 mg/kg; glycopyrrolate 0.005 to 0.02 mg/kg.
Onset of Action
• Atropine 1-2 minutes IV, 5 to 10 minutes IM;
• Glycopyrrolate 3-4 minutes IV, 5-15 minutes IM. Glycopyrrolate generally takes slightly longer than atropine but onset for both drugs is slowed by poor muscle blood flow secondary to hypotension and by patient hypothermia.
• Onset may take longer when administered SQ and this route is not recommended to TREAT bradycardia but can be used when attempting to PREVENT bradycardia.
Duration of Action
Atropine 60 to 90 minutes (up to 3 hours); glycopyrrolate 2 to 4 hours (up to 6 hours).
Effects
Increased heart rate, increased viscosity (thickness) of saliva and respiratory secretions.
Side/Adverse Effects
Tachycardia; can cause or exacerbate arrhythmias; increases cardiac work and oxygen consumption; may cause a decrease in volume of respiratory, GI and oral/

nasal secretions; slowing of GI motility; decreases bladder and ureter contractions; can cause dysphoria or sedation (atropine only since only atropine crosses the blood brain barrier).

Clinical Use

• Anticholinergics are used to prevent or treat vagally-mediated bradycardia (meaning bradycardia due to vagus nerve stimulation). There are other causes of bradycardia [e.g., severe hypothermia] that are not vagally mediated and would not be affected by this class of drugs.

• Both are also used to treat some bradycardic arrhythmias like atrio-ventricular (AV) block (see ECG in Chapter 10) and atropine is used to eliminate vagal tone when treating cardiac arrest.

• Anticholinergics have been used to 'dry up' salivary secretions to make intubation easier and decrease the incidence of saliva occluding the airway or endotracheal tube. However, anticholinergics decrease the water content of saliva, causing it to become thicker. This can actually increase the potential for airway obstruction. Excessive salivation is more likely to occur with ketamine than with other anesthetic drugs.

Precautions

Check the heart rate first! Do not administer anticholinergics if the heart rate is already high for that patient.

Absolute Contraindications

Do not use anticholinergics for patients with tachyarrhythmias (like ventricular premature contractions)!

CRITICAL POINT!

Although not an absolute contraindication, anticholinergics should NOT be administered to patients with most types of heart disease unless absolutely necessary. The increase in heart rate and increased oxygen demand can exacerbate the disease and even cause heart failure.

Tips for Clinical Use

Anticholinergics are best used to TREAT bradycardia when it occurs. Routine premedication with atropine or glycopyrrolate to PREVENT bradycardia is used by some veterinarians and this is acceptable as long as not ALL patients are premedicated with these drugs. Patients that are premedicated with an alpha-2 agonist, those that have an abnormally high heart rate prior to premedication and those that have cardiovascular disease should NOT receive an anticholinergic. A better approach is to withhold the anticholinergic and measure blood pressure. The anticholinergic can always be administered if the heart rate decreases and causes a decrease in blood pressure.

IMPORTANT REMINDER
If the heart rate is low but **BLOOD PRESSURE IS NORMAL OR HIGH**, do not 'treat' the heart rate - it doesn't need treatment! The blood pressure is more important than the heart rate for oxygen delivery to the tissues. Bradycardia with high blood pressure is a very common scenario following the administration of alpha-2 agonists - the heart rate drops but the blood pressure is HIGH because of vasoconstriction caused by the alpha-2 agonist. There is no need to administer an anticholinergic in this situation.

TIP FOR CLINICAL USE
It is best to anticipate the need for anticholinergics and to administer them IM. When administered IV, profound tachycardia can occur. Tachycardia increases the work of the myocardium (heart muscle), which increases the oxygen use of the muscle. Failure to meet the new oxygen demand can cause ischemia (lack of oxygen to the tissue) which can cause arrhythmias and/or myocardial damage.

SPECIAL SITUATION TIP FOR CLINICAL USE
Neonates may need anticholinergics because they have a decreased amount of contractile tissue in the myocardium (when compared to adults) and are 'heart rate dependent' for maintenance of adequate blood pressure.

Drug Specific Comments
- Heart rate increase following administration of glycopyrrolate is not as profound as the increase following atropine so glycopyrrolate is often preferred since the higher the heart rate, the greater the increase in cardiac muscle work.
- When administered IV, especially at low dosages, atropine often causes a paradoxical bradycardia and AV block prior to an increase in heart rate. Glycopyrrolate is much less likely to cause this effect.
- Atropine should be administered if the patient has experienced a cardiac arrest because the drug crosses the blood-brain barrier (glycopyrrolate does not cross), thereby treating both central (in the brain) and peripheral (at the heart) causes of bradycardia that might have led to the arrest.
- Because it crosses the blood-brain barrier, atropine can cause central effects and both sedation and agitation have been reported. Although not proven, these atropine-mediated effects may contribute to dysphoria in recovery.
- Atropine also crosses the placental barrier, which may be useful if Stage II labor ('active' labor) has been prolonged and fetal distress is expected, but may not be good if fetuses are normal and don't need an increased heart rate.
- Glycopyrrolate is a more potent antisialogogue, which means that it is better at decreasing the volume of saliva produced. Remember, this is caused by making the saliva thicker.
- Atropine is the least expensive of the two anticholinergics.

Tachycardia

Tachycardia can cause hypotension secondary to decreased cardiac output but it is not the rate that is the problem, it is the stroke volume (remember that cardiac output = heart rate x stroke volume [the amount of blood ejected by each 'stroke' or beat of the heart]). If the heart rate is extremely high, the ventricles of the heart do not have time to fill with blood before the heart contracts so there is less blood ejected with each beat. Tachycardia can be caused by cardiac disease but in anesthetized patients is most likely caused by an underlying problem, like pain, an excessively light plane of anesthesia, hypovolemia, hypoxemia and/or hypercarbia. Pain is a common cause of tachycardia in patients undergoing surgery. If the increase in heart rate occurs during a painful stimulus, the patient should receive analgesic drugs like opioids, local anesthetic drugs, ketamine, etc. Analgesia is covered in Chapter 7. If the patient is indeed too lightly anesthetized and not just responding to pain, administer a low dose of an injectable anesthetic drug or turn up the gas slightly but don't make the patient too deeply anesthetized as this can cause profound adverse effects, as discussed in the first section of this chapter. For all other tachycardia causes/treatment see Chapter 10.

Blood Pressure Support: Circulating Fluid Volume
Mary Albi, LVT

Support of circulating fluid volume through administration of IV fluids will ensure proper hydration of the patient, replace fluid losses and provide blood pressure support. The fluids that are administered can include crystalloids, colloids, blood and/or plasma.

IMPORTANT POINT
Intravenous fluid administration will support blood pressure if low circulating volume is the main contributor to hypotension (and it often is), but once volume is corrected, ongoing hypotension should be treated by other means.

Reasons for Fluid Therapy
The main reasons to deliver fluids are to replace fluid losses (like those occurring from dehydration, hypovolemia, hemorrhage, or shock); to restore and maintain adequate circulating volume, which will help to support blood pressure and maintain organ perfusion; and to correct electrolyte & acid-base imbalances. In addition, having a patent IV catheter in a patient is a great safety net in case the patient has complications and needs IV drugs. The most effective and efficient way to maintain a patent catheter is to administer fluids through the catheter.

Routes of Fluid Administration

For rapid response to therapy, fluids should be administered intravenously (IV) or intraosseously (i.e., in the bone marrow - used in patients that are so small that IV access is not possible) in anesthetized patients. Subcutaneous delivery of fluids may be acceptable in patients where IV or IO access is not possible but the fluids should be administered at least one hour before anesthesia so that they can be absorbed into the circulation. This route is more commonly used to treat dehydration in patients NOT scheduled for anesthesia. Not all fluids can be administered subcutaneously because some can cause tissue damage. Other routes that are used in patients not scheduled for anesthesia include orally by mouth or by feeding tube and intraperitoneally (i.e., in the abdomen). The latter option is useful only in very small patients like 'pocket pets'. Fluids should not be administered orally to anesthetized patients because they can't swallow and might breathe fluids into their lungs (or 'aspirate').

Types of Fluids

Along with the choice of routes for fluid delivery, we must also choose the most appropriate type of fluid to use based on the patient health status and the goal of fluid therapy. The main categories of fluids include crystalloids and colloids.

• Crystalloids are fluid solutions that readily cross the capillary membranes and diffuse into the tissues, thus treating both loss of fluids from the vasculature and tissue fluid loss (dehydration). Crystalloids are often called 'replacement' fluids because they are used primarily to replace losses, like fluid lost from dehydration, evaporation from an open body cavity or in the production of urine and sweat. Commonly used crystalloid solutions include lactated Ringer's solution (LRS), Plasma-Lyte and 'normal' or 'physiologic' saline (0.9% sodium chloride [NaCl]).
• Colloids are fluid solutions that contain large molecular weight substances (proteins or starches) that do not readily cross capillary membranes, thus allowing the molecules to stay primarily in the circulation. Colloids are often called 'perfusion fluids' because they are used primarily to support blood pressure and, thus, perfusion of organs. Commonly used colloids include voluven (VetStarch®), hetastarch & plasma.
• Whole blood can be considered in a fluid therapy discussion since loss of blood = loss of fluid. Loss of whole blood may require a blood transfusion. Transfusions are not covered in this chapter.

Composition, Distribution and Effects of Crystalloids vs Colloids

Before discussing specific crystalloid and colloid solutions, it is important to review a little physiology. The decision to use crystalloids or colloids depends, in part, on our knowledge of where the fluids go once they enter the body and what they do when they get to that location. Remember that the body is primarily water!

(Figure 6-1) In fact, total body water **(TBW; in liters)** is 60 to 70% of the total body weight (in kilograms). This percentage is increased in neonatal/pediatric animals and decreased in geriatric and obese animals. The discussion of TBW and the specific differences in crystalloids and colloids may seem complicated - but it is critical to understand what we are doing to our patients when we administer fluids. Fluids can have both positive and negative effects. We want to maximize the positive and minimize the negative effects.

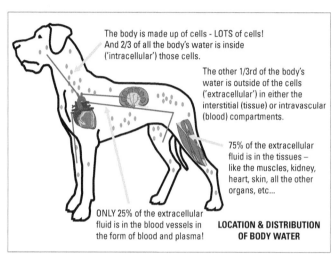

The body is made up of cells - LOTS of cells! And 2/3 of all the body's water is inside ('intracellular') those cells.

The other 1/3rd of the body's water is outside of the cells ('extracellular') in either the interstitial (tissue) or intravascular (blood) compartments.

75% of the extracellular fluid is in the tissues – like the muscles, kidney, heart, skin, all the other organs, etc...

ONLY 25% of the extracellular fluid is in the blood vessels in the form of blood and plasma!

LOCATION & DISTRIBUTION OF BODY WATER

Figure 6-1. Proportion and location of body fluid.

• Total body water **(TBW)** is divided into two main locations: the intracellular fluid **(ICF)** and the extracellular fluid **(ECF)**. Most of the body's water (⅔) is inside the cells (ICF) and only ⅓ is outside the cells (ECF).
• The ECF is further divided into two locations: the interstitial fluid (the fluid in the tissues like muscle, internal organs, skin and bone) and the intravascular fluid (blood and plasma inside the blood vessels). The interstitial fluid is 75% of the ECF and the intravascular fluid (all that blood and plasma) is only 25% of the ECF.

▌IMPORTANT POINT
Fluids are primarily administered to replace losses in the ECF. RARELY would we want fluids to enter the ICF. The cells can control their own water content and that process should not be disrupted - it can lead to cell swelling and death. Thus, fluids that enter the cell (hypotonic fluids) are very rarely used and then only for very specific problems.

Fluid is distributed throughout all of these locations and distribution is determined in part by the type of fluid and in part by the membranes separating the locations (e.g., the cell membrane separates the inside of the cell from the outside, the capillary membrane separates the inside of the blood vessels from the tissues around it). Pure water is freely permeable to all locations and will distribute throughout the body until pressure forces across the membranes are equal (meaning that there is the same amount of water on both sides of the membrane). But medical fluids that are administered to patients are not pure water, they have other components (e.g., electrolytes, large molecules.) that affect which membranes they can cross.

Crystalloids

Crystalloids **(Table 6-3)** are described by their tonicity, electrolyte composition and buffering capability (i.e., ability to change acid/base balance). There are three categories of crystalloids based on tonicity (hypotonic, isotonic and hypertonic). Tonicity is the concentration of solutes in the fluid. Solutes include things like electrolytes (sodium, potassium, calcium and chloride) and glucose. The tonicity of the fluid affects its movement through the body (including movement into and out of cells). Tonicity is often used interchangeably with osmolarity, although the terms are slightly different. Fluids are isotonic if tonicity is within or near the normal tonicity range for plasma (280 to 310 mOsm/L), hypotonic if tonicity is lower than that of plasma, and hypertonic if tonicity is higher than that of plasma.

Crystalloids are also classified by the electrolytes that are in the solution and sodium is generally the most abundant electrolyte, which is also true in plasma. The sodium is combined with chloride plus/minus a variety of other electrolytes that may include potassium, magnesium, and calcium. The most commonly used crystalloids are called 'balanced' electrolyte solutions and they have an electrolyte profile similar to that of plasma. Examples include Plasma-Lyte and LRS. Normal saline (0.9% NaCl) is not a balanced electrolyte solution because it contains only sodium and chloride, and both of these electrolytes are at a much higher concentration in normal saline than in plasma.

Finally, fluids are either alkalinizing (i.e., used to treat an acidotic patient) or acidifying (i.e., used to treat an alkalotic patient). Alkalinizing solutions (LRS and Plasma-Lyte) contain a buffer (a compound that can be turned into bicarbonate) and the buffer is different between solutions. Normal saline (0.9% NaCl) is acidifying because it will cause a dilution of plasma bicarbonate.

The specific composition of the crystalloid will determine which fluid is most useful in patients with various conditions or diseases. The most commonly used fluids in medicine are isotonic, balanced-electrolyte, alkalinizing crystalloids like LRS and Plasma-Lyte.

Isotonic Crystalloids

As stated, the most commonly used fluids in medicine e.g., (LRS, Plasma-Lyte) have a tonicity similar or equal to the tonicity of normal plasma and contain sodium and chloride, and often potassium, in concentrations similar to plasma. Isotonic fluids are used for rehydration, resuscitation, and replacement.

Table 6-3
Composition of Commonly Used Fluids Compared to the Composition of Plasma

Solution	Na⁺	Cl⁻	K⁺	Ca⁺⁺	Mg⁺⁺	Lact	Acet	Gluc	pH	Osm
Plasma	144	107	5	5	1.5				7.5	290
LRS	130	109	4	3	-	28			6.5	273
Plasma-Lyte A	140	98	5	-	1.5		27	23	7.4	294
0.9% NaCl	154	154	-	-	-				5.0	308
7.5% NaCl	1283	1283	-	-	-				5.0-5.7	2567
5% Dextrose	-								4.0	252

The concentrations of sodium (Na⁺), chloride (Cl⁻), calcium (Ca⁺⁺), magnesium (Mg⁺⁺), lactate (Lact), acetate (Acet), and gluconate (Gluc) are presented as mEq/L (milliequivalents per liter). Osmolarity (or tonicity) is presented as mOsmol/L (milliosmoles per liter).

LRS and Plasma-Lyte differ slightly in their electrolyte composition but both are balanced electrolyte solutions. They also differ in the buffer that they contain. LRS contains lactate and Plasma-Lyte contains acetate. Both are effective buffers but lactate must be metabolized by the liver to become a buffer and this may be impaired in patients with liver disease. However, total inability to convert lactate to a buffer would likely only occur with severe liver disease so LRS is an appropriate fluid for most patients. However, if there is concern about hepatic function, Plasma-Lyte can be administered since acetate does not need hepatic transformation. These fluids should be administered to patients with conditions that cause acidemia or acidosis. Most conditions cause acidemia/acidosis and it is encountered more often than alkalemia/alkalosis. Examples include hemorrhage, shock and most gastrointestinal conditions). Sodium chloride (NaCl) is also an isotonic fluid, but does not contain electrolytes other than sodium and chloride nor does it contain a buffer. NaCl causes dilution of plasma bicarbonate, which makes the solution acidifying, Therefore, NaCl is a good choice in patients that are losing acid and becoming alkalotic (e.g., high [near the stomach] gastrointestinal obstruction with vomiting of stomach contents).

A major point to understand about crystalloids is that they move or 'redistribute' rapidly out of the vasculature (within 30 to 60 minutes after administration) and into the tissues, which makes these fluids ideal for treating dehydration but may limit their impact on improvement of hypotension, especially after all fluid losses have been replaced.

Hypertonic Crystalloid Solutions
These solutions generally contain only sodium and chloride at high concentrations (3%, 5%, 7%, and 7.5% NaCl) which means that they can cause an electrolyte imbalance if used excessively. A concentration of 7.5% NaCl is most commonly used in veterinary medicine. All have a tonicity greater than that of plasma which makes them hypertonic.

Hypertonic solutions provide rapid expansion of the intravascular fluid volume and increase the intravascular volume more than the amount of fluid actually administered (i.e., if 1 liter of hypertonic saline is administered IV, the intravascular volume will increase by MORE than 1 liter). This is because hypertonic solutions draw fluid from body tissues and cells into the intravascular space. The increase in circulating fluid volume is usually quite dramatic and almost immediately noticeable, but does have a short duration (1 to 3 hours).

Hypertonic solutions are resuscitation fluids for patients that need a very rapid increase in circulating fluid volume in order to maintain blood pressure and for large animal patients that have a very large fluid compartment that can be difficult to rapidly hydrate with conventional fluid therapy. Hypertonic saline is usually administered as a bolus of 2.5 to 5 ml/kg total dose. Isotonic crystalloids should be administered concurrently with hypertonic saline to replace the fluid that was pulled from the tissues and cells. Most recommendations state that hypertonic saline should not be used if the patient is dehydrated since the tissues and cells are already depleted of fluid and further depletion could cause tissue damage. However, hypertonic saline administration is acceptable in patients that are only mildly dehydrated. Hypertonic saline should only be used if there are no other options in patients that are actively hemorrhaging (bleeding). This is because the rapid increase in fluid volume and blood pressure induced by the hypertonic saline can make the hemorrhage worse.

Hypotonic Crystalloids
These fluids (0.45% NaCl, 5% Dextrose in water) have a tonicity lower than that of plasma, so they provide more water than electrolytes and the free water can move intracellularly, which is generally not desired. These fluids have low sodium, and as such are suggested for use in patients with cardiac disease but the need for this is controversial and hypotonic crystalloids are not currently recommended for anesthetized patients, even those with cardiac disease. These fluids may also be used in some patients for long-term maintenance delivery of fluids. These fluids are rarely used in anesthesia.

Colloids
These are fluid solutions that contain large molecular weight substances (starches in synthetic colloids and proteins in natural colloids) that do not readily cross capillary membranes, thus allowing the molecules to stay primarily in the circulation. This allows a smaller volume of fluid to be administered for support of circulating volume and means that the increase in circulating volume will last longer than it does after the administration of crystalloids. Colloids generally stay in the vasculature for up to 24 hours. Colloids should be used when the patient is hypoproteinemic, hypotensive in spite of adequate crystalloid administration and when the patient has cardiac disease that limits the amount of fluid that the heart can effectively pump. Crystalloids should be administered with colloids since, like hypertonic solutions, colloids 'pull' some fluid from the tissues into the vasculature and this fluid has to be replaced. The patient will need crystalloids to replace fluid 'losses' like urine and evaporation of fluid from the airway (that's where all that fluid comes from that you see in the breathing hoses at the end of the anesthetic procedure).

Synthetic Colloids
These include hetastarch and voluven. Synthetic colloids have an impact on clotting factors and should be used with caution, or not at all, in patients with clotting disorders. Voluven has less of an impact on clotting factors than hetastarch and is the colloid type that we highly recommend. Most voluven products are made for humans but Vetstarch® is a veterinary product and our recommended synthetic colloid. Colloids have been associated with increased risk of renal complications in humans. This appears to be uncommon in dogs and only associated with multiple days of colloid administration. This has not been reported in cats.

Natural Colloids and Blood

Plasma is a natural colloid that is often used to provide clotting factors (synthetic colloids do not contain clotting factors or protein) and to support colloid osmotic pressure. Whole blood or packed red blood cells are used in cases of excessive hemorrhage and anemia (See Chapter 10).

Volume of Fluids to Administer to Anesthetized Patients

Fluids are generally more helpful than harmful but excessive fluid delivery (or 'volume overload') can cause problems like edema, excessive load on the heart and even death. Also fluids can cause specific fluid-related problems, like hypertonic saline can cause hypernatremia (excessive sodium) and colloids can cause allergic reactions. Think of fluids the same way you think of drugs. They are helpful, but CAN CAUSE ADVERSE EFFECTS.

Volume of Crystalloids

Guidelines for the administration of crystalloid fluids have changed radically over the past several years, with a focus on decreasing the volume of fluids administered in order to prevent overhydration and fluid accumulation (edema) in the tissues and organs. Currently the American Animal Hospital Association (AAHA; Davis et al. 2012) recommendations for maintenance fluid rates during anesthesia are < 10 ml/kg/hr for most patients. The recommendation is to start at a calculated volume of fluids and gradually reduce that volume by 25% each hour until the maintenance rate of 3-4 ml/kg/hour for cats or 5 ml/kg/hour for dogs is achieved. To simplify: for most healthy (ASA I-II) anesthetized patients that are not expected to have major blood loss during surgery, isotonic balanced-electrolyte crystalloids should be administered at 10 ml/kg (dogs) or 8 ml/kg (cats) for the first hour of anesthesia and 5 ml/kg (dogs) or 3-4 ml/kg (cats) for subsequent hours of anesthesia. This will provide the patient's basic requirement for fluids and will replace minor fluid losses. The fluid rate for patients that are anesthetized for non-surgical procedures can be the same as those just described or simply 5 ml/kg (dogs) or 3-4 ml/kg (cats) for the entire procedure since the losses in these patients are usually minor (because they aren't hemorrhaging and don't have open body cavities for evaporation of fluids). Patients that are ASA III-V because they have underlying disease that causes hypovolemia, are dehydrated at induction to anesthesia, are hemorrhaging intraoperatively or have major losses through open body cavities should have their needs carefully calculated. Most of these patients will likely require a higher fluid rate. For patients that are presented with severe hypovolemia or shock, fluid rates as high as 1 blood volume per hour have been utilized but this high rate is generally not recommended during anesthesia (but may be necessary for stabilizing the patient prior to anesthesia) because it can lead to fluid overload. A blood volume is roughly 90 ml/kg in the dog and 60 ml/kg in the cat.

Fluid rate for patients with cardiac disease should be tailored to meet, but not exceed, the fluid losses. Fluid rates can be as low as 3-5 ml/kg for the first hour with 2-2.5 ml/kg for subsequent hours. A low volume of colloids may be a better option in these patients.

Boluses of crystalloids can also be used to increase the circulating volume within the vasculature which will in turn increase blood pressure. A 3 to 20 ml/kg (exact volume depends on health of cardiovascular system, degree of dehydration and volume of ongoing losses) crystalloid bolus may be delivered during anesthesia to aid in the treatment of anesthetic induced hypotension. This amount may be repeated once if the patient is hydrated or as needed if the patient is dehydrated or is experiencing major ongoing losses. Once hydration is corrected, continuing to bolus high volumes of IV fluids will not improve low blood pressure so other measures must be instituted (see Chapter 10). However, IV crystalloid fluids should be continued to replace losses, even if other measures are being used to improve low blood pressure.

IMPORTANT POINT
Intravenous fluid administration will support blood pressure if low circulating volume is the main contributor to hypotension (and it often is), but once volume is corrected, ongoing hypotension should be treated by other means (See Chapter 10).

Volume of Colloids
Synthetic colloids may be administered at 5 to 10 ml/kg IV, with a current recommendation of no more than 20 ml/kg/day for hetastarch but up to 50 ml/kg/day for voluven in dogs. The total volume is slightly lower in cats since they have a smaller blood volume (15 ml/kg/day for hetastarch and 30 ml/kg/day for voluven).

IMPORTANT POINT
Although the volume of colloids needed to improve blood pressure is lower than the volume of crystalloids needed to improve blood pressure, the volume can still be dangerous for patients in which volume overload could be detrimental - like patients with heart disease. Use low dosages (e.g., 1 to 3 ml/kg) in these patients!

Specific Fluid Choices based on Individual Patient Needs
Balanced-electrolyte isotonic fluids are the most commonly used fluids in medicine. However, specific patient diseases may dictate specific fluid choices. For instance,

Plasma-Lyte might be better than LRS for patients with hepatic disease and 0.9% NaCl would be better than either Plasma-Lyte or LRS in patients with alkalosis. In addition, many compounds can be added to IV fluids to treat specific conditions. For instance, sodium bicarbonate can be administered to treat metabolic acidosis, glucose can be administered to treat hypoglycemia, calcium can be added to treat hypocalcemia or potassium can be added to treat hypokalemia. See more information on fluid additives in Chapter 8.

How to: Administer Fluids to an Anesthetized Patient:

For administration of fluids to the patient, first determine the type or types of fluids to be administered and the volume to be delivered, then choose the appropriate drip and extension sets. Calculation examples are available in Chapter 8.

> ### CRITICAL TIP!
> It is VERY easy to volume overload small dogs and cats so be VERY CAREFUL with the volume of fluids that are administered to these patients. Ideally, a syringe pump, some type of volume control device (e.g., Buretrol; Figure 6-2) or even fluids drawn up in a syringe and administered intermittently by the anesthetist should be used to administer fluids in very small patients.

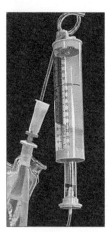

Figure 6-2. The Buretrol device used for volume control when administering fluids to small patients.

Monitoring Fluid Therapy

Any fluid has the potential to cause volume overload. The patient should be closely observed during fluid therapy. Signs of volume overload that need to be monitored during anesthesia are numerous, but are parameters you should be monitoring normally. Abnormalities to watch for include prolonged capillary refill time, blueish mucous membrane color, increased heart rate (sometimes followed by rapid decrease in heart rate), increased respiratory rate, harsh or 'crackly' lung sounds, edema (especially noticeable on the face and paws), low body temperature, low PCV/TP, low BUN, high blood pressure and low SpO$_2$. Changes in any of these may be concerning and should be further investigated.

Support of the Respiratory System: Gas Exchange

The respiratory 'system' includes everything from the nares to the alveoli. Anesthesia can negatively impact this system in a variety of ways. For instance, many anesthetic drugs (especially the inhalant anesthetics) can cause inadequate ventilation through either decreased respiratory rate or tidal volume, with a subsequent decrease in oxygen delivery to the tissues. These adverse effects are magnified in patients with disease that could also impact the respiratory system, which includes patients with brachycephalic airway syndrome, laryngeal paralysis, collapsing trachea, pneumonia, pneumothorax (and any other foreign material in the thorax) or diaphragmatic hernia. Although not truly airway disease, breathing can be impaired by anything obstructing normal movement of the thorax (e.g., fractured ribs, surgeons leaning on the patient or very tight table ties that cross the thorax) or anything affecting diaphragmatic movement (e.g., advanced pregnancy or GI distension from stomach dilation). Don't forget that faulty equipment can also affect normal respiratory function (e.g., endotracheal tube plugged with mucous or kinked, breathing hoses kinked, pop-off valve closed, one-way valves stuck, oxygen flow insufficient or carbon dioxide absorbent exhausted), which is one of the many reasons that thorough knowledge and frequent assessment of your equipment is very important (See Chapter 3)! Support of the respiratory system includes maintenance of normal oxygenation and adequate respiratory rate and tidal volume to insure normal values of carbon dioxide (see Chapter 5).

Oxygen and carbon dioxide are gases and 'gas exchange', which is the inhalation of oxygen coupled with the exhalation of carbon dioxide, is controlled by both respiratory rate and tidal volume (the volume of air that moves into/out of the lungs with each breath). Adequate oxygen delivery to the cells and carbon dioxide elimination from the body are crucial for normal body function.

Most sedative and anesthetic drugs cause some degree of respiratory depression (decreased respiratory rate, decreased tidal volume, or both). Respiratory depression can lead to low oxygen levels in the blood (hypoxemia) and decreased oxygen delivery to the cells (hypoxia). Oxygen is the fuel needed by all cells in the body so if oxygen is low, cells cannot function normally. If hypoxemia affects a large number of cells, organ dysfunction may occur. The organs most commonly affected by hypoxemia include the kidneys, myocardium, brain and liver, but any organ can be impacted.

Respiratory depression can also lead to high carbon dioxide levels in the blood (hypercarbia) and failure to eliminate carbon dioxide from the cells. Carbon dioxide (CO_2) is a normal product of cell metabolism, but failure to eliminate CO_2 from the cells after it is produced can lead to respiratory acidosis (i.e., low pH), which can cause cell dysfunction. All cells/organs in the body can be negatively impacted by abnormal pH.

Oxygenation

The effects of anesthesia-induced respiratory depression on oxygenation can often be overcome by increasing the percent of oxygen that the patient inhales. This is easy when patients are anesthetized with inhalant anesthetics because the inhalants are delivered in oxygen. But don't forget that patients anesthetized with injectable anesthetics - and even many patients that are just deeply sedated - may experience respiratory depression and would benefit from supplemental oxygen.

▌IMPORTANT POINT

All anesthetized patients (regardless of whether it is injectable or inhalant anesthesia) should receive supplemental inhaled oxygen.

▌IMPORTANT TIP

If you are unsure whether or not the patient needs oxygen, check the SpO$_2$ with the pulse oximeter. If it is < 90%, provide oxygen.

Delivering Supplemental Oxygen

There are several ways to supplement, or increase, the percent of inhaled oxygen. The patient can be intubated and the oxygen delivered through the endotracheal (ET) tube, or oxygen can be delivered through a mask placed over the patient's muzzle **(Figure 6-3)** or delivered through the breathing hose from the anesthesia machine by placing the end of the hoses near the patient's nostrils (called 'blow by' oxygen; **Figure 6-4**). "Blow by" oxygen allows supplementation of oxygen but not delivery of 100% oxygen. Remember that room air contains only 21% oxygen, and 'blow by' oxygen may increase the inspired percentage to about 30% - which is often just enough to improve the SpO$_2$. HOWEVER, if the patient is really ventilating poorly, consider intubating the patient and delivering 100% oxygen, and consider breathing for the patient (if necessary).

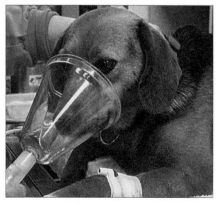

Figure 6-3. Oxygen delivery using a face mask.

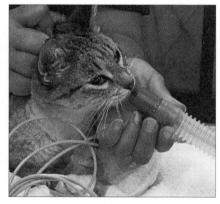

Figure 6-4. Oxygen delivery using the 'blow by' method.

Preoxygenation

Some patients are prone to rapid desaturation (i.e., SpO_2 of < 90%) at induction.
Desaturation can be prevented by delivering oxygen by face mask before the
patient is even anesthetized (called 'preoxygenation'). The patient can be preoxygenated while the sedatives are taking effect. The IV catheter can be placed during
this time. Oxygen can be delivered by placing a mask over the patient's nose and
mouth and using 1 to 2 liters of oxygen flow, or by using 'blow by' oxygen. Delivery
of 100% oxygen for as little as 3 minutes prevents desaturation (SpO_2 of < 90%) for
up to 5 minutes in hypoventilating patients (McNally et al. 2009).

Post-operative Oxygenation

Also remember that inhalant anesthetics are potent respiratory depressants and
their effects will linger into recovery, especially if the patient is deeply anesthetized. Just because the vaporizer is turned off doesn't mean the inhalant gasses
are gone! All patients should be maintained on oxygen for at least 5 minutes after
turning off the gas and any patient that is sick, geriatric or neonatal might need to
stay on longer, especially if they were not breathing and/or oxygenating well intra-
operatively. Some patients may need to receive oxygen in recovery and may even
need to be in an oxygen cage. Don't stop the oxygen until the patient can maintain
SpO_2 > 90% on room air!

IMPORTANT POINT
Delivering oxygen through the anesthesia machine immediately postoperatively has the added benefit of allowing the exhaled inhalant gas to be evacuated into the scavenging system rather into the room, allowing human exposure.

Carbon Dioxide Elimination

The effects of anesthesia-induced respiratory depression on carbon dioxide elimination can almost always be overcome by increasing respiratory rate, tidal volume or both. However, equipment malfunction can contribute to hypercarbia and, if increasing ventilation does not immediately decrease the CO_2, start checking the equipment for expired CO_2 absorbent, inadequate oxygen flow, non-functional one-way valves and kinks or obstructions in the ETT tube or breathing hoses. More information is available in Chapter 3.

Maintaining Normal Ventilation

Young, healthy patients at an appropriate depth of anesthesia will generally breathe adequately on their own (both adequate respiratory rate and tidal volume; See Chapter 5 for normal values). Normal support in all patients, including those breathing well on their own, does include the delivery of a deep breath or 'sigh' **(Table 6-4)** every 15 to 30 minutes. Sighing helps keep the alveoli (the air sacs in the lung) open and maximizes gas exchange (gas exchange = oxygen in, carbon dioxide out).

Table 6-4
How to: Perform a 'Sigh'

- Press down on the pop-off button or close the pop-off valve;
- Squeeze the reservoir (rebreathing) bag until the peak inspiratory pressure (PIP) on the airway manometer (described in Chapter 3) reads 15 cm H_2O in a medium to big dog or 10 cm H_2O in a cat or small dog;
- Hold the pressure for 2 to 3 seconds;
- Release the pressure;
- Release the pop-off button or open the pop-off valve.

Older patients or patients with disease will often NOT ventilate adequately and ventilation (both respiratory rate and tidal volume) may need to be assisted or controlled. Assisting can mean anything from administering 1 to 2 breaths every 5 minutes to administering 1 to 2 breaths every minute, depending on how much the patient is breathing on its own. To deliver the breaths, use the guidelines for administering a 'sigh' but with an inspiratory time of only 1 to 2 seconds.

Patients that won't breathe at all may need controlled ventilation (from a person breathing for the patient or from a mechanical ventilator), which requires approximately 10 breaths/min in most dogs and 15 breaths/min in toy breed dogs and cats. Peak inspiratory pressure (PIP) is critical and should not exceed 10 to 15 cm H_2O in most patients but PIP of 20 cm H_2O **(Figure 6-5)** may be appropriate in large patients. Guidelines for controlled ventilation are presented in **Table 6-5**.

Ideally, the patient should be ventilated to an end-tidal CO_2 of 35 to 45 cm H_2O **(Figure 6-6)**. If an end-tidal CO_2 monitor is not available, use the guidelines above for setting a normal respiratory rate and PIP and assume that this will provide an end-tidal CO_2 of 35 to 45 cm H_2O (See Chapter 10).

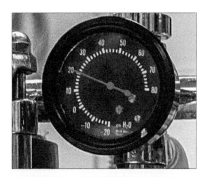

Figure 6-5. Airway pressure manometer indicating 20 cm H_2O.

Table 6-5

Guidelines for Controlled Ventilation
(by mechanical ventilator OR by person squeezing the rebreathing bag to breathe for the patient)

Patient	Respiratory Rate (breaths/min)	Peak Inspiratory Pressure (cm H_2O)	Tidal Volume (ml/kg)	End-tidal CO_2 (cmH$_2$O)
Cat or Small Dog	15	10-15	10-15	35-45
Medium-Large Dog	10	15-20	10-15	35-45

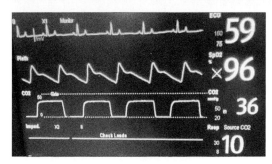

Figure 6-6. Anesthetic monitor screen indicating an end-tidal CO_2 of 36 cmH$_2$O (bottom), the saturation of oxygen as measured by pulse oximetry of 96% (middle) and the heart rate from the ECG of 59 beats/min (top).

Body Temperature Support
Janel Bingman LVT, VTS (Anesthesia/Analgesia)

Anesthesia can cause abnormalities in body temperature which can lead to adverse effects. Hypothermia is by far the most common anesthesia-induced temperature abnormality but hyperthermia can also occur.

Hypothermia (Low Body Temperature)

Anesthetized patients can develop hypothermia very quickly and the cause of the drop in body temperature is multifactorial. Some contributing factors include, direct suppression of the thermoregulatory activity of the hypothalamus (which is a region of the brain) by general anesthetic drugs; impaired patient thermoregulatory activity as may occur in geriatric or neonatal patients or patients with certain diseases (e.g., hypothyroidism); anesthesia-drug induced vasodilation, which causes a redistribution of warm blood from the body's core to the skin where heat is released; anesthesia induced muscle relaxation (muscle tone and movement help to maintain normal body temperature); evaporation of surgical scrub solutions from the body surface; equilibration of core body temperature with ambient temperature through open body cavities; duration of anesthesia (longer=colder); and delivery of cold anesthetic gases to the large surface area of the alveoli.

Small patients are particularly susceptible to development of hypothermia since they have a large body surface area for their weight - which means they have a large surface to lose heat from. They are also likely to be on a nonrebreathing system, which means that a high volume of cold air will be delivered to their lungs (See Chapter 3).

> **TIP**
> Core body temperature (using a rectal or esophageal thermometer) should be monitored in all anesthetized patients! And body temperature should be rechecked during recovery because the temperature often goes down before it goes up!

Although it was once thought that keeping the surgery room cold was good for the patient because bacterial growth was reduced in a cold environment, we now know that a cold operating room (OR) = a cold patient and HYPOTHERMIA IS NOT BENIGN. In fact, hypothermia can cause a variety of complications, some of which put the patient at high risk for adverse events **(Table 6-6)**. The complication that we usually notice is prolonged recovery time. Other complications include clotting dysfunction, tissue hypoxia, acidosis, abnormal myocardial electrical conduction and myocardial ischemia (Clarke-Price 2015; Noble 2006). Ironically infection rates are actually higher in hypothermic patients (even if the bacteria count in the OR is lower) because hypothermia impairs the patient's immune system. Hypothermia also causes cerebral effects that decrease the patient's anesthetic needs. Unfor-

Table 6-6
Adverse Effects of Hypothermia

Adverse effects of hypothermia include:
- PROLONGED RECOVERY from anesthesia.
- Impaired drug metabolism due to altered metabolic processes and enzymatic activity (adds to prolonged recovery & decreased elimination of drugs which can lead to relative overdose).
- Decreased need for anesthetics due to CNS dysfunction (adds to the prolonged recovery and can lead to relative overdose).
- Immune system depression (increases infection rate and impairs healing).
- Coagulation dysfunction due to decreased activity of enzymes associated with the clotting cascade and impaired platelet function (may cause excess bleeding).
- Increased blood viscosity and sludging of blood in vessels (causes poor blood flow which decreases organ perfusion).
- Decreased cardiac contractility, hypotension and arrhythmias.
- Decreased heart rate which may lead to hypotension and is often resistant to treatment with anticholinergics (i.e., the heart rate will not increase).
- Shivering which causes increased oxygen consumption.
- Respiratory impairment (decreased oxygen delivery, respiratory acidosis).
- Vasoconstriction (decreased oxygen delivery to the tissues).
- Increased morbidity and potentially mortality.

tunately, the decreased anesthetic need is not always recognized and the delivery of anesthesia is not changed, resulting in an over-dosage of anesthetic drugs. Although shivering in recovery may increase the body temperature, the intensive muscle movements associated with shivering causes discomfort and significantly increases oxygen consumption (how much oxygen the body uses). In fact, in human medicine, prevention of shivering in the postoperative period is a major concern and should be a major concern for our veterinary patients as well.

CRITICAL POINT!
Animals commonly get very cold during anesthesia. Anesthetic gas delivery should be decreased during profound hypothermia, but this is often overlooked.

Tips for Warming (Table 6-7)
The normal body temperature of dogs and cats is 100°F to 102.5°F (about 37.8°C to 39.2°C) and the body temperature should be maintained as close to normal as possible (Table 6-7). Body temperatures below 98°F (39.2°C) can cause adverse effects. Make sure the patient is warm BEFORE induction since preoperative hypothermia is a predictor of intraoperative hypothermia.

Prevention of hypothermia is much more effective than treatment of hypothermia so measures should be taken to keep the patient warm as soon as the patient is induced to anesthesia. The biggest drop in body temperature occurs in the first hour of anesthesia (Clarke-Price 2015).

Table 6-7
Tips for Prevention/Treatment of Hypothermia and Complications of Hypothermia

To prevent/treat hypothermia and complications of hypothermia:
- Monitor core temperature - esophageal temperature probe or rectal thermometer.
- Monitor ambient temperature of the rooms (induction, surgical and recovery rooms) and keep the areas as warm as possible.
- Use active warming devices and techniques to minimize heat loss:
  - Forced warm air (Baja Breeze®, Bair Hugger®);
  - Hot water pads (not as good as warm air blankets);
  - Specialized electric heat blanket (HotDog®) but NOT a regular electric heating pad;
  - Heated surgical table;
  - In-line fluid warmers;
  - Warmed and humidified breathing hoses;
  - Socks, latex gloves, or fleece wraps on paws;
  - Plastic wrap or bubble wrap around body parts not involved in procedure during surgery;
  - Warmed blankets during pre-op and post-op;
  - Warmed irrigation fluids (i.e., fluids used to irrigate or 'lavage' body cavities or wounds).
- Decrease anesthetic time.
- Supplement oxygen to meet metabolic requirements (shivering).
- Monitor for relapse hypothermia in recovery - this is very common!
- If hypothermia is severe, consider:
  - Administration of 10ml/kg of warm isotonic fluids rectally;
  - Lavage urinary bladder with warm fluids.

CRITICAL POINT!
Body temperature starts dropping as soon as the patient is induced to anesthesia so preventive warming should begin at the same time. If a hypothermic patient is scheduled for anesthesia, warming should begin BEFORE induction.

Forced air warmers (like the Baja Breeze® or Bair Hugger®; **Figure 6-7**) are more effective than circulating water blankets and both forced air and circulating water blankets are MUCH safer than regular electric heating pads, the latter are highly likely to burn the patient and SHOULD NOT BE USED IN ANESTHETIZED PATIENTS. The exception is the highly insulated HotDog® warmers **(Figure 6-8)** with temperatures that automatically cut off before they reach a temperature that would burn the patient. Warm the ambient temperature (the air around the patient). This can mean warm the whole surgery room or just warm the patient's immediate area by covering it with warm towels and blankets and putting warmed devices (like rice bags and water bottles) under the towels and blankets, BUT NOT IN DIRECT CONTACT WITH THE PATIENT'S SKIN. Make sure the patient has a warm recovery room or recovery cage to come to postoperatively. Use minimal scrub solution - scrub only the surgical site - don't douse the entire patient with wet scrub solution. Use fluid warmers, socks on paws, anything that might help maintain body temperature.

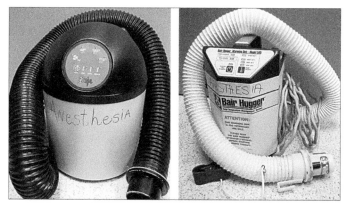

Figure 6-7. Forced air warmers like the Baha Breeze (left) or Bair Hugger (right) are the most effective patient warming devices. The end of the hose on the left in both photos can be attached to a specially made blanket or can be placed under a regular blanket that is covering the patient.

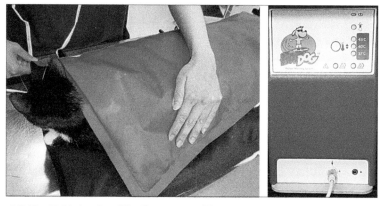

Figure 6-8. The highly insulated Hot Dog warmer (the actual blanket on a cat in the picture on the left; the heating unit in the picture on the right), that automatically cuts off before reaching a temperature that would burn the patient, is also effective. **A towel should be placed between the patient and the warming blanket to prevent burns.**

Some studies show these are not effective when used alone but combining them with other warming devices certainly helps!

CRITICAL POINT!
BE SURE TO USE TOWELS BETWEEN THE PATIENT AND HEATING PADS OR HEATED RICE BAGS OR WATER BOTTLES. All of these products can cause serious thermal burns if the patient is in direct contact with them. Heated air blankets are the least likely cause thermal burns.

CRITICAL POINT!
DO NOT USE REGULAR ELECTRIC HEATING PADS FOR ANESTHETIZED PATIENTS. They are very likely to burn the patient.

Finally, keep anesthesia time as short as possible. The longer a patient is anesthetized, the more likely it is to get cold!

CRITICAL POINT!
KEEP ANESTHESIA TIME TO A MINIMUM. The duration of anesthesia is a MAJOR CONTRIBUTOR to hypothermia.

Hyperthermia (High Body Temperature)

Hyperthermia (body temperature > 103°F) is not very common in anesthetized patients but when it does occur, the patient may need to be actively cooled **(Table 6-8)**. Temperatures < 104°F (40°C) may be 'self-limiting' (meaning the body temperature will decrease without treatment) but any warming devices should definitely be removed. Active cooling should be instituted if the body temperature is > 104°F (40°C) and aggressive therapy may be required if the temperature is > 105 to 106°F (40.6 to 41.1°C). Active cooling can include fans blowing on the patient, cool water or ice packs in areas of large superficial veins (jugular and inguinal areas), cold IV fluids and alcohol on the pads (dogs only).

As the patient is being cooled MONITOR THE BODY TEMPERATURE CLOSELY. DO NOT make the patient hypothermic. Stop cooling when the patient's body temperature reaches 103° F (39.7°C) so as not to overshoot the normal temperature and cause hypothermia.

Causes of Hyperthermia
• Warm weather, especially if the clinic is also overly warm or the patient came in slightly overheated;
• Heavy coated and giant breed dogs (just more likely to over-heat, nothing; specific with breeds or genetics);
• Excitement or stress;
• Over use of warming devices;
• Reaction to pure mu opioids in cats;
• Sepsis, endotoxemia, viremia, bacteremia (systemic infection);
• Febrile transfusion reaction;
• Heat generated during low flow anesthesia (which is not commonly used);
• Malignant hyperthermia (which is caused by a rare genetic mutation).

Attention to Basic Husbandry

General comfort of the patient should be considered preoperatively, intraoperatively and postoperatively. The patient should be kept warm and dry and pain should be controlled. Intraoperatively don't forget that abnormal positioning (like legs stretched out and tied with ropes to the table) and lack of padding on a cold, hard surgical table can cause sore muscles and joints, especially in older patients with painful osteoarthritis. Be as gentle as possible with positioning and be sure that the table has some padding. Postoperatively, be sure that the patient has a chance to urinate. We often confuse the need to urinate with postoperative dysphoria or even pain. If the patient is restless postoperatively and you have addressed pain, walk it outside and let it empty its bladder! Also consider species-specific needs, like housing cats away from barking dogs and giving them a box to hide in as they are recovering from anesthesia (but keep a hole in it so you can watch them!).

No matter how good we are at all of the complicated aspects of veterinary medicine, if we don't address basic husbandry, we are not meeting the needs of our patients.

Summary

Anesthesia causes changes that can lead to complications if the impact of those changes is not minimized by using basic support techniques like attention to anesthetic depth, provision of analgesia, and support of the cardiovascular, respiratory and thermoregulatory systems. All anesthetized patients should receive supplemental inhaled oxygen. Intravenous fluids are highly recommended for most patients, and required for patients that are sick, traumatized, hemorrhaging, geriatric, or have any other condition that might result in hypovolemia. Maintenance of normal body temperature is often overlooked as a critical part of support but hypothermia can lead to many complications and can make recovery from anesthesia very slow and potentially dangerous. Finally, basic husbandry is an important support mechanism and should not be overlooked.

References

Clark-Price S. Inadvertent Perianesthetic Hypothermia in Small Animal Patients. Vet Clin North Am Small Anim Pract. 2015;45(5):983-94.

Davis H, Jensen T, Johnson A, Knowles P, Meyer R, Rucinsky R, Shafford H; 2013 AAHA/AAFP fluid therapy guidelines for dogs and cats. American Association of Feline Practitioners; American Animal Hospital Association. J Am Anim Hosp Assoc. 2013 May-Jun; 49(3):149-59.

McNally EM, Robertson SA, Pablo LS. Comparison of time to desaturation between preoxygenated and nonpreoxygenated dogs following sedation with acepromazine maleate and morphine and induction of anesthesia with propofol. Am J Vet Res. 2009 Nov; 70 (11):1333-8.

Noble KA. Chill can kill. J Perianesth Nurs. 2006 Jun; 21(3):204-7.

Chapter 7
Pain and Analgesia

Shelley Ensign, LVT, CVPP

Tamara Grubb, DVM, PhD, DACVAA

Importance of Analgesia

The relief of pain is one of the most important things that we can do for our patients, but it isn't always easy since we are still battling the myth that animals don't feel pain and/or that they don't need analgesia. In reality, they do feel pain and provision of analgesia provides major medical benefits to the patient. But recognition of pain can be difficult since animals are very good at hiding pain and treatment selection can be complicated when the effects and adverse effects (or 'side effects') of drugs are unknown - or misunderstood - by the person designing treatment protocols. Thus, a thorough knowledge of drugs is important for anyone involved in pain management.

The Technician's/Nurse's Role in Pain Management

A major component of good pain management is NURSING care. From recognizing changes in behavior, to following monitoring trends under anesthesia to being a VOICE for the patient, technicians, or veterinary nurses, play a major role in the recognition and treatment of pain in animals (Table 7-1).

Do Animals really feel Pain?

Of course animals feel pain! Scientifically we know that all mammals have a similar neuroanatomic (anatomy of the nervous system) pain pathway (Figure 7-1). Pain starts when the peripheral pain receptors (called 'nociceptors') are activated in a process called 'transduction'. The painful impulse is passed along the peripheral nerves ('transmission') to the spinal cord where the signal is changed or 'modulated' ('modulation'). Finally, the pain impulse reaches the brain and the patient perceives the pain (called 'perception'). Since this pain pathway is similar in humans, dogs, cats, rabbits, horses, cows, goats, gerbils, etc., we can scientifically say that all mammals feel pain and that, if something is painful to a human, it is painful to an animal. The problem is that animals have very good reasons to hide pain and often don't show pain until it is too intense to hide.

Table 7-1
Importance of the Technician/Nurse in Pain Management

Technicians are generally the most likely person in the practice to recognize the patient's pain. This is because TECHNICIANS/NURSES:
- often know the patient better than anyone else in the hospital - and are thus most likely to recognize changes in behavior that may indicate pain.
- monitor the patient during painful procedures (e.g., surgery or wound repair) and are the most likely to recognize intraoperative changes in physiologic parameters that may indicate pain.
- are also most likely to be observing the patient after analgesic treatment and often understand the clinical effects/adverse effects of the drugs in that patient better than other people in the practice.
- are the 'voice' of the patient and should advocate for pain relief, just as human nurses do for human patients.

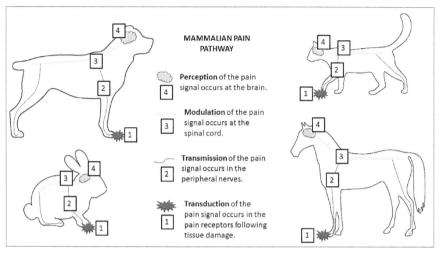

Figure 7-1. The Mammalian Pain Pathway.

I Heard that Pain is Good because it Keeps an Animal from Moving around after Surgery. Is that True?

Pain can be good because it is a protective response and sudden, moderate to severe pain should cause the animal to withdraw from, or stop doing, something that is painful to avoid injury. This beneficial pain component is called 'protective pain' or 'physiologic pain'. However, unless injury is actively occurring, protective pain should be absent and the patient shouldn't feel pain all the time. Lingering moderate to severe pain that is present beyond the protective response is called 'pathologic pain' because it serves NO PROTECTIVE PURPOSE and because it creates more problems for the animal. Pathologic pain initiates a stress response, which can impair patient healing and cause a negative impact on the patient's quality of life. Pathologic pain can actually make the animal really restless because it is hard to find a comfortable position to rest if they are painful. A painful patient is more likely than a comfortable patient to circle around in its cage, get up and down a lot, not be able to find a comfortable way to sleep and may even cause damage to the initial site of injury and/or surgical repair by being overactive or by chewing/excessively licking at the injury/surgery site. So the answer is no, pain does not keep an animal still and can actually cause adverse effects that may make the patient's condition worse. The exception is excruciating pain that is so severe that the animal cannot move. Any animal that is in this much pain must be treated immediately.

The goal of analgesia is to provide quality of life and improve healing by decreasing pathologic pain without eliminating protective pain. This is a very easy goal to meet because we don't actually have any analgesic drugs (other than local anesthetics - and they have a very short duration of action) capable of eliminating protective pain - it will still be there even if we do GREAT analgesia. The problem with animals is that they don't always 'listen' to protective pain and take care of themselves so we need to be good caregivers and restrain or even sedate patients that are too active. It is okay to medicate over-active patients with calming or sedating drugs! But it is NOT okay to leave pathologic pain, with all of its negative medical effects and its contribution to patient suffering, untreated.

IMPORTANT POINT
Protective pain may not be recognized by a really active dog or cat so we may need to use crates, kennels, small rooms, leashes, and even tranquilizers to control patients while they are healing.

What Happens if we Don't Treat Pain?
Even if animals don't show pain, we can use our medical knowledge of the fact that animals have a pain pathway that is similar to ours to identify the fact that if something would hurt us, it would hurt them. And if something hurts, it produces a stress-response in the patient and stress, from any cause, can lead to a multitude of adverse effects (**Table 7-2**).

In addition to the pathologic changes in the organ systems that can be caused by pain, pathologic changes can actually occur in the pain pathway itself, especially if pain is moderate to severe and is left untreated. These changes exacerbate the pain sensation for the patient, which further decreases the quality of life and impairs healing, and, because the pain is worse, causes even more of the changes in the organ systems that we just described. Two changes that often occur are:

• **Peripheral sensitization,** which occurs at the site of the injury or surgical incision. The damaged cells at the site release chemical compounds that cause inflammation and lower the threshold of the pain receptors ('nociceptors'), meaning that they are more 'sensitive' to stimuli. When this happens, stimuli that are normally mildly painful become much more painful (**'hyperalgesia'**) and stimuli that are normally NOT painful can cause pain to the patient (**'allodynia'**). In addition, as cells are damaged and leak the chemical compounds, they damage cells that are close to them, which then leak their chemical compounds, which then damage more cells, which leak their chemical compounds…, and you can see that this is an ongoing process that spreads the pain to a larger area, which means more pain for the patient and more pain signals sent to the central nervous system, which can lead to central sensitization.

• **Central sensitization,** which occurs in the central nervous system. Central sensitization is an increase in the excitability of neurons within the central nervous system, which is often started by the increased input from the periphery but becomes an actual change in the fibers, synapses and neurons in the nervous system. This results in a system that has a hyperreactive response to pain signals and further contributes to allodynia and hyperalgesia. In addition, the sensation of pain can

Table 7-2
A Few Examples of the Adverse Effects and Consequences Caused by Pain

System Affected	Adverse Effects	Consequences
General	Insomnia, anorexia, cachexia (overall deterioration or 'wasting')	All of these can impair healing and can lead to other health problems.
Behavior	The patient can become aggressive or may hide (see more below under recognizing pain)	Changes in behavior can alter the human-animal bond and can even lead to abandonment and/or euthanasia.
Gastrointestinal	Anorexia, gastric ulcers, nausea, vomiting, altered GI motility, ileus	Anorexia, nausea and vomiting can all decrease food intake - which further impairs healing. Gastric ulcers can add to the pain. Ileus can be a very serious condition that requires treatment and can further add to pain as gas builds up and stretches the intestinal wall.
Cardiovascular	Tachycardia, hypertension, arrhythmias	These changes can exacerbate, or even cause, cardiovascular problems.
Pulmonary	Tachypnea, hypoxemia, oxygen deficit, respiratory alkalosis or acidosis	Anytime oxygenation is impacted, numerous adverse effects can occur since all tissues and organs require oxygen for fuel. Also, acidosis and alkalosis can cause further complications since normal body function requires normal pH.

now be spread through the nervous system to areas that were not impacted by the original source of pain. This is the reason that sometimes we feel pain all over and not just at an injury site - and the reason that a patient might not want to be petted on any part of their body, even though they have a localized source of pain (like an incision or a wound, or even a really painful joint as might occur in osteoarthritis).

REVIEW: Why should we Prevent Pain when Possible and Treat Pain when it does Occur?
(Tables 7-3 and 7-4)

Table 7-4
Oaths Taken by Veterinarians and Veterinary Technicians

Veterinarian's Oath	Veterinary Technician's Oath
Being admitted to the profession of veterinary medicine, I solemnly swear to use my scientific knowledge and skills for the benefit of society through the **protection of animal health and welfare,** the **prevention and relief of animal suffering,** the conservation of animal resources, the promotion of public health, and the advancement of medical knowledge. I will practice my profession conscientiously, with dignity, and in keeping with the principles of veterinary medical ethics. I accept as a lifelong obligation the continual improvement of my professional knowledge and competence.	I solemnly dedicate myself to aiding animals and society by **providing excellent care and services for animals,** by **alleviating animal suffering,** and by promoting public health. I accept my obligations to practice my profession conscientiously and with sensitivity, adhering to the profession's Code of Ethics, and furthering my knowledge and competence through a commitment to lifelong learning.

Analgesia Decreases the Negative Medical Impact of Pain

Analgesia improves our medical success rate because adequate analgesia improves healing and allows a decreased incidence of postoperative stress-related complications **(Table 7-2)**. Pain initiates a fairly profound stress response and a sympathetic nervous system response. Stress and autonomic imbalance (an imbalance of the sympathetic and parasympathetic nervous systems) are not benign and can induce a cascade of adverse effects, including gastrointestinal (GI) ileus, GI ulceration, clotting dysfunction, hypertension, tachycardia, tachyarrhythmias, and many others. Furthermore, stress and pain cause a fairly marked increase in cortisol release and a substantial increase in energy requirements, the latter of which may lead to a negative nitrogen balance and both of which impair and/or delay healing. If we want our patients to heal quickly and completely, we have to treat pain!

Analgesia for Acute Pain Can Improve Long-Term Patient Outcome

Inadequate pain management at the time of intense pain (like surgery or trauma) can increase the potential that the patient will develop chronic pain because moderate to severe pain can create long-term pathologic changes in the neural components of the pain pathway. Prevention of these changes with analgesic drugs can alleviate or eliminate the incidence of chronic pain syndromes related to the initial surgery, injury or disease.

Analgesia Improves Anesthetic Safety

Analgesia increases anesthetic safety by decreasing the dose of anesthetic drugs necessary to keep the patient asleep. Most anesthetic drugs, including the inhalant anesthetic drugs, block the brain's <u>response</u> to pain but don't actually block pain. If the pain is severe enough, the brain can still respond and make the animal appear to be inadequately anesthetized. The result is that the vaporizer is turned up and the brain ceases to respond, but the patient is now too deeply anesthetized and can be at a very dangerous physiologic plane of anesthesia. A more appropriate response would be to decrease the pain with analgesics and maintain the patient at a light, safe depth of anesthesia.

We Promised to Provide Analgesia

Finally, veterinarians and veterinary technicians/nurses promised to abide by their respective oaths which, among other things, state that we pledge to provide excellent care of animals, that we will protect animal welfare and that we will prevent or relieve animal suffering. All of these promises can be defined to include the relief of pain, so, ethically, we committed to relieving pain when we joined this profession **(Table 7-4)**.

CRITICAL POINT!

For all of the reasons listed above, pain relief is both the ethically 'right thing to do', AND the medically 'right thing to do'.

How do we know when a Patient is in Pain? Isn't it Really Easy to Tell?

It is actually very hard to know whether or not an animal is in pain. Animals exhibit prey/predator behaviors (even our domesticated pets exhibit these behaviors) and they instinctively hide any 'weakness' that might make them prey instead of predator. Pain could be perceived as a 'weakness' in this scenario. We know that animals hide pain from humans - there are several studies where animals were videoed after painful surgeries and, without people present, they exhibited pain behavior signs, but the behavior stopped as soon as a person came into view. Because animals try to hide pain when at all possible, it is likely that once an animal is exhibiting pain, the pain is severe and the central sensitization process has probably begun - and pain will be more difficult to treat.

So we have to LOOK for pain. We aren't good about looking for pain - but we definitely won't find what we don't look for. We also need to 'ask' them if they feel pain by using assessment tools and by treating what we presume to be pain while observing the patient's response to the treatment. Primarily, we should use common sense - if we do something painful, we should treat for pain. And we should not presume that the animal will show us pain if we don't look.

The Importance of Pain: the 5th Vital Sign:

Pain is called the 5th vital sign in human medicine (vital signs: heart rate, respiratory rate, arterial blood pressure, body temperature, pain) and is one of the main reasons that humans seek medical care. Why is pain the '5th vital sign'? Because pain has a major impact on the health of the patient (See Table 7-2)

Why do we care in veterinary medicine? Because, as already stated, our patients feel pain too and pain is often called the 4th vital sign in veterinary medicine (because we don't often measure blood pressure in a routine physical exam). Perhaps pain is not the main reason that animals 'seek' veterinary care, but the importance of unrecognized pain is the same in our patients as it is in human patients and we should evaluate pain just as we evaluate all other vital signs.

How to: Assess Pain

We should treat pain as a vital sign and pain should be assessed in all patients using pain scoring tools. A pain score should be written in the patient's record. Pain scoring systems are not perfect, but they make us really look at - and interact with - the patient, making it more likely that we will detect pain. By using physiologic, physical and behavioral signs of pain, especially when combined in a pain scoring system, we are more likely to identify patients that need analgesic therapy and can more accurately monitor response to analgesic therapy.

Looking for Pain

Let's go back to the vital signs. We don't 'ask' the patient to 'tell' us the other vital signs, so why would we 'ask' them to 'tell' us their pain level? We must LOOK for pain. We can use the other vital signs to aid in pain assessment. Since pain is a stressor, we can look for physiologic signs of stress (tachycardia, tachypnea, hypertension, arrhythmias). A partial list of signs that might indicate pain are listed in **Table 7-5**. But the vital signs can also be changed by stress from causes other than pain (e.g., the heart rate is often increased due to stress of hospitalization or a barking dog in the cage next door) so they should be included in the pain assessment but shouldn't be the only thing we look at.

Vocalization is sometimes used to indicate the presence of pain, and this can be useful, but vocalization is often breed specific (e.g., Husky dogs and Siamese cats) and, in the postoperative setting, can be due to dysphoria, so it isn't always indicative of pain. Vocalization can include barking (dogs), growling (dogs and cats)

Table 7-5
Examples of Signs that Might Indicate Pain in Dogs and Cats

Physiologic Signs	Behavior Signs	Vocalization	Body position	Gait (Locomotion)	Other
Tachycardia	Any change in behavior	Howling (dog)	Head down	Lame	Failure to groom
Tachypnea, Panting	Aggression	Whimpering (dog)	'Hunched' body or 'tucked' abdomen	Reluctant to move	Excessive grooming of painful site
Hypertension	Hiding/ avoidance	Excessive barking (dog)	Tail down	Stiff or abnormal gate	Failure to go outside to urinate or defecate
Arrhythmias	Seeks comfort, won't leave owner	Growling (dog or cat)	Ears 'flat' or out to side (cat)	Walking with more weight on front or back legs	Failure to use litter box
Dilated pupils	Guards painful area - may snap if painful area touched Won't lie down, won't sleep	Hissing (cat) Purring (cat)	Lying in straight position rather than curled (cat)	Pacing	Change in facial 'expressions' Anorexia

or hissing (cats) and, of course, is more specific for pain if the vocalization occurs following a painful event - especially if the patient didn't bark, growl or hiss before the painful event.

Changes in posture and gait can often be quite specific for pain. Changes in posture like 'tucked' abdomen or 'hunched' back usually indicate pain. Head down, neck stretched, ears back or flat and tail down are also all signs that could indicate pain. Body posture while lying down is equally important. For instance, cats generally sleep 'curled' and cats that are laying stretched out may be experiencing pain, but again this should be linked to a potential painful condition or event, not just a happy cat stretched out in the sun. Of course, lameness is usually indicative of pain, although mechanical lameness can occur if healed fractures or articular injuries cause abnormal anatomical changes to the limb. But lameness should always be investigated. Lameness may become worse with exercise (pain of unstable joints) or worse with sedentary activity (like old dogs with musculoskeletal pain that are more painful after a night's sleep) so it is important to get a history from the owner regarding the timing of the animal's lameness. Walking with a very stiff or abnormal gait, even if not actually lame, may also occur with pain, especially with more generalized pain.

Changes in eating, grooming or defecation/urination habits may also be linked with pain. For instance, cats that are litter box trained but suddenly stop using the box for defecation/urination may have pain that keeps them from climbing into the box, especially if the box has really high sides or deep litter. Of course, all other sources of changes in defecation/urination (e.g., urinary bladder infection, gastrointestinal disease, new cats in the house) must be ruled out.

Changes in facial 'expressions' have recently been linked with pain and the ability to relate facial expressions in animals to levels of pain (the scales are called 'grimace scales') has now been validated by research in numerous species. Facial expressions that might be related to pain include eye squinting or holding the eyes tightly closed and ears out to the side (instead of upright) in cats or held really flat against the head in dogs. Changes in whisker position (cats) and brow 'furrowing' (dogs) are also useful.

Change in behavior is one of the most specific signs of pain. Of course, we can't be sure that a change in behavior necessarily means pain, but a change in behavior that coincides with a painful event (surgery or trauma) or disease (like osteoarthritis) is highly likely due to pain. Animals that were friendly may become aggressive or defensive and those that were solitary may seek human companionship and comfort. The animal's behavior may even seem normal until the painful area is approached or touched and then fear or aggression may be exhibited. Animals that don't have normal sleep behavior, especially those that don't want to lie down and sleep after a painful surgery, are very likely painful. This goes back to the fact that **pain often makes patients restless** and the myth that pain keeps patients from moving is wrong.

Pain Scoring Systems/Scales

The best way to detect and to monitor pain is to use pain scoring systems or scales, especially systems or scales that combine the physiologic, physical and behavioral signs just discussed **(Figure 7-2 A)**. There are several advantages to using pain scores over just looking at the patient but not writing anything down **(Table 7-6)**, including the fact that it is much easier to follow trends in pain and response to pain treatment if descriptors of the patient are actually documented. It is almost impossible to be consistent with pain therapy without writing some type of score in the patient's record at each assessment time.

Table 7-6
Benefits of Using Pain Scores

Pain scoring systems:
• Provide a means to assess changes in pain level and follow trends;
• Allow us to assess response to analgesia and develop treatment plans based on response;
• Allow more consistent patient evaluation, even if different people are assessing the patient.

No pain scoring system or scale is perfect, especially since we have to rely on a human's perception of what the animal is feeling - or what the animal is trying to hide. There are many scoring systems so each clinic can choose the one that works best for them. Ideally, the same person will score the animal before and after a painful procedure (like surgery) or before and after pain relieving treatment. Using the same person to score the patient improves the accuracy of the scoring system, but using a good scoring system with descriptors of what the patient looks like improves the accuracy even if multiple people need to score the patient. Scoring systems are available for both acute and chronic pain. Several pain scoring examples are provided here, including very easy to use scales developed at Colorado State University which are available free on the internet for both dogs and cats **(Figure 7-2 B & C)**.

Owners know the normal behavior of their pets better than anyone and owners see their pets in an environment very different from the stressful environment of the animal hospital. Thus, we should get a good history of the animal's behavior from the owner when investigating pain. And, especially with chronic pain, the owner should be asked to participate in an evaluation of their pet's pain - and pain relief. Assessment systems like those in **Figure 7-2 D** can easily be used by pet owners.

Finally, the most useful way to determine whether or not an animal is in pain, is to 'ask it' - pharmacologically of course! We 'ask' the patient by administering an analgesic drug and evaluating the response to the drug. For acute pain, an opioid is often the best option because of the rapid onset and profound potency of the drug. For chronic pain, an NSAID is often the best choice, but a dose of an opioid can be

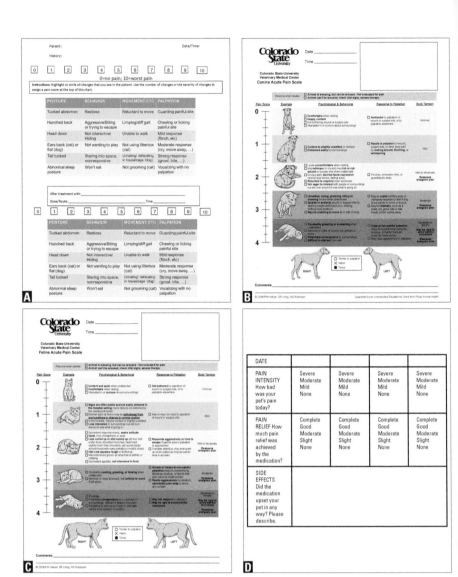

Figure 7-2. A pain scoring system for evaluating acute pain and response to analgesic treatment (**A**). The pain scales/scoring system developed at Colorado State University for dogs (**B**) and cats (**C**). Example of an assessment system for chronic pain level and response to treatment that can be used at home by the pet owner (**D**).

used to make a rapid decision if necessary. If the patient's behavior returns to normal after treatment, then the diagnosis has been made - PAIN, and now we can move on to developing a treatment plan that will provide the patient with pain relief. If the patient's behavior does not return to normal but pain is still a likely diagnosis, try another dose of the analgesic drug PLUS a drug from another drug class (for example, use opioids and NSAIDs together). Relief of severe pain requires multimodal therapy

222

and may require higher than expected drug dosages. Lack of response to aggressive analgesic therapy can be used as a diagnostic tool since continued abnormal behavior would unlikely be due to pain if analgesic therapy is adequate but the patient doesn't improve. Pain is then ruled out and further diagnostics are begun.

IMPORTANT POINT
If you are unsure if a patient is in pain, 'ask' it! Of course that means asking it with a dose of analgesic drugs and monitoring the patient's response. Generally opioids are used for this 'question' since they are fast acting, potent analgesic drugs. If you are wrong (you probably won't be!) and the patient isn't in pain, the effects of the opioids can be reversed, if necessary. 'Asking' the patient is the best way to know for sure if the patient is experiencing pain.

Prevention/Treatment of Pain
Safe anesthesia is **not possible** without the inclusion of analgesia. The three principles of pain management (see below) should be followed when designing anesthetic/analgesic protocols and analgesic drugs should be incorporated into the different phases of anesthesia.

Basic Prinicples of Pain Management
We may not all use the same analgesic drugs but we should all use the 3 basic principles of pain management when designing analgesic protocols. These principles together are termed 'preventive' or 'balanced' analgesia and this should be the goal of treatment for EVERY painful patient **(Table 7-7)**.

Table 7-7
The Three Principles of a Good Pain Management Protocol

The three principles of pain management are:
• Utilize preemptive analgesia;
• Utilize multimodal analgesia;
• Don't quit until pain quits!

Preemptive Analgesia
Analgesia provided prior to the pain stimulus ("pre-emptive analgesia") is more effective than analgesia provided once pain has occurred because it prevents or decreases the likelihood that hypersensitization of the pain pathways (central sensitization) will occur. Preempting pain will decrease the overall intensity of the pain sensation and will increase the effectiveness of analgesic drugs.

IMPORTANT POINT
It is much easier to prevent pain than to treat pain so preemptive analgesia is an important component of a balanced analgesic protocol.

Multimodal Analgesia

Using a variety of analgesic drugs, techniques and routes of administration ("multimodal analgesia") capitalizes on the additive or synergistic effects of analgesic drugs and promotes pain relief that is more intense and/or of longer duration than relief provided with any one drug or technique used alone. For example, the use of an NSAID with an opioid typically provides more profound analgesia that lasts longer than the analgesia provided by either an NSAID or opioid used alone. In part, this is due to the fact that different analgesic drugs or drug classes act at different sites in the pain pathway (**Figure 7-3**).

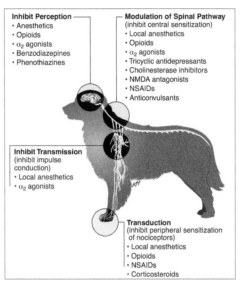

Figure 7-3. Sites of action of drugs in the pain pathway, use drugs that work at different sites for multimodal analgesia. (From Tranquilli WJ, Grimm KA, Lamont LA. Pain Management For The Small Animal Practitioner, Figure 1-3. Teton New Media, 2000. (Adapted from Tranquilli, WJ, Grimm KA, Lamont LA, Figure 1-2. Teton New Media 2000).

Don't Quit Until Pain Quits

Finally, pain must be addressed not only postoperatively but even after the patient has been discharged from the hospital. It is a misconception that that animals do not need analgesic drugs once they have left the hospital just because the patients often do not show pain at home. However, as we have said, animals instinctively hide pain and that pain, even from elective procedures, does not just magically go away once the animal is no longer in the hospital. Instead, the pain decreases gradually over a period of days to weeks (depending on the severity of the disease, injury or surgery) and the pain that the animal experiences in that time should be addressed. Even if the animal appears 'okay', we know that, depending on the source of the pain, nerves were cut or damaged, tissue was traumatized, and/or inflammation was induced. These sources of pain will undoubtedly cause some discomfort that does not cease as the patient exits our hospital door. So don't quit until pain quits! Or at least don't quit until the patient is comfortable and that lingering pain, if present, isn't negatively impacting the patient's quality of life.

Analgesic Drugs

For treatment of acute pain, we commonly utilize 3 major classes of analgesic drugs (opioids, local anesthetics and nonsteroidal anti-inflammatory drugs [NSAIDs]) and two 'adjunctive' classes, alpha-2 agonists and N-methyl-D-aspartate [NMDA] receptor antagonists (ketamine and amantadine). Other drugs that may be utilized in acute pain include maropitant and gabapentin. In addition to discussing the drugs themselves, the way the drugs are used or 'analgesic techniques' are important and will be discussed.

Opioids

Opioids provide moderate to profound analgesia, have a very high safety margin, are reversible, and many are inexpensive. Furthermore, opioids provide sedation (at least in dogs) and are versatile, meaning they can be administered PO, IM, IV, SQ, transdermally, as a CRI (constant rate infusions), in the epidural space, or in the intra-articular space. The adverse effects of this class are largely over-rated, uncommon in most patients receiving appropriate dosages and sometimes annoying (like the vomiting) but very unlikely to be serious. Furthermore, the adverse effects are reversible. The adverse effects can include nausea, vomiting, slowing of GI motility, excessive sedation, excitement, and dysphoria. Because opioids are commonly administered pre-operatively, there is a large volume of basic information on this drug class in Chapter 4. The information in this chapter will focus on the clinical use of opioids.

There are 3 main categories of opioids based on their binding to the mu and kappa opioid receptors: full opioid agonists that bind to and activate both mu and kappa receptors; agonists-antagonists that bind to and activate kappa receptors but bind to and antagonize (or reverse) opioid effects at the mu receptor; and partial agonists that bind to and partially activate the mu receptors.

Full Opioid Agonists

Morphine, hydromorphone, fentanyl, methadone, and oxymorphone are full opioid agonists. This is the most potent class of opioids and should be considered any time that pain occurs, especially if pain is moderate to severe. Clinically, these should be the main opioids used in practice because they are potent and because they are affordable for the practice and the client. Both morphine and hydromorphone are inexpensive in the U.S. and methadone is inexpensive in many other countries. Opioids in this class can be used as boluses, infusions, in the epidural space, and in the joint space. Fentanyl can be administered transdermally and methadone can be administered on the oral mucosa (called 'oral transmucosal' or 'OTM' administration).

> ## TIP
> Use a full opioid agonist as the standard opioid in your practice since they are potent and many are inexpensive. A partial agonist or agonist-antagonist is appropriate if the pain is mild to moderate.

> ## TIP
> Utilize a variety of routes of administration for differing effects. This includes IM or IV bolus for quick onset for pre-operative use; transdermal for long duration postoperative use; epidurally for long duration analgesia with minimal systemic effects; as a constant rate infusion for minute-to-minute control over delivery; or OTM (oral transmucosal) as a convenient, easy way for owners to medicate their pet at home.

Agonist-antagonists

Butorphanol and nalbuphine are agonist-antagonists. These drugs provide only mild to moderate analgesia and both have a very short duration of action. They should be reserved for treatment of mild to moderate pain and should always be used as part of a multimodal protocol. Because of the low potency and short duration, these drugs should not be used alone for pain from surgical procedures or trauma. The time to onset is < 5 minutes and the duration of action is 45 (dogs) to 90 (cats) minutes, which is not long enough to effectively control pain from most surgeries. Butorphanol provides mild to moderate sedation, which can be an advantage when administered preoperatively. Nalbuphine causes mild to no sedation.

> ## TIP
> Use butorphanol for sedation but not for analgesia for most procedures because of the short duration of action.

Partial Agonists

These currently include only buprenorphine. Buprenorphine is not as potent as the full opioid agonists and should be part of a multimodal protocol for surgical or trauma pain. The duration of action is longer than that of most other opioids but not as long as once presumed and is dependent on both dose and severity of pain. It has a slow onset so is not ideal for immediate control of pain unless combined with a faster acting drug (like dexmedetomidine). The time to onset is 10 to 20 minutes and the duration of action is 4 to 8 hours. The exception is the FDA-approved buprenorphine (Simbadol®) that is specifically for cats and has a time to onset of 1 hour and a duration of action of 24 hours. Buprenorphine is not very sedating which can be an advantage postoperatively if sedation is not needed or desired. Buprenorphine is absorbed when administered on the oral mucosa but the absorption from this route is much lower and less predictable than originally thought. Thus the dose should be higher than the dose for IM administration. The current recommendation is that the OTM (oral transmucosal dose) should be roughly double the IM dose (so 0.03-0.06 mg/kg). The dose of Simbadol® is 0.24 mg/kg. However, we commonly use 50-75% of that dose in sick, geriatric and pediatric cats.

TIP

Oral transmucosal (OTM) administration of buprenorphine is a reasonable route of administration that allows pet owners to deliver buprenorphine once their pet has come home from the hospital. However, recent evidence proves that buprenorphine administered OTM does NOT reach the same serum concentrations and the serum concentrations are not as predictable compared to IV or IM administration. Thus the OTM buprenorphine dose is HIGHER than the IM/IV dose and the OTM route should not replace injections in hospitalized patients.

Special Note on Tramadol

Tramadol is called an 'opioid like' drug because a portion of its effects are mediated through the opioid pathway. In addition to having some opioid effects, tramadol is a norepinephrine and serotonin reuptake inhibitor **(SNRI)**. Drugs in the SNRI class are primarily used as antidepressants but do have some weak analgesic properties. There are several problems with tramadol, especially in dogs.

• The bioavailability (which means the amount of drug 'available' in the body to produce effects) is INCREDIBLY variable, which means that some dogs probably absorb enough drug to have an analgesic effect while others get next to nothing.
• The drug is cleared 4x faster in dogs than in humans, so it has a very short duration of efficacy.
• Dogs (and most animals except for humans) don't make an intermediate metabolite when the drug is metabolized by the liver. Unfortunately, it is that intermediate metabolite that provides most of the tramadol-mediated analgesia.
• The tramadol-mediated analgesia in animals, especially in dogs, is more likely due to the WEAK SNRI effects rather than opioid effects.
• Tramadol bioavailability is higher in cats than in dogs but, like dogs, cats don't make the intermediate metabolite and often become dysphoric on tramadol.
• Tramadol has a very, very bitter taste - once an animal has tasted it, that animal will have a strong aversion to the drug. Cats HATE it.

Because there may be mild analgesia from the SNRI pathway, tramadol maybe an effective 'add on' drug since even a little analgesia from tramadol PLUS analgesia from some other drug provides multimodal pain relief. Tramadol may be more appropriate for multimodal analgesia in mild to moderate chronic pain than in acute post-surgical pain (which can be fairly severe). The highly variable bioavailability, inadequate formation of the active intermediate metabolite and short duration of action (only lasts 2 to 6 hours) makes it inappropriate for use as a sole drug for postoperative pain. The dose is 2 to 10 mg/kg BID every 4-8 hours. The starting dose is commonly 2-5 mg/kg. Lower dosages are less likely to cause sedation, but also less likely to provide analgesia.

Non-Steroidal Anti-Inflammatory Drugs (NSAIDs)

NSAIDS are one of the few classes of drugs available that actually treat the source of the pain (inflammation) as well as the pain itself. Because of this impact on the pathology (inflammation) that is causing the pain, NSAIDs should be administered any time that pain of inflammation is present, unless they are contraindicated in the patient. Remember, most of the painful conditions that we treat, like surgery, trauma, osteoarthritis and cancer, involve some degree of inflammation. It is important to use drugs that are FDA-approved in each species. FDA-approved NSAIDs include: carprofen, meloxicam, deracoxib, robenacoxib, firocoxib and grapiprant for dogs, and meloxicam and robenacoxib for cats. The individual drugs have been covered in detail in other publications so we don't have a lot of information on NSAIDs in this book, but we do use NSAIDs in almost every patient (unless they are truly contraindicated) for both acute and chronic pain.

• The advantages of the NSAID class of drugs include: One of the few drug classes that treat pain at its source (i.e., inflammation), relatively long-lasting analgesia, easy to administer, and not controlled so no extra record keeping.
• The disadvantages of the NSAID class of drugs include: Not suitable for patients with some pre-existing diseases (e.g., renal or hepatic disease, bleeding disorders) and may cause GI upset, GI ulceration, platelet abnormalities and renal or hepatic dysfunction.
  • The renal and hepatic effects of NSAIDs are often the most serious, but they are also the most rare. GI ulceration is also serious and is slightly more common than renal and hepatic effects.
  • Mild GI upset (nausea, vomiting, decreased appetite, maybe mild abdominal discomfort) is THE MOST COMMON adverse effect of NSAIDS, so the MOST COMMON adverse effects should not be ignored, but would rarely cause serious problems. In fact, based on the number of NSAIDs dosed every day compared to the number of serious adverse effects that occur, NSAIDs are a very safe class of drugs (when dosed appropriately, of course).
  • Sometimes it seems that there is a high percentage of adverse effects, but that is only because we dispense a lot of NSAIDs - more than any other drug class - so we may see more adverse effects just because there are more patients on the drugs. Because of its mechanism of action, grapiprant causes fewer adverse effects than traditional NSAIDs.

IMPORTANT POINT
When dosed appropriately to patients that have no contraindications, NSAIDS are a fairly safe class of drugs. It only seems like there are more adverse effects because we have so many patients receiving NSAIDs!

Can NSAIDs be administered to Cats?

YES! We can and we should administer NSAIDs to cats! Although we don't know everything about NSAIDs and cats, we do know that cats have pain of inflammation and NSAIDs are approved for use in cats. Both injectable meloxicam (approved in the US) and injectable carprofen (approved in other countries but not the US) are used as a one-time injection to treat acute pain in cats. Oral meloxicam is approved in MANY countries other than the US for use for chronic pain. Robenacoxib is approved for oral and/or injectable administration for up to 3 days in the US and 6 days in other countries. Oral robenacoxib is approved for treatment of chronic pain in cats in countries other than the US.

Although it is true that cats may be a little more 'sensitive' than dogs to the adverse effects of NSAIDs, the main reason for the NSAID-related adverse events and subsequent fear of NSAIDs in cats occurred because WE overdosed cats. The US label dose for meloxicam in cats is extremely high (0.3 mg/kg) compared to the label dose in other countries (usually 0.05-0.1 mg/kg) and dosages recommended in the literature (often as low as 0.01-0.03 mg/kg). Thus to appropriately use NSAIDs in cats, the DOSE must be correct! We recommend using meloxicam at a lower dose than the label dose or using robenacoxib at the label dose (it is not too high!).

Should NSAIDs be Administered Preoperatively or Postoperatively?

NSAIDs can be administered EITHER preoperatively or postoperatively depending on the patient, the reason for administering the NSAIDs and the comfort level of your practice. Like most analgesic drugs, NSAIDs are more effective if administered preemptively. So for efficacy, give preoperatively. But what about safety? Prostaglandins (chemical compounds in the body that control many body functions) control the blood flow to many organs, including the kidneys, by controlling blood vessel diameter. If blood flow - usually determined by measuring blood pressure - is adequate, the prostaglandins don't need to do anything. But if the flow is low, for instance in a patient that is dehydrated, losing a lot of blood, or hypotensive due to anesthesia, the prostaglandins become very important in normalizing blood flow. Since NSAIDs block prostaglandins, they eliminate this protective effect. So if the patient is likely to become hypotensive under anesthesia, postoperatively may be best.

Based on that Information, When should we Administer NSAIDs?

• Preoperatively in hydrated, healthy patients admitted for elective surgical procedures in which moderate to profound hypotension or hemorrhage is unlikely.
  • If patients in your practice are commonly hypotensive under anesthesia, first we should fix the anesthesia protocol!
• Postoperatively in patients that would benefit from IV fluids or blood pressure stabilization or patients that could potentially experience moderate to profound hemorrhage during surgery.

- POSTOPERATIVELY DOES NOT MEAN START TOMORROW!
- Start with injectable NSAIDs as soon as you are comfortable with the fact that the patient won't become hypotensive. So administer just before or just at the time the vaporizer is being turned off (since the biggest contributor to hypotension is the inhalant!)
- Then have the owner start the next day with oral NSAIDs.
- Waiting too long to start the NSAID will allow all of the perioperative analgesia to wear off and we have to start our analgesic plan all over, now with a patient in pain.
  - Preemptive analgesia works - but balanced analgesia is the goal - once preemptive wears off, pain will resume, and it is much harder to treat pain than prevent pain.
- Discharge the patient with NSAIDs for the duration of expected pain that needs to be treated. Probably somewhere between 4-10 days for most mild to moderate soft tissue pain and 7-21 days for orthopedic and severe soft tissue pain.
- Because cats may be more 'sensitive' to the adverse effects of NSAIDs, some veterinarians prefer to use postoperative administration in all cats, healthy or not. This is not a wrong decision - especially if it means that the clinic is more comfortable with administration of the drug and cats get NSAIDs!

Recommendation for Perioperative NSAID Administration in Cats and Dogs

Use injectable NSAIDs for perioperative pain and send the patient home on the oral formulation of the same NSAID.

TIP
For Starting NSAIDs postoperatively, Don't wait! Administer an injectable NSAID as soon as the vaporizer is turned off! Turning off the vaporizer will allow the inhalant dose to decrease - and the inhalant contribution to hypotension is dose dependent.

Local Anesthetic Drugs

Local anesthetic drugs are inexpensive, easy to administer and very effective. Local anesthetics are a highly under-utilized class of drugs, mainly because not everyone realizes the advantages of using local anesthesia when the patient is under general anesthesia. Local anesthetic drugs block pain impulses in the peripheral nerves and prevent the impulses from reaching the central nervous system. This effect alleviates or even eliminates the sensation of pain for the duration of the block and allows a decrease in the dosages of drugs used to provide general anesthesia, thereby improving anesthetic safety by decreasing the likelihood of dose-dependent adverse effects. This effect also decreases the likelihood that 'wind-up' or central sensitization will occur, so the overall sensation of pain will be less than it might have been without the use of local blocks. The only real disadvantage of local anesthetics is that they have a relatively short duration of action when compared to the duration of the pain, but that is easily compensated for with the use of multimodal analgesia.

The most commonly used local anesthetic drugs are bupivacaine, ropivacaine and lidocaine. The newest local anesthetic drug is NOCITA®, which is a liposome-encapsulated bupivacaine with a duration of action of up to 72 hours.

> **TIP**
> Use local anesthetic blocks in EVERY patient if at all possible.

Alpha-2 Adrenergic Agonists

All of the alpha-2 agonists provide reversible dose-dependent sedation AND analgesia, with medetomidine and dexmedetomidine providing better analgesia than some of the other alpha-2 agonists (xylazine). The disadvantage of the alpha-2 agonists is that they can cause cardiovascular changes that are not significant in patients with healthy hearts, but not appropriate for patients with most types of cardiovascular disease. See more in Chapter 4.

> **TIP**
> Include alpha-2 agonists as part of a multimodal protocol both pre- and post-operatively in dogs and cats. The post-operative 'rescue' dose is one of our favorite uses of alpha-2s.

NMDA Receptor Antagonists

Ketamine is the only NMDA-receptor antagonist that we currently use for acute pain (amantadine is an NMDA-receptor antagonist used to treat chronic pain). Ketamine is not a true analgesic drug when administered on its own but is used as part of a multimodal protocol to prevent or treat central sensitization or 'wind-up'. However, this effect is not achieved with induction doses of the drug but by a low-dose CRI. Ketamine is inexpensive so infusions are very economical for the practice.

> **TIP**
> Add ketamine to the IV fluids anytime that central sensitization may be a component of pain. Central sensitization is most likely to occur in patients that are painful before surgery (so more likely in a patient anesthetized for a fracture repair than in a patient anesthetized for an ovariohysterectomy [OHE or 'spay']) and those that have a lot of damage to the skin (burns, extensive abrasions or lacerations) since the skin is very highly innervated, meaning that skin damage can be very painful.

Maropitant

Is a drug that is actually approved to control vomiting but also likely has a role in pain management, especially the management of visceral pain, when used as part of a multimodal analgesic protocol. It is often administered as part of the premedications to control vomiting associated with the patient's disease and/or vomiting from drugs like the potent opioids. In addition to the maropitant-induced analgesia, the decrease in vomiting adds to the patient's overall comfort. Patients that receive maropitant also return to normal eating after surgery more quickly than patients that don't receive maropitant and normal nutritional intake is a very important part of healing.

Gabapentin

Is a drug that is not FDA-approved in animals but is very commonly used to treat pain, especially chronic pain. Gabapentin is used to treat a specific type of pain called 'neuropathic pain', which means pain from pathology of the nervous system. Examples of neuropathic pain include intervertebral disc disease, tumors that involve the nervous system, and damage to nerves from trauma. Neuropathic pain can also be caused by cutting nerves in surgery, especially large nerves like those cut during amputations. Pain from osteoarthritis (OA) can develop a neuropathic component due to changes in the pain pathway and OA pain can often be controlled with gabapentin used along with an NSAID to control the pain of inflammation. Cancer pain commonly has a neuropathic component.

The main adverse effect of gabapentin by far is sedation, although diarrhea can occur (not common). Ataxia can also occur, especially in older dogs with decreased muscle strength. The drug does not cause renal or hepatic damage but is partially metabolized by the liver (at least in dogs) and partially excreted unchanged by the kidney so hepatic or renal disease can slow elimination of gabapentin. Thus, in patients with dysfunction of either of those organs, a decreased dose may be necessary to compensate for drug accumulation.

Although no research manuscripts are available regarding the use of gabapentin in dogs and cats for the treatment of chronic pain, this is a common recommendation:

• The dosage generally ranges from 3-20 mg/kg/dose PO BID to QID but dosages as high as 50 mg/kg have been anecdotally reported.
• Generally, gabapentin therapy is initiated at 5 mg/kg BID (3-10 mg/kg depending on pain level and health of patient).
• The dose should be increased by about 25% every 3-7 days (3 days for severe pain, 7 for mild pain) until the patient gets relief from pain or gets sedate. IF THE PATIENT DOESN'T GET RELIEF OR SEDATION, YOU HAVEN'T REALLY TRIED GABAPENTIN!
• If the patient becomes sedate with the first 1-3 doses, decrease the dose and start again. Gradually increasing the dose over time often decreases the incidence of sedation.
• If the patient becomes sedate at higher dosages, back down to the last dose that was not sedating and maintain treatment for 2-4 weeks, then reassess efficacy of the drug.
• If the patient becomes ataxic at any dose, back down to the last dose that did not cause ataxia and maintain treatment for 2-4 weeks, then reassess efficacy of the drug.
• If the patient is to be removed from gabapentin therapy (e.g., the patient is

'cured' or the gabapentin is not working), the drug should be gradually withdrawn over a period of one to three weeks (depending on the duration of therapy and the dose administered) to prevent rebound hyperalgesia.

Analgesic Techniques

A discussion of pain management should not be limited to a discussion of drugs, but should also include a discussion of ways to use the drugs and ways to provide analgesia that does not include drugs. Of course, bolus injections of drugs are commonly used, as are constant rate infusions (CRIs) and local/regional blockade.

Constant Rate Infusions (CRIs)

CRIs of analgesic drugs are an excellent way to manage pain in all species in which IV access can be obtained. A CRI of analgesic drugs has several advantages over multiple repeated injections for pain relief, including: A more stable plane of analgesia with less incidence of break-through pain (which can be difficult to treat); A lower drug dosage delivered at any given time, resulting in a lower incidence of dose-related side effects; Greater control over drug administration (easy to change the dose); Decreased need for stimulation of resting patients to administer drugs; and Decreased cost (when compared to technician time, needles and syringes required for repeat injections). Drugs that are useful for CRIs include fentanyl, hydromorphone, morphine, methadone, butorphanol, ketamine, lidocaine, dexmedetomidine and a myriad of combinations of these drugs.

Local and Regional Blockade

This is an effective, easy and inexpensive way to make a profound impact on a patient's pain. Commonly used local anesthetic blocks include: incisional, maxillary, mandibular, digit, brachial plexus, intercostal, testicular and many others. Local anesthetics can also be used in the epidural and articular spaces. Regional blockade includes epidurals. Opioids, like morphine, should be used for epidurals because of the long duration of action with minimal to no systemic effects or motor blockade.

Non-Pharmacologic Therapy

Nonpharmacologic therapy can also be used to decrease post-operative pain and is commonly used to treat chronic pain. Therapies that could be considered as multimodal additions for treatment of acute and chronic pain include (but are not limited to): Thermotherapy (heat or ice), acupuncture, physical therapy and rehabilitation including light exercise (like walking or swimming), low-level laser and transcutaneous electrical nerve stimulation (TENS). Non-pharmacologic therapies can be very effective and we highly recommend them.

Incorporating Analgesic Techniques into Surgical Protocols

Anesthesia is divided into 4 separate and equally important phases (preanesthesia, induction, maintenance and recovery). Analgesia should be divided into those same four phases, although analgesia is not usually addressed during induction (Figure 7-4).

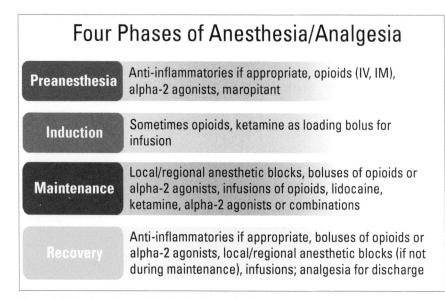

Four Phases of Anesthesia/Analgesia

Preanesthesia	Anti-inflammatories if appropriate, opioids (IV, IM), alpha-2 agonists, maropitant
Induction	Sometimes opioids, ketamine as loading bolus for infusion
Maintenance	Local/regional anesthetic blocks, boluses of opioids or alpha-2 agonists, infusions of opioids, lidocaine, ketamine, alpha-2 agonists or combinations
Recovery	Anti-inflammatories if appropriate, boluses of opioids or alpha-2 agonists, local/regional anesthetic blocks (if not during maintenance), infusions; analgesia for discharge

Figure 7-4. The four phases of analgesia for surgical pain are the same as the four phases of anesthesia.

Preanesthesia Phase
Use boluses of opioids, alpha-2 agonists, maropitant and NSAIDs. Consider starting a CRI and/or applying transdermal fentanyl for patients with moderate to severe pain.

Induction Phase
Not the most common phase for addressing analgesia but boluses of opioids (often fentanyl because of its rapid onset) can be part of induction.

Maintenance Phase
Can repeat boluses of opioids or alpha-2 agonists. Use local and regional blocks and/or use CRIs. Analgesia in the maintenance period improves anesthetic safety by allowing a decrease in the need for inhalant anesthetic drugs. Analgesia in the maintenance phase can also make the patient more comfortable in the recovery phase, in part because central sensitization is a lot less likely to occur if adequate analgesia is provided at the time of most intense pain.

Recovery Phase

PAIN MUST BE ADDRESSED in recovery. That doesn't necessarily mean that the patient needs analgesia, but the patient should be assessed for pain and the duration of analgesic drugs that have been administered need to be considered. The analgesic effects from the drugs administered preoperatively are generally decreased by the time the patient is in recovery. We are often asked, 'how can you tell pain from post-operative dysphoria'? The answer is that we can't always tell AND pain itself can cause dysphoria - so, if in doubt, TREAT FOR PAIN!

CRITICAL POINT!

It can be very difficult to differentiate pain from dysphoria in the postoperative period - especially since pain can be a cause of the dysphoria! If post-operative excitement occurs for 30-60 seconds, it is probably just a brief dysphoric episode and can be left untreated. IF THE EXCITEMENT LASTS LONGER THAN THIS BRIEF PERIOD, IT SHOULD BE TREATED. It doesn't matter if it is pain OR dysphoria, prolonged and/or profound excitement in recovery is NOT ACCEPTABLE. Treat with a low dose of an alpha-2 agonist for sedation AND analgesia. Consider a dose of opioids if the analgesic effects of the opioid administered pre- or intra-operatively have likely diminished. Base this decision on your knowledge of the duration of action of opioids. And remember that response to analgesia is VERY individual so even if you think the opioid should still be effective - it might not be effective in this patient so don't be afraid to re-dose! The effects of both alpha-2 agonists and opioid are reversible so you can treat pain/dysphoria when it occurs and reverse the effects later, if necessary.

Postoperative Treatment Options/Considerations Include:

• Repeated boluses of opioids and/or alpha-2 agonists.
• Continued CRIs (or may need to start a CRI if one was not used intra-operatively).
• Administration of 24-hour duration FDA-approved buprenorphine to cats.
• Application of transdermal fentanyl to dogs or cats.
• Administration of NSAIDs (if not administered preoperatively).
• Prescription of drugs/techniques to be utilized after discharge from the hospital. NSAIDs are commonly used postoperatively.
• Initiation of non-pharmacologic therapy both in the immediate recovery period and for continued treatment at home. Post-operative techniques that the owners can do at home include icing incisions, simple flexion/extension exercises, light massage, and controlled leash walking.

IMPORTANT TIP

Don't forget to send home analgesic drugs for the owner to administer for several days after the surgery. Pain does not end just because the patient left the hospital and pain is not absent just because the pet doesn't show pain at home (it may be HIDING pain)!

Sample Perioperative Analgesic Protocols

Sample perioperative analgesic protocols are listed in **Table 7-8** and more protocols are presented in Chapter 9. Remember, it is important to use the 3 principles of pain management when designing analgesic protocols (use of preemptive analgesia, use of multimodal analgesia, don't quit until pain quits) and to address pain in all phases (except maybe induction) of anesthesia.

Summary

Safe anesthesia **cannot be done** without effective analgesia and failure to treat pain adequately can lead to major adverse events. Analgesic drugs and techniques should be added into the premedication, maintenance AND recovery phases of anesthesia. Major drug classes that are commonly used to control pain include opioids, NSAIDs and local anesthetic drugs. Adjunctive drugs/drug classes that are commonly used to control pain include ketamine and the alpha-2 agonists. Maropitant and gabapentin may also be used. The three principles of pain management (use of preemptive analgesia, use of multimodal analgesia, don't quit until pain quits) should be followed when designing analgesic protocols.

Table 7-8
Analgesic Protocol Suggestions for a Variety of Painful Procedures in Dogs and Cats. Protocols are Based on the Three Principles of Analgesia: Use Preemptive Analgesia, Use Multimodal Analgesia, Don't Quit Until Pain Quits!

Surgery	Species	Considerations	Preemptive/Multi-modal	Intraoperative	Postoperative
OHE or Castration	Dog	These surgeries are PAINFUL. We call them 'routine' because the surgery is easy, not because they don't cause pain.	-Hydromorphone (0.1 to 0.2 mg/kg), morphine (0.5 mg/kg) or methadone (0.3-0.5 mg/kg) -Alpha-2 agonist for sedation AND analgesia 0.003 to 0.010mg/kg dexmedetomidine; -NSAID? More effective if administered preemptively. Choose from the NSAIDs FDA-approved for preoperative use. Consider injectable NSAIDs.	-Testicular block with local anesthetics for neuter, -Ovarian ligament block or peritoneal lavage with local anesthetics for OHE.	-NSAIDs for 4+ days -Tramadol or other adjunctive? Perhaps. Especially with OHEs and especially if tissue handling is 'rough' or prolonged. Exact level of pain is unknown.
OHE or Castration	Cat	Same comment as for the dog.	-Hydromorphone (0.1 mg/kg), morphine (0.2 to 0.3 mg/kg) or methadone	-Testicular block with local anesthetics for neuter,	-0.01 to 0.03 mg/kg OTM buprenorphine BID x 4 days OR

Table 7-8 continued

			(0.3 mg/kg); Buprenorphine (0.03 mg/kg) IM may be sufficient for castration if multimodal analgesia used; Simbadol buprerphine can be administered at 0.24 mg/kg -Alpha-2 agonist for sedation AND analgesia, dexmedetomidine (0.008 to 0.015 mg/kg IM); - NSAID? More effective if administered preemptively. 0.1 mg/kg meloxicam or 2 mg/kg oral or SQ robenacoxib.	-Ovarian ligament block or peritoneal lavage with local anesthetics for OHE.	Simbadol buprenorphine at 0.24 mg/kg SID x 3 days AND/OR - NSAIDs - continue oral robenacoxib for 2 more days, could continue meloxicam at 0.05 mg/kg OFF LABEL
Orthopedic Procedure	Dog	More painful than OHE, need more analgesia.	-Hydromorphone (0.2 mg/kg), morphine (1.0 mg/kg) or methadone (0.5 to 1.0 mg/kg) Consider applying a fentanyl patch.	-CRI (e.g., morphine, lidocaine, ketamine)	-NSAIDs for 7 to 14 days; -Add gabapentin, codeine, etc., if transdermal fentanyl was not utilized or until fentanyl patch

Orthopedic Procedure					
			Patches take 12 hours for onset in the dog. Provides analgesia for 3 days. --Alpha-2 agonist for sedation AND analgesia; -NSAID? More effective if administered preemptively. Choose from the NSAIDs FDA-approved for preoperative use. Consider injectable NSAIDs.	-Local or regional blockade (i.e., epidural analgesia for procedures on rear legs, brachial plexus block for procedures of the forelimb, etc.). Consider using NOCITA.	is fully effective (ie, for first 12 hours after patch placement).
	Cat	Same comment as for the dog.	-Use the most potent opioids listed in the OHE protocol and use the high end of the dose. Consider applying a fentanyl patch. Takes 6 hours for onset in the cat, provides analgesia for >3 days.	-Same as for dog but might not use lidocaine for the CRI. Consider using NOCITA.	-NSAIDs as described for OHE -If fentanyl patch not used OTM buprenorphine 0.02 to 0.05 mg/kg BID-TID for +/- 7 days OR -Simbadol buprenorphine as described above

Table 7-8 continued

| Abdominal Exploratory | Dog or Cat | More painful than OHE and often done in sick patients. Pain can cause further complications and impair healing. | Exact drugs & dosages depend on health of patient -OPIOIDS for sure - may need to use low end of dose -Alpha-2s depend on cardiovascular status -NSAIDs more likely to use postop if at all, depends on underlying disease | -CRI (e.g., morphine, lidocaine, ketamine); -Local or regional blockade (i.e., epidural analgesia, incisional blockade, etc.) Cat specific: can omit lidocaine from the CRI | Depends on health status -Continue CRIs postoperatively -Send home on opioids -NSAIDs if appropriate |

OHE- ovariohysterectomy or 'spay'; OTM - oral transmucosal; BID - twice a day; TID - three times a day; CRI - constant rate infusion

Although large animal species are covered elsewhere, we wanted to make the point here that the same principles apply regardless of the species! Here are just a few thoughts on analgesic protocols for large animals.

Surgery	Species	Considerations	Preemptive/ Multimodal	Intraoperative	Postoperative
Castration	Horse	These surgeries are PAINFUL. We call them 'routine' because the surgery is easy, not because they don't cause pain.	-Butorphanol; -Alpha-2 agonist: Xylazine, detomidine or romifidine; -NSAIDs - flunixin meglumine, phenylbutazone or firocoxib.	-Intratesticular injection of local anesthetics	-NSAIDs

Disbudding, dehorning	Goat or calf	This surgery hurts and will cause the patient to decrease feed intake for several days.	-Butorphanol or buprenorphine; -Alpha-2 agonist (could use small animal alpha-2 agonists for better analgesia); -NSAIDs	-Local anesthetic blockade around horn buds - be careful with dosages since kid goats are very small and overdosing is unfortunately easy.	-NSAIDs
Orthopedic Procedure	Any	More painful than soft tissue proce-dures.	-Appropriate opioid for the patient -Alpha-2 agonists -NSAIDs	-Constant rate infusion (e.g., morphine, lidocaine, ketamine); -Local or regional blockade. Consider using NOCITA.	-Continue NSAIDs; -May need to add other drugs or continue CRIs or local blocks

Local and Regional Anesthesia Blocks

This topic is one of the most important in the book because local/regional anesthesia (also called local/regional analgesia and local 'blocks') is a major component of effective analgesia. This topic is also important to technicians/nurses because these blocks should/can be done by technicians/nurses in most practices. Most state veterinary guidelines do not mention anything about pain management but many do specify that licensed technicians can administer SQ and IM injections and most of the local blocks fall into that category. It is generally more efficient and more effective for the technicians/nurses to do the blocks as they are preparing the patient for a procedure than to wait for the veterinarian to do the blocks immediately before inducing pain.

Benefits of Local/Regional Blocks

• Local anesthetic drugs are extremely effective, inexpensive and easy to use. They have a high safety margin, can be used in most, if not all, species and are cost effective, which can increase profits to the clinic.

• Local anesthetic drugs provide profound analgesia. In fact, they are the only drug class that can cause complete loss of sensation - which is why they are called 'anesthetics'! All of the other analgesic drugs make the patient more comfortable but do not eliminate all pain.

• In addition to the local analgesia at the site of the pain, the local anesthetic drugs prevent pain impulses from reaching the central nervous system. This has several positive effects:

  • Because pain impulses don't get to the brain, the anesthetized patient is not stimulated by pain and is less likely to wake up during painful procedures. This means that the dose of anesthetic drug (usually an inhalant drug) needed to keep the patient asleep is reduced. Decreasing the dose will decrease the likelihood that dose-dependent cardiovascular and respiratory depression from the inhalants will occur, thus making anesthesia safer.

  • The likelihood that 'wind-up' or central sensitization will occur is greatly decreased because the portion of the pain pathway called 'transmission' is blocked. Transmission involves the conduction of pain impulses from the peripheral nociceptors (pain receptors) to the dorsal horn neurons in the spinal cord. The neurons in the dorsal horn are responsible for central sensitization. By blocking input to these neurons, central sensitization, or "wind-up", pain is reduced or eliminated. This increases patient comfort in the postoperative period and can decrease the need for postoperative pain medications.

Adverse Effects Caused by Local Anesthetic Drugs

With ALL drugs, it is just as important (or maybe even more important!) to know a drug's adverse effects as it is to know the drug's positive effects. Adverse effects from local anesthetic drugs are extremely rare but can include:

• Central nervous system effects are the most common adverse effects of lidocaine over dosage. Effects include muscle tremors and fasciculations, and, with profound overdose, seizures and coma.

- An over-dosage of bupivacaine is most likely to cause cardiac effects (arrhythmias, hypotension and even cardiac 'collapse' or complete dysfunction). This is most likely if the bupivacaine is administered as an IV bolus, thus, it should NEVER BE ADMINISTERED IV.

CRITICAL POINT!
ONLY LIDOCAINE CAN BE SAFELY ADMINISTERED IV. All other local anesthetic drugs can cause severe adverse effects or even death if injected IV. Some IV uptake may occur following injection of the drug into the tissues, just be sure to aspirate before you inject so that you don't inject a bolus into the bloodstream!

- Local tissue effects such as swelling, bleeding and inflammation can occur and should be anticipated with the injection of ANY drug into the tissue.
- Allergies are REALLY RARE, especially with the group of local anesthetics that are commonly used. This is the 'amide' group and includes lidocaine and bupivacaine.
- Methemoglobinemia (damaged hemoglobin) appears to occur in cats only, is VERY RARE and clinically insignificant so this DOES NOT LIMIT the use of local anesthetics in cats.

Most Commonly Used Local Anesthetic Drugs
(Table 7-9)
- Lidocaine has a very fast onset of action (starts working almost immediately) and about a 90-minute duration of action. Use lidocaine for procedures in which pain will be of very short duration. Lidocaine - and only lidocaine - can be administered IV for a constant rate infusion.
- Bupivacaine (some people call this drug 'marcaine') has a slightly slower onset of action (starts within 5 minutes but time to full block is a little longer) and about a 4-hour duration. Bupivacaine should be the local anesthetic used for most procedures since most pain caused by surgery and wound repair is likely to last several hours. The slower onset shouldn't be a problem if you plan ahead. One common technique is to do a rough scrub of the area to be blocked, inject the bupivacaine and then finish the scrub. For dental blocks, inject the bupivacaine before cleaning the teeth, then go back to do the painful procedures like extractions. By injecting the bupivacaine early in the preparation for the procedure, the drug has plenty of time to take effect prior to the painful stimulus without compromising the duration of analgesia.

Special note on mixing lidocaine and bupivacaine
Some people mix lidocaine and bupivacaine thinking that the lidocaine will cause fast onset while the bupivacaine will provide long duration. This might work, but the evidence is mixed. Some studies indicate that the mixture might cause too much dilution of the bupivacaine so that it does not provide the long duration. Our recommendation is to use straight bupivacaine whenever possible and to inject it as early as possible.

Table 7-9
Commonly used Local Anesthetic Drugs in Veterinary Medicine

DRUG	ONSET of ACTION	DURATION of ACTION	CLINICAL DOSE
Bupivacaine (Marcaine)	5 (up to 10 for full onset in very large nerves)	4-6 hours	1-2 mg/kg dog 0.5-1 mg/kg cat
Bupivacaine, liposome encapsulated (NOCITA®)	2-5 minutes	72 hours	5.3 mg/kg dog 10.6 mg/kg cat
Lidocaine	1-2 minutes	1-2 hours	4-6 mg/kg dog 2-4 mg/kg cat
Mepivacaine (Carbocaine)	2-5 (up to 10) minutes	2-3 hours	4-6 mg/kg dog 2-4 mg/kg cat
Ropivacaine	Slightly faster than bupivacaine	Slightly shorter than bupivacaine	1-2 mg/kg dog 0.5-1 mg/kg cat

• Nocita® is a liposome-encapsulated bupivacaine that provides 72-hours of analgesia. It is approved for blockade of incisions for stifle surgery in dogs and peripheral nerve blocks in cats. However, it can be used for almost any incision, wound block or peripheral nerve block. The drug should be injected at closure of the wound or incision. If injected before incision, the scalpel blade can disrupt the liposomes and cause rapid release of the bupivacaine, so the block does not last 72 hours. For a preemptive block, regular bupivacaine can be used prior to incision followed by NOCITA at closure. NOCITA can be used preemptively to block nerves that are not at the incision site (e.g., for the RUM block described in the next section).
• Mepivacaine is sometimes called carbocaine. It has an onset and duration of action that are between those of lidocaine and bupivacaine. It is most commonly used for diagnostic blocks in equine lameness but can also be used as a routine local anesthetic drug for local/regional blocks.
• Ropivacaine is very similar in onset and duration of action to bupivacaine, but a little less likely to cause blockade of motor nerves or adverse cardiovascular adverse effects. It can be used in place of bupivacaine at the same dose as bupivacaine (Table 7-9).

General Rules for using Local Anesthetic Drugs
• Calculate the total dosage of local anesthetic drugs that the patient can receive before you start injecting. More than one site often needs to be blocked and the total dose should be calculated and divided between the sites. CALCULATE ALL DRUG DOSAGES ON LEAN BODY WEIGHT!

CRITICAL TIP!
Don't overdose the patient! The local anesthetic drugs have a high safety margin when dosed and administered correctly. Always calculate the maximum dose that the patient can receive and do not exceed that dose.

• Look up the landmarks for the block, identify the landmarks on the patient - and prepare to INJECT!

IMPORTANT POINT
Trust your knowledge of anatomy! Use the guidelines in this or other books, find the anatomical location where the nerve(s) should be and INJECT! The local anesthetic drugs diffuse through tissue fairly readily and will reach the nerve if your injection is close. You have nothing to lose except the patient's pain by trying, as long as the dose is right. Nocita® injection is slightly different. Due to the liposomes, it has to be injected exactly where you want the bupivacaine to be released.

• Use good injection technique by inserting the needle directly into the tissue and backing out slightly to redirect if necessary (don't 'dig around' in the tissue with the needle) and ASPIRATE before every injection.

CRITICAL POINT!
Always aspirate before injecting! Most local anesthetic drugs have a very narrow safety margin when injected IV. Aspirate and make sure you don't inject into a blood vessel!

General Tips for using Local/Regional Blocks
• For most blocks, use a 22- to 25-gauge one-inch needle and a syringe large enough to hold the calculated volume of drugs. This will be appropriate for most of the blocks described in this chapter. If different equipment is required, it will be mentioned in the description of the block.

• For many blocks, the volume of local anesthetic calculated for the patient exceeds the volume that can be physically injected at the block site. This is not a problem because, for a block, the drug only needs to work locally - right where you inject it - and a lower volume will be effective as long as your injection site is fairly close to the nerve to be blocked. This is different from drugs that are administered systemically where the whole dose is required because the drug will need to circulate throughout the body. HOWEVER, the total drug dose that the patient can receive should always be calculated so that it is not exceeded if multiple sites are to be blocked. Where appropriate, volumes to be injected for specific blocks are mentioned in the description of the block.

• Occasionally, less volume is calculated using the mg/kg dose than is needed to cover the entire area to be desensitized. The local anesthetic drug can be diluted with saline if the calculated dose does not provide enough volume to cover the area that you want to block. This might be necessary if the area to block is large (a very big wound). Dilution of the local anesthetic is also often necessary for safe use in very small patients (e.g., 'pocket pets') because the calculated volume of the full strength drug will be very low.

IMPORTANT POINT
Small volume is NO EXCUSE for withholding local blocks in small patients (small cats and pocket pets). DILUTE the drug with saline so that you achieve an appropriate volume for injection and USE LOCAL BLOCKS!

• Local anesthetics, especially lidocaine, often 'sting' on injection because they are acidic drugs. Adding bicarbonate to the local anesthetic will decrease the sting. The rule for lidocaine is to add 1 part bicarbonate for every 9 parts of lidocaine. A 1 ml injection will be 0.9 mls lidocaine and 0.1 mls bicarbonate. Bupivacaine may cause less sting than lidocaine and less bicarbonate can potentially be used. Dilutions as low as 0.005:1 are reportedly effective. That means that for every 1 ml of bupivacaine, only 0.005 mls of bicarbonate are required.

IMPORTANT TIP
Bicarbonate should be added to lidocaine administered to conscious patients to decrease the 'sting' caused by the drug. In anesthetized patients, the sting is not intense enough to cause a reaction and the bicarbonate is not necessary.

• The addition of adjunctive analgesic drugs, like opioids or alpha-2 agonists, to the local anesthetics for peripheral nerve blocks may (the evidence is mixed) enhance and prolong the analgesia provided by the block (Brummett and Williams 2011). However, the evidence is fairly strong for the efficacy of dexmedetomidine (0.0001 mg/kg) and for buprenorphine (0.003-0.004 mg/kg) added to the local anesthetic.
• The addition of epinephrine to the local anesthetics may prolong the analgesia provided by the shorter acting local anesthetic drugs (lidocaine). However, concern for epinephrine-induced tachycardia and epinephrine-induced vasoconstriction with subsequent decreased blood flow to the area that is blocked may outweigh the benefits of prolonged analgesia.

Commonly used Local/Regional Blocks in Veterinary Medicine
General Blocks
'Line' Blocks
(also called 'incisional', 'infiltrative' or 'field' [as in the 'field' of surgery or injury] blocks):
As the title suggests, local anesthetic drugs are injected directly into, or around, an incision site or a wound. These blocks are extremely easy, and very important since the skin is highly innervated (meaning lots of nerves!) and may be the primary source of pain for many procedures. Line blocks can be used for any procedure that will have an incision or for repairing wounds.

Technique
• Insert the needle subcutaneously (no need to go too deep - unless the muscles are injured and are part of the pain source) at the site of the incision or wound. Inject local anesthetic as you advance the needle (or you can insert the needle to its full length and inject as the needle is pulled out of the tissue) **(Figure 7-5 A)**.
• Reinsert the needle and inject as many times as necessary to cover the entire surgery site or wound. For each injection, insert the needle into tissue that is already blocked (so that there is no pain from the needle stick) and then advance into unblocked tissue **(Figure 7-5 B)**.
• Volume: If the incision site or wound is large, the local anesthetic may be diluted with saline to allow for coverage of the entire painful site without exceeding the maximum drug dose. There is no guideline on how much saline you should add, but the key is to add just enough to increase the volume of drug so that the painful site can be covered but not so much that you make the drug too dilute as this may decrease effectiveness.
• If using Nocita® for this block, inject the Nocita® at closure, not before the incision.

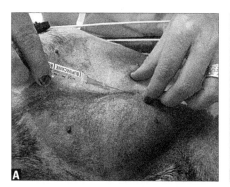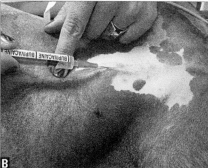

Figure 7-5. Injection of local anesthetic as a 'line' or incisional block on the midline of the abdomen. Inject local anesthetic subcutaneously as the needle is advanced, or the length of the needle can be inserted and the drug injected as the needle is withdrawn. The needle is inserted at a very 'flat' angle so that only the subcutaneous tissue is penetrated **(A)** and is reinserted and the drug injected as many times as necessary to cover the entire surgery site or wound **(B)**.

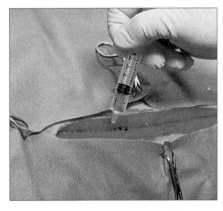

Figure 7-6. For a 'splash' block, the local anesthetic is sprayed or dripped onto the wound or incision. It is done after the deep layers of the incision are closed but before the skin is closed. It is not as effective as a block done before the incision is made.

Contraindications or Precautions

If the surgery site is for tumor removal, be sure that the block is made far enough away so that no needles are inserted into the tumor. There is the potential that needles inserted into tumors can spread the tumor cells to other sites that the needle penetrates.

Wound Diffusion Catheters (also called 'soaker' catheters) or Nocita®

Wound diffusion catheters and Nocita® are easy to use to deliver profound analgesia (local anesthetics are POTENT!) with no systemic effects (remember to calculate the right dose!) for several days. Pain from the incision or wound can be the biggest contributor to the overall level of pain that the patient is feeling so blockade of that source of pain for several days can be very beneficial for pain control **(Figure 7-7)**.

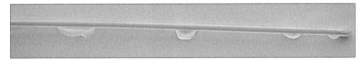

Figure 7-7. A wound diffusion catheter or 'soaker' catheter showing fluid exiting from all the small holes (fenestrations) along the distal end of the catheter. The section with the holes must be buried in a wound or incision so that local anesthetic will diffuse into the painful tissue.

• WHEN TO USE: The catheters or Nocita® (not together - one or the other) can be used for any large or deep incision or wound. Examples include: Limb amputations (fore or hind), mastectomies, large mass removal, large wounds, thoracotomies and ear canal ablations.
• EQUIPMENT LIST: Wound diffusion catheter, injection cap, pump (if you plan on continuous administration), a syringe large enough to hold the calculated volume of local anesthetic, bupivacaine or lidocaine +/- adjunctive drugs. For Nocita®, supplies include the drug, a syringe and a needle. The needle should be 25-G or larger to prevent disruption of the liposomes that might occur if they were squeezed through a very small needle.
  • Wound diffusion catheters can be purchased commercially or hand-made in

your clinic. MILA catheters are made specifically for veterinary patients, come in different lengths and can be purchased with a pump.

Technique
Have the surgeon:
• Incorporate the fenestrated portion of the catheter (the portion with holes) into the wound or incision before closure **(Figure 7-8 A)**.
• Place the catheter into the deepest part of the wound or subcutaneously.
• Be sure all of the fenestrations are in the wound or incision or the local anesthetic may exit the holes that are outside the skin rather than the holes that are in the tissue.
• Close the incision or wound.
• Suture the catheter in place and put the injection cap on the catheter **(Figure 7-8 B)**.

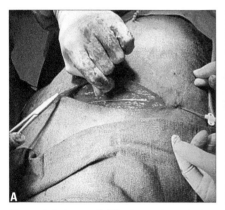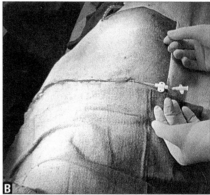

Figure 7-8. A wound diffusion catheter being incorporated into a large incision **(A)**. The incision is closed, the fenestrated portion of the catheter is buried in the tissue and local anesthetic is administered through the injection port at the top of the incision **(B)**.

Have the surgeon or other person responsible for analgesia:
• Inject a standard dose of lidocaine (2 to 6 mg/kg; lower end in cats) or bupivacaine (1 to 2 mg/kg; lower end in cats). Repeat that dose 2 (lidocaine) or 4 (bupivacaine) hours after the first dose, then start increasing the time between doses if the patient is comfortable.
• The volume of local anesthetic can be increased by diluting the drug with saline or sterile water.
• Extension of the dosing interval beyond the expected action of the drugs is possible because 1) multimodal analgesia is being used - any patient with a diffusion catheter will also be receiving systemic drugs and 2) the level of pain decreases over time.
   • By keeping the patient's incision from contributing to the overall pain sensation, the patient is much more comfortable, which means that the patient requires less analgesic drug(s).
• Alternatively, use a pump for continuous infusion. The pumps are specific for the

catheters and are very small so that they can be attached to a collar or harness.
• Leave the catheter in as long as necessary to keep the patient comfortable. Usually 1 to 5 days with 72 hours being the average, but catheters have been left in for as long as 2 weeks.
• Although not on the label, Nocita® can be redosed 72 hours after the first dose.

Contraindications/Precautions
None, other than general considerations for placement (not near a tumor) and wound management. Calculate the dose carefully so that the patient is not overdosed. In a study on complications of diffusion catheters used in veterinary patients, the most common complication was disconnection of the catheter from the diffusion pump. One patient got a seroma and one showed signs of local anesthetic toxicity. The infection rate with the catheter in place was no different than the incisional infection rate with no catheter (Abelson et al. 2009). This could be due to the fact that local anesthetic drugs have mild antimicrobial (ie, antibacterial) properties.

Blocks for Structures on the Head
Maxillary and Mandibular Blocks
These blocks are easy and provide analgesia not only for dental procedures but also for surgeries or wound repair on oral or nasal structures. Uses other than dentistry include maxillary and mandibular fracture repairs, tumor removal, mandibulectomies, maxillectomies, rhinoscopies and nasal biopsies. Because there are so many uses other than dentistry, these blocks should be called 'oral blocks' or 'maxillofacial' blocks (as in human medicine) rather than 'dental blocks'!

Infraorbital Block
This block will desensitize the tissues that are in front of ('rostral to') the infraorbital foramen to the midline on the same side as the injection. Tissues blocked include roots of the teeth (including the front 4th premolar roots), part of the upper lip and the nasal passages, and the nostrils.

• WHEN TO USE THE INFRAORBITAL BLOCK: Use for any procedure in the area desensitized including dentistry on the premolars and incisors, laceration repair on the lip or nose, tumor removal from the lip or nose, and surgery on the nares.

Technique
• The infraorbital nerve exits the infraorbital foramen **(Figures 7-9, 7-10 A-B)**, which can be palpated as a depression in the oral mucosa above the 3rd premolar in the area where the gingiva on the maxillary bone 'folds over' to become the gingiva on the inside of the lip.
• There are two techniques
    • Inject local anesthetic under the gingiva just rostral to (or 'in front of') the foramen **(Figure 7-10 C)**.

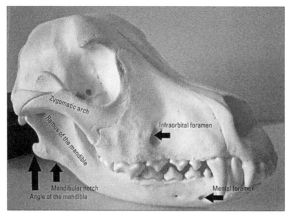

Figure 7-9. A dog skull with landmarks for maxillary and mandibular local blocks.

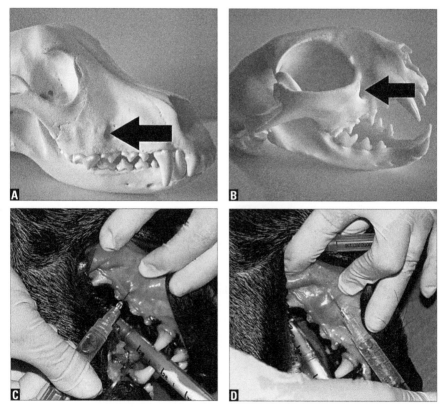

Figure 7-10. The infraorbital nerve exits the infraorbital foramen In a dog **(A)** and a cat **(B)**. Subgingival injection right in front of the infraorbital foramen of a dog **(C)**.The technique is the same in the cat. Local anesthetic injected into the infraorbital foramen of a dog **(D)**. This injection site generally allows a more caudal migration of the drug. The needle and syringe are almost parallel to the mandible. If the needle and syringe are angled away from the mandible, it will be difficult to insert the needle into the foramen.

- Or insert the tip of the needle into the infraorbital foramen (**Figure 7-10 D**) and inject.
- Injecting into the foramen insures more caudal ('backwards') spread of the block but is not necessary if the oral surgery site is rostral to the foramen (for example, surgery of the canine tooth).
- Also, the foramen can be difficult to locate or to enter in small dogs and cats but injection rostral to the canal is still useful, even if the surgery is caudal to the injection site, since there will be some caudal migration of the local anesthetic into the infraorbital canal.
- Because the distance between the foramen and the boney orbit is really short in cats and brachycephalic dogs, some people recommend that the needle not be placed in the foramen in these patients in order to avoid potential injury to the eye. We are comfortable with placing the needle in the foramen in these patients but just the TIP of the needle. You can do whichever technique you are comfortable with.

TIP
Applying pressure with your finger at the injection site may help force the anesthetic back into the foramen, which increases the likelihood that tissues caudal to the injection site are desensitized.

- **Volume:** For cats and small dogs 0.1 ml per side is adequate. For medium to large breed dogs 0.1 up to 0.5 mls per side is adequate.

Contraindications/Precautions
See comment about injecting into the foramen in small dogs and cats above.

Maxillary or 'Caudal Maxillary' Block
This block will desensitize the tissues from the site of the injection to the ipsilateral (ie, same side) midline, including tooth roots, soft tissue, the hard and soft palate, and much of the nasal passage and sinuses.

WHEN TO USE THE CAUDAL MAXILLARY BLOCK: Use for anything painful on the maxilla or in the nasal passage, sinuses and nares, as well as for dentistry. We prefer this block (any of the three approaches described below) to the infraorbital block in medium to large dogs since the distance from the infraorbital foramen back to the point that the maxillary nerve enters the the infraorbital canal is fairly long and the drug might not diffuse all the way to that site if injected at the infraorbital foramen. Remember, the farther back the nerve is blocked, the more tissues are desensitized! Because the distance from the infraorbital foramen to the site where the maxillary nerve enters the boney cavity in the skull is VERY short, the infraorbital injection site is most commonly used in cats and the caudal techniques may not be necessary.

Technique
There are 3 approaches: extraoral from the zygomatic arch, extraoral from the orbit, and intraoral.

EQUIPMENT: For the caudal extraoral block, a 1.5 inch needle is best in medium to large dogs, 1 inch can be used in all other patients. No special equipment is required for the other blocks.

• For the **caudal extraoral approach from the zygomatic arch** palpate the angle between the zygomatic arch (the bone under the eye) **(Figure 7-9)** and the ramus of the mandible (the part of the mandible that is vertical). This spot will be roughly 0.2 to 0.5 cm straight down from the lateral canthus of the eye (the outside corner of the eye), depending on the size of the patient. At this point, if the ramus of the mandible can't be palpated, the site can still be confirmed because the zygomatic arch starts to curve down (if you are palpating from back to front). Insert the needle at this location and keep the needle <u>parallel</u> with the maxilla as you aim the tip of the needle towards the premolars or the nostril on the opposite side of the head. This insures that the needle will not be anywhere close to the eye. When the needle hits bone or is completely buried in the muscle, aspirate and inject **(Figure 7-11 A & B)**.
• For the **extraoral from the orbit approach**, cover the eye with the lower eyelid and GENTLY push the eye back into the socket a few millimeters (alternatively, you can pull the lower eyelid out so that you can see the conjunctiva). Insert a 1.0 to 1.5 inch needle (depending on the size of the patient) at the midpoint of the ventral rim of the bony orbit and insert straight down between the globe and the bone. Aspirate and inject when the half (small dogs and cats) or all (medium to large dogs) of the one-inch needle is completely buried in the tissue **(Figure 7-11 C & D)**.
• When using an **intraoral approach**, open the patient's mouth as wide as possible. With cats, it can be difficult to open the mouth wide enough to get the needle and syringe in the oral cavity but this technique is fairly easy in most dogs. Insert the needle just caudal to and slightly towards the lingual (tongue) side of the most caudal maxillary molar. The needle should be inserted perpendicularly to the palate and the depth should be about 1-3 mm depending on body size. In other words, it is a very short distance from the gingiva to the site where the nerve will be blocked! Aspirate (there is a large vessel here!) and inject **(Figure 7-11 E & F)**.
• **Volume:** For all approaches, approximately 0.1 to 1.0 mls per site is usually sufficient in the in the dog, depending on size. The extraoral caudal maxillary block may require up to 2.0 mls per site in big dogs. For cats 0.1mls per site is sufficient.

Contraindications/Precautions
• For the extraoral caudal approach, BE SURE THAT THE NEEDLE IS KEPT PARALLEL TO THE MAXILLARY BONE. If the needle is aimed up, underneath the zygomatic arch towards the eye, it could cause blockade of the optic nerve and temporary blindness. This is a major deviation from the location of the block and is not a general concern, but has been reported in patients where the block was done incorrectly (REALLY incorrectly).
• For the intraoral approach, be sure to aspirate since injection of the drug into the palatine artery could occur.
• For the extraoral orbital approach, be gentle with the eye as it is pushed back into the socket as corneal ulcers could be caused by rough handling of the eye.

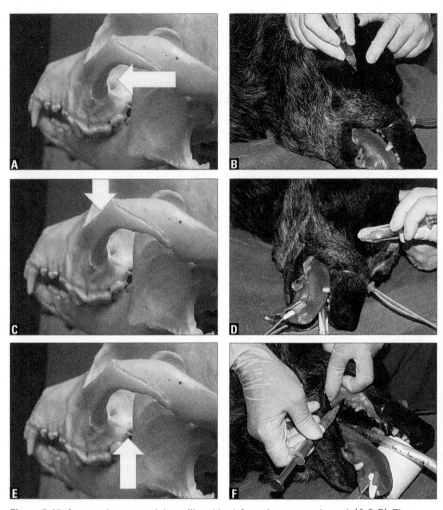

Figure 7-11. Approach to a caudal maxillary block from the zygomatic arch **(A & B)**. The arrow shows the location of the needle as it enters the angle formed by the zygomatic arch and the ramus of the mandible. The needle is several centimeters below the lateral canthus of the eye and both the needle and syringe are <u>parallel</u> to the maxillary dental arcade with the tip of the needle aimed at the nostril on the opposite side of the head so that it stays below the eye during the block. The needle is buried to the hub (or until it hits bone) in the masseter muscle. Approach to the caudal maxillary block from the rim of the orbit **(C & D)**. Location of the needle (arrow) as it enters the skin at the rim of the orbit. The eye is being gently and slightly pushed out of the way of the needle. The needle is inserted straight down inside the boney orbit to a depth where the needle is about half way between the rim of the orbit and the molars. Intra-oral approach to the caudal maxillary block from behind the last molar **(E & F)**. Location of the needle (arrow) as it enters the gingiva. The needle is inserted intra-orally behind the last molar to a depth of 1 to 3 mm. In each photo on the left, notice the maxillary foramen (the large 'hole') just on the rostral (front) edge of the zygomatic arch. The most efficient way to desensitize large areas of the skull is to block the maxillary nerve branches before they enter that foramen.

Pressure on the globe could also cause bradycardia.

Mandibular Block

This block desensitizes all soft and boney structures of the mandible from the site of the injection to the midline of the mandible (the 'symphysis') on the same side as the injection.

WHEN TO USE THE MANDIBULAR BLOCK: Use for any painful procedure on the mandible, including tooth extractions, mandibular fracture repair, mandibulectomy, tumor removal and biopsies.

Technique

There are two techniques: intraoral and extraoral. For both techniques, the tip of the needle needs to be near the mandibular foramen which is on the lingual (tongue) side of the mandible on a line from the last molar to the angle of the jaw (meaning the curve at the back of the mandible where the direction changes from horizontal to vertical; **Figure 7-12 A**).

- **For an Intraoral Approach (Figure 7-12 B):**
  - Place a soft mouth gag (a roll of tape or a foam hair curler, for example) that will hold the mouth gently open. Don't use rigid mouth gags that force the mouth to stay fully open. This is especially important in cats since holding the mouth fully open can cause compression of the artery that supplies blood to the cat's retina and some brain structures and can cause blindness and/or neurologic problems (Stiles et al. 2012; Barton-Lamb et al. 2013; Martin-Flores et al. 2014; Scrivani et al. 2014). In cats, a foam (disposable!) hair curler makes a great mouth gag!
  - Palpate the lingual side of the mandible behind the last molar. The nerve can sometimes be palpated behind the mandibular foramen on an imaginary line from the last molar to the angle of the jaw and will feel like a string or a stretching rubber band.
  - If the nerve can be palpated, inject the local anesthetic directly over the nerve.
  - If the nerve cannot be palpated inject the local anesthetic about ½ way between the angle of the jaw and the last molar. This will be really close to the nerve and the drug will diffuse to the nerve - trust your landmarks, aspirate, and inject!

- **For an Extraoral Approach:**
  - Palpate the mandibular notch from outside the mouth. It is a depression on the inside of the mandible just in front of the angle of the mandible **(Figure 7-9)**.
  - Place a mouth gag that gently keeps the mouth open, remembering not to use a rigid mouth gag in cats. Put your index finger in the mouth with the tip of your finger over the site where you feel the nerve or where you expect the nerve to be (same location as that described in the intraoral approach). It is not necessary to clip and scrub the skin - this is the same as a subcutaneous injection.
  - From outside the mouth, place the needle through the skin on the lingual side of the mandible at the mandibular notch and slide the needle under the gingiva

until you can feel the tip of the needle with your finger that is in the mouth (**Figure 7-12 C & D**). The exact location of insertion of the needle through the skin is not critical, what is critical is that you aim the TIP of the needle towards the spot where you expect the nerve to be (where your finger is!).

• Aspirate and inject the local anesthetic when you feel the tip of the needle in the correct location.

• Volume: Approximately 0.1 to 0.2 mls per side is usually sufficient in the cat and from 0.1 to 2.0 mls per side is usually sufficient in the dog, depending on size.

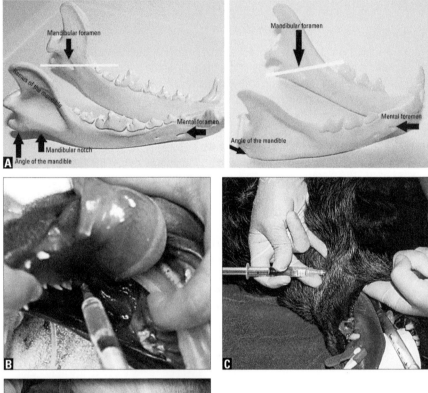

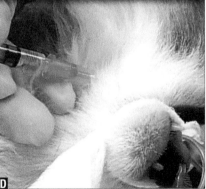

Figure 7-12. Mandibular block: Dog *(left)* and cat *(right)* mandibles with landmarks, including the mandibular foramen **(A)**, and the imaginary line between the angle of the mandible and the last mandibular molar on which the mandibular foramen can be found (yellow line). The intraoral approach **(B)** is commonly used in medium and large dogs and the extraoral approach is often used in small dogs **(C)** and cats **(D)**.

Contraindications/Precautions

There is a myth that a dog will 'chew its tongue off' during recovery from anesthesia if both sides of the mandible are blocked. We have never seen this. If you do happen to see a dog chewing its tongue as it recovers, sedate the dog until the block wears off. This myth has not been described for cats since cats don't generally hang their tongues out of their mouths in recovery.

Mental Block (Block of Middle Mental Nerve)

This block desensitizes the mandible, teeth and lip rostral from the mental foramen to the symphysis on the same side as the injection.

WHEN TO USE THE MENTAL BLOCK: Use for symphyseal (the junction of the two halves of the mandible on the midline) fracture repair and extractions of lower incisors, although the entire incisor root may not be blocked if the tooth root is healthy and firmly rooted in the bone.

Technique

• Palpate the mental foramen, which is on the outside of the mandible between the 1st and 2nd premolars in the dog and ½ way between the first premolar that you can see (which is actually the 3rd premolar) and the lower canine tooth in cats. It is very small and feels like a small depression rather than a hole **(Figure 7-9 and Figure 7-13)**.
• Insert the needle near the foramen (the needle tip does not need to enter the foramen), aspirate and inject enough local anesthetic to form a 'bleb'.
• The needle can be inserted either through the skin or, with the lip pulled out slightly, directly through the gingiva.
• Volume: 0.1-1.0 ml (depending on size of patient) per side.

Contraindications/Precautions

None

Auriculotemporal and Great Auricular Nerve Blocks

These blocks are used together to desensitize the external ear canal and the base of the pinna.

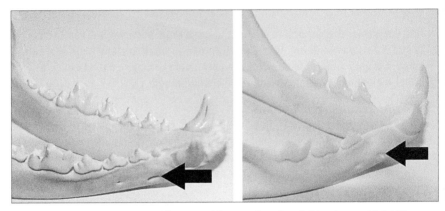

Figure 7-13. Mental nerve block: The mental foramen in a dog *(left)* and a cat *(right)*. The nerve can be blocked as it exits the foramen to desensitize from this location to the midline by either injecting the local anesthetic through the skin or into the gingiva along the mandible. Insertion of the needle into the foramen is not necessary for this block.

WHEN TO USE THE AURICULOTEMPORAL/GREAT AURICULAR NERVE BLOCKS:

Use for procedures involving the ear including, lancing of aural hematomas, total ear canal ablations, ear trauma repair and ear cleaning. However, these blocks (as with most blocks) must be part of a multimodal protocol because they will not block the deepest part of the canal and ear canal ablation and deep ear cleaning may still cause pain. The pinna is also not completely blocked.

Technique
• The site of injection to desensitize the auriculotemporal nerve is located cranial to the vertical ear canal and can be identified by palpating the zygomatic arch caudally towards the ear until you feel a 'V' shaped 'canal' between the vertical ear canal and caudal end of the zygomatic arch **(Figures 7-14 A & B)**.
  • Aspirate and inject the local anesthetic subcutaneously at that 'canal'.
• The site of injection to desensitize the greater auricular nerve is located caudal to the vertical ear canal and can be identified by palpating between the wing of the atlas (the first cervical [neck] vertebra) and the caudal aspect of the ear canal, where you will feel a 'V' shaped canal **(Figures 7-14 C & D)**.
  • Aspirate and inject the local anesthetic subcutaneously at that 'canal'.

Contraindications/Precautions
The blink response may be absent for several hours after the block, lubricate the eye until the blink returns. Use multimodal analgesia, especially for surgeries on the deep structures of the ear because this block will not desensitize those structures.

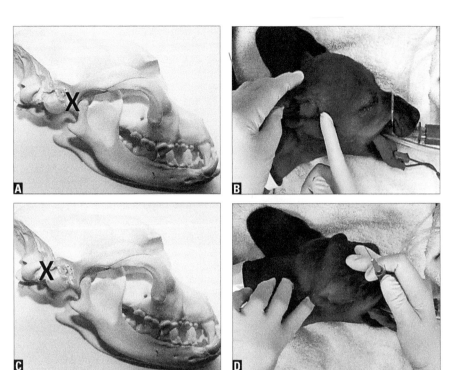

Figure 7-14. The site of injection to desensitize the auriculotemporal nerve is cranial to the vertical ear canal and identified by palpating the zygomatic arch caudally towards the ear until you feel a 'V' shaped 'canal' between the vertical ear canal and the caudal end of the zygomatic arch **(A, B)**. The site of injection to desensitize the greater auricular nerve is caudal to the vertical ear canal and identified by palpating between the wing of the atlas (first cervical vertebra) and the caudal aspect of the ear canal, where you will feel a 'V' shaped canal **(C, D)**. For both blocks, insert the needle subcutaneously, aspirate and inject.

Thoracic, Abdominal and Genito-urinary Blocks

Testicular Block
This is an easy and effective block to desensitize the testicles and spermatic cord.

• **WHEN TO USE THE TESTICULAR BLOCK:** Use for castration in all species. It can be used in addition to general anesthesia (common method in dogs, cats, horses) or instead of general anesthesia (common method in many farm animals).

Technique
• Complete the first scrub of the testicles.
• Insert a 22- to 25-gauge one-inch needle starting from the bottom of one of the testicles and aiming towards the spermatic cord (towards the body of the patient) or directly into the middle of the testicle **(Figure 7-15 A & B)**.
• Aspirate.

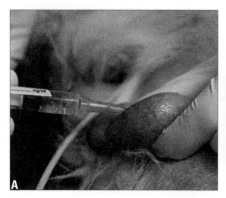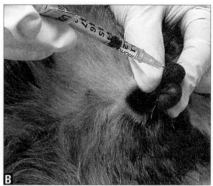

Figure 7-15. Testicular Blocks: Insert a 22 to 25-gauge one-inch needle starting from the body of the testicle. The procedure is the same for both dogs **(A)** and cats **(B)**. The skin at the incision site should also be blocked.

- Inject lidocaine or bupivacaine into the body of the testicle until you feel the testicle become turgid (firm) or when ½ of the calculated dose has been injected.
- Repeat the injection in the other testicle.
- The drug will migrate up the spermatic cord within about 3 minutes for lidocaine (probably slightly longer for bupivacaine) so that the part of the procedure that will cause the most pain (crushing of the spermatic cord) will be desensitized.
- For incisions directly over the testicle (cats), continue infiltrating as the needle exits the testicular body so that the skin and subcutaneous tissue will be blocked.
- For incisions in other locations (dogs), inject local anesthetic in the skin and subcutaneous tissue at the site of incision and finish the scrub.
- By the time scrubbing is finished, the testicles and spermatic cord will be desensitized!
- Volume: Calculate a dose of 0.5-1 mg/kg bupivacaine or 2-4 mg/kg lidocaine (generally lower end dosages for cats, higher end for dogs). The actual dose that is injected may be volume limited due to the size of the testicular tissue. The volume that will result in a palpable increase in testicular volume is about ½ of the calculated volume. This will generally be 0.25 to 2.0 mls (depending on body size) per testicle in dogs and 0.1-0.2 mls in cats.

TIP
Don't forget cats! This is an easy, effective, inexpensive way to provide analgesia for cats.

Contraindications/Precautions
Be SURE to aspirate because the testicle is densely vascularized (lots of blood vessels!). If you get blood, redirect the needle and try again. Because of the high vascularity, some people are more comfortable using lidocaine than bupivacaine since lidocaine can be administered IV and is unlikely to cause adverse effects if some of the drug is absorbed IV. We are comfortable with both drugs, but use what makes YOU comfortable!

Ovarian Blocks

These are easy and effective blocks to desensitize the mesovarian ligament and potentially other structures depending on the block chosen. The blocks are done intra- operatively by the surgeon.

WHEN TO USE THE OVARIAN BLOCK: Use for ovariohysterectomy in all species.

Abdominal Lavage Technique (Carpenter et al. 2004; Benito et al. 2016)
This is the easiest of the two techniques and is commonly used in humans for hysterectomy surgery. This may be the more effective technique because both the uterine stump and the ovarian ligaments will be exposed to the local anesthetic.

• Calculate the dose of lidocaine or bupivacaine to be administered and use a small portion of the drug to block the incision site in the skin. Note that the dose of drugs for this technique is higher than the dose used for peripheral nerve blocks. In cats, we recommend 2 mg/kg bupivacaine. The lidocaine dose is 2-4 mg/kg. In dogs, we recommend 4 mg/kg bupivacaine. The lidocaine dose is 4-8 mg/kg.
• **Dilute the remaining drug** with saline, if necessary. The total volume of the local anesthetic/saline combination should be roughly 0.4-0.6 ml/kg. This seems like a lot but the volume of the abdomen is large and the local anesthetic needs to perfuse the entire abdomen.
  • Adequate volume is important because the entire abdomen needs to be 'bathed' in the local anesthetic/saline mixture.
  • This step can be done intraoperatively by the surgeon with a sterile syringe OR the technician can administer the mixture into the abdomen (without touching any tissue with the non-sterile syringe) as the surgeon holds the incision open.
• Ideally, the local anesthetic/saline mixture is administered into the abdomen (literally 'squirted, in) as soon as the abdomen is open but administration just prior to closure is also acceptable. The former is preferred because it provides preemptive analgesia but the latter may be easier for the surgeon since there won't be extra fluid in the abdomen during the surgical procedure. The mixture will settle into the dependent areas, which includes areas of pain like the mesovarian ligament and the uterine stump. The abdomen is closed as usual.

IMPORTANT TIP
The local anesthetic/saline mixture can be 'squirted' into the abdomen but may be more effective if divided equally into three parts. The three parts would be instilled near the right and left ovarian ligaments and the caudal uterus. This is most easily done if a small IV catheter is connected to the syringe containing the drug mixture.

Mesovarian Ligament Injection Technique
This technique is a little more time consuming and only blocks the mesovarian ligament (no other sources of pain) but is preemptive. The pulling on and breaking of the mesovarian ligament (the attachment of the ovary to the body wall) is highly

stimulating so this is an important area to block.
- Block the incision site in the skin.
- The surgeon will then:
  - Begin the ovariohysterectomy and, once the abdomen is open, identify the mesovarian ligament.
  - Draw the dose of local anesthetic into a sterile syringe.
  - Elevate the ovary and infiltrate the mesovarian ligament OR infiltrate the ligament without elevating the ovary OR merely place local anesthetic on the mesovarian ligament in situ to be absorbed (this is easily done by attaching a red rubber catheter or an IV catheter to the syringe and placing the tip of the catheter into the abdomen down to the site of the ovarian ligament). The latter technique is easier than injecting the mesovarian ligament in small dogs and cats (Zilbersetin LF et al 2008).
  - Elevate the opposite ovary, infiltrate the mesovarian ligament.
  - Return to the first ovary blocked and remove, remove the second ovary, proceed with the ovariohysterectomy.

Contraindications/Precautions
None, but, as with all blocks, be sure to calculate the dosages correctly.

Lumbosacral (LS) Epidural Analgesia
Injection of analgesic drugs in the epidural space at the lumbosacral (LS) junction provides analgesia from about the thoracolumbar region (the junction of the thorax and the lumbar regions), or more cranially if an epidural catheter is placed, to the tip of the tail. Most of the commonly used drugs are taken up from the epidural space by the blood VERY slowly so there is little to no measurable drug from the epidural injection in the blood stream, thus there are minimal to no systemic adverse effects.

WHEN TO USE A LUMBOSACRAL EPIDURAL: Consider using for any painful procedure or condition in the abdomen, rear limbs, tail or perineal region of the patient. Examples include, rear limb soft tissue or orthopedic surgery, abdominal exploratory and bladder surgeries, cesarean sections and surgeries on the tail or perineal region.

Choosing Drugs
- Opioids (Table 7-10) are most commonly used for epidural analgesia because of their long duration of action (up to 20-24 hours with morphine).
  - The time to onset of action is slow (can be as long as 30 to 45 minutes with some drugs) which is one of several reasons that local anesthetic drugs, which have a rapid onset of action, are generally added to the opioids.
  - Opioids do not cause motor dysfunction (the patient can still walk).
  - Morphine provides longer duration analgesia than any other opioid.
    - Preservative-free (PF) morphine is the gold standard opioid injected into the epidural space and is the safest product since there is some concern that preservatives can cause tissue damage.

Table 7-10
Opioid Doses for Epidural Injection in Dogs and Cats

DRUGS	DOSAGES (mg/kg)	TIME TO ONSET (minutes)	DURATION OF ACTION (hours)
Preservative-free (PF) morphine	0.1	20-45	12-24
Morphine	0.1	20-45	12-24
Methadone	0.1-0.3	10-20	6-12 (maybe 18)
Hydromorphone	0.1-0.2	10-20	6-12 (maybe 18)
Fentanyl	0.004	5-10	0.5
Buprenorphine	0.01-0.02	30-60	10-24*

* Results differ among studies, minimal information available.

- HOWEVER, many practices use 'regular' morphine (with preservatives) and other drugs containing preservatives and this is generally considered to be safe. SO, don't let the fact that you don't have PF morphine keep you from doing epidurals!
- Local anesthetic drugs are commonly added to the opioid.
  - The duration of analgesia provided by local anesthetic drugs is the same duration as injecting local anesthetics in any other tissue, meaning about 90 minutes for lidocaine and 4 hours for bupivacaine.
  - The time to onset is the same onset as injecting the local anesthetics in any other tissues, meaningr about 2 minutes for lidocaine and 5 to 15 minutes for bupivacaine.
  - The local anesthetics can cause motor dysfunction, meaning the patient may have difficulty using its rear legs for a short time.
    - Lidocaine is more likely to cause motor dysfunction than bupivacaine but the duration of lidocaine is shorter so, either way, motor dysfunction is unlikely to be present by the time the patient regains consciousness and needs/wants to walk.
    - Ropivacaine is a newer local anesthetic that is even less likely to cause motor dysfunction than bupivacaine (although motor blockade with either drug is uncommon).
  - Vasodilation with subsequent hypotension can occur following local anesthetic administration into the epidural space so patients that may be prone to hypotension, for example patients in shock, should receive only epidural opioids and no epidural local anesthetics.
- The calculated opioid dose should be drawn into a syringe and diluted with local anesthetic (sterile water or saline can be used if a local anesthetic is not desired) to a TOTAL VOLUME of 1 ml of drugs per every 4.5 kg [or 10 lbs] of patient body weight or 0.2 mls/kg [or 2.2 lbs]. A total volume limit of 8 mls per patient no matter the size of the patient has been suggested but this is controversial and not used by

our group for opioids diluted with saline or water, but is used if local anesthetics are included. This is because there is some concern that the local anesthetics could spread far enough cranially to affect the nerves that control the diaphragm, which might impair breathing.

> ## TIP
> When calculating the total volume for an epidural injection, first calculate the DOSE of opioid and draw that up. THEN dilute that opioid with local anesthetic or saline to a TOTAL VOLUME of 1 ml/4.5 kg. Example: A 15 kg patient needs 0.1 mg/kg of 1 mg/ml morphine. The total volume of morphine is 1.5 mls ([15 kg x 0.1 mg/kg] ÷ 1 mg/ml). The dog needs a VOLUME of 3 mls (15 kg ÷ 4.5 kg). So 3 mls total - 1.5 mls morphine = 1.5 mls local anesthetic or saline.

Organizing Supplies
Supplies should be organized ahead of time so that the epidural can be completed efficiently. Supplies include sterile gloves, an epidural needle, syringes of several sizes, saline to test the needle location, and the analgesic drug to be injected **(Figure 7-16)**. The epidural needle size is important.

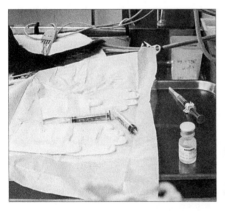

Figure 7-16. Epidural supplies include sterile gloves, an epidural needle, syringes of several sizes, saline to test the needle location, and the analgesic drug to be injected.

• Epidural needles are most commonly 22-G for dogs and cats, although 20-G can be used in large dogs.
• The length of the needle should be sufficient to reach through the skin, subcutaneous tissue and fat, past the vertebral processes and into the epidural space.
• Recommended needle lengths:
  • 1.5 inch in small dogs and cats
  • 2.5 inch in medium to large dogs
  • 3.0+ inch in giant breed or very fat dogs
• A needle that is 'too long' is fine, just be sure that the needle is stabilized at all times and NOT FLOPPING AROUND! A needle that is 'too short' can be a problem because it might not reach all the way to the epidural space.

Drugs for the epidural injection can be drawn up prior to starting the procedure or once the person doing the epidural has put on the sterile gloves.

Injection Technique

Place the anesthetized patient in sternal or lateral recumbency.

- There are two ways to place the patient in sternal recumbency.
  - The legs can be pulled forward along the patient's side (this curves the spine in such a way that the lumbo-sacral space is widened slightly; **Figure 7-17 A**).
  - or 'frog legged' out behind the patient (this makes the space much easier to palpate, especially in overweight or large patients; **(Figure 7-17 B)**.

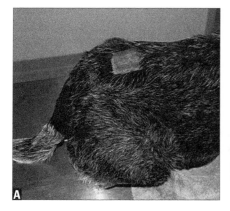
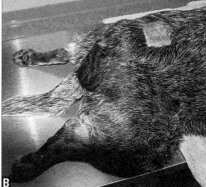
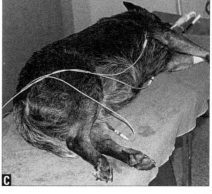

Figure 7-17. Patient positioning for a lumbo-sacral epidural injection: sternal recumbency with legs pulled forward **(A)**; sternal recumbency with legs pulled out behind **(B)**; lateral recumbency **(C)**. These options are used for dogs, cats and other small mammals.

- When injuries prevent sternal recumbency or if lateral recumbency is your preference, place the patient in lateral with the hind limbs pulled slightly forward **(Figure 7-17 C)**.
- To find the LS space, palpate the spinal column between the wings of the ilium (the highest point of the hip bones). The LS space is on midline, generally directly in line with the wings of the ilium or slightly caudal to the wings. The space is identified as a large 'divet' between the fairly tall dorsal spinous processes of the lumbar vertebrae and the much shorter dorsal spinous processes of the sacrum **(Figure 7-18 A & B)**.

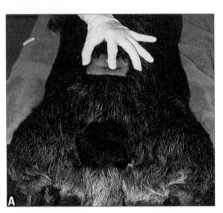
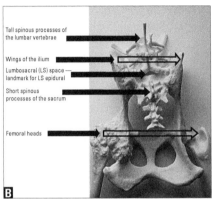

Tall spinous processes of the lumbar vertebrae

Wings of the ilium

Lumbosacral (LS) space — landmark for LS epidural

Short spinous processes of the sacrum

Femoral heads

Figure 7-18. The lumbosacral **(LS)** space is the injection site for a lumbosacral epidural and is on midline, usually directly in line with or slightly caudal to the wings of the ilium **(A)**. It is identified as a large 'divet' between the fairly tall dorsal spinous processes of the lumbar vertebrae and the shorter dorsal spinous processes of the sacrum **(B)**. Note the profound osteoarthritis in the left coxofemoral joint of this dog skeleton.

- Clip and scrub over the space **(Figure 7-19 A & B)**.
- Put on sterile gloves. Consider a sterile drape over the area if the site is hard to locate and may require extensive palpation.
- Take the cover off the spinal needle and note the direction of the bevel. Most spinal needles have a notch in the needle hub which indicates the location of the bevel. In most cases, the needle should be inserted so that the bevel points cranially. This is necessary because cranial spread of the opioids is necessary so that they can bind to opioid receptors in the spinal cord and produce analgesia.
- Place finger ON MIDLINE **(Figure 7-19 C)** as a landmark for needle insertion.
- Insert the needle through the skin ON MIDLINE in the LS junction in a 60 to 90 degree angle with the spine **(Figure 7-19 D)**.

IMPORTANT TIP
Placement of the needle on MIDLINE is critical for success! If the needle is not on midline, it will never hit the space.

- Advance the needle through the skin and first layer of muscle.

- STABILIZE THE NEEDLE with your non-dominant hand (your left hand if you are right handed and vice-versa), remove the stylet **(Figure 7-19 E)** and drip saline into the needle hub until you can see a drop at the top of the hub **(Figure 7-19 F)**. This will be used for the 'hanging drop technique' for confirmation of correct needle placement.

NOTE
The hanging drop technique will not work in patients in lateral recumbency because the saline drop will not stay in the needle hub.

- Continue advancing the needle into the lumbosacral epidural space **(Figure 7-19 G)** until the saline solution in the needle is aspirated (or 'pulled') into the space (hanging drop technique) or until the needle penetrates the ligamentum flavum (this is the ligament on the top of the epidural space, it is tough so a 'pop' may be felt as the needle penetrates the ligament).
- Commonly, the needle will hit bone instead of the space between the vertebrae. This is normal - do not be concerned about hitting bone. Bone is actually a landmark that will let you know how deep the needle is!
- If the needle does hit bone, withdraw the needle a few millimeters and redirect the tip of your needle a few degrees more 'cranially' or 'caudally' (meaning a little steeper or a little flatter). DON'T MAKE BIG MOVEMENTS - just small movements or the space might be missed.

CRITICAL POINT!
In this process, you are not just moving the needle around hoping you get lucky and hit the space. You are using your needle as a PROBE to locate the space. So probe carefully and methodically!

- Advance again. If you hit bone again, repeat the process. Make 3-5 movements in one direction (e.g., cranially). If you don't hit the space, go back to where you started and make 3-5 movements in the other direction (e.g., caudally), each time moving only a small distance. Make all cranial moves first followed by all caudal moves (or vice-versa). In other words, be organized with your movements - you are 'searching' for the space - not moving erratically and hoping you get lucky.
  - This is called 'walking off the bone' since you are 'walking' the needle using small movements.
  - You will know that the space has been entered when the needle no longer hits bone but can be inserted deeper than the depth of the bone.
- If you still haven't entered the epidural space after moving the needle both cranially and caudally, stop and be sure that the needle is at the LS space and that the needle is on midline. If the answer is no to either question, fix the problem.
- If everything looks correct, repeat the entire process again. If the space is still not entered, consider providing analgesia with a CRI (or other choice) so that you don't keep sticking the patient with a needle and don't cause too much of a delay for surgery.
- **STOP** advancing as soon as the space is entered. **How do you know the space was entered?**

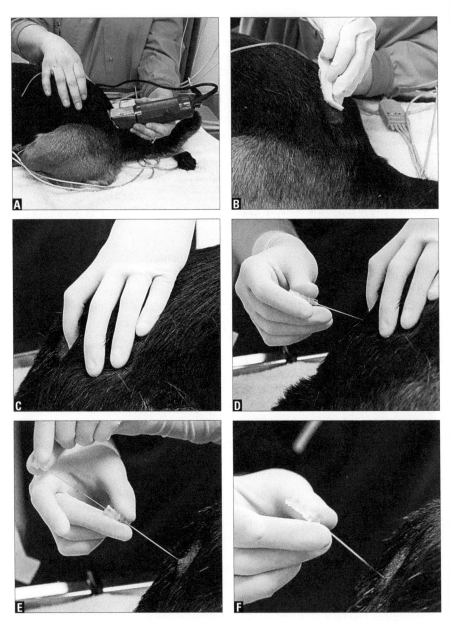

Figure 7-19. lumbosacral epidural: clip and scrub over the lumbosacral space **(A, B)**. Place a gloved finger on the midline **(C)**. Insert the needle through the skin **(D)**.STABILIZE THE NEEDLE, remove the stylet **(E)**, and drip saline into the needle hub to create (the 'hanging' drop) **(F)**.

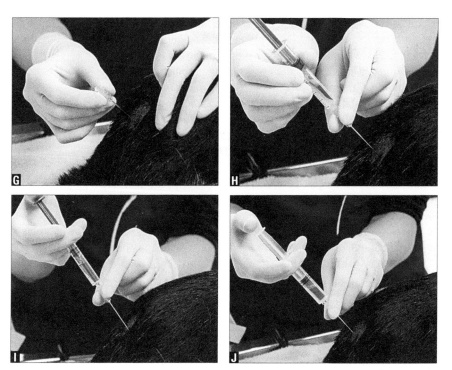

Figure 7-19 Continued. Advance the needle into the lumbosacral space **(G)**. Connect a syringe with 2 mls of saline and 1 ml of air to the needle **(H)**. Stabilize the needle and inject some saline **(I)**. Take your thumb off the syringe plunger, the fluid should continue to flow into the space. **(J)**.

- Watch the hanging drop - if it is pulled into the needle, the needle is in the space. This doesn't work all the time (only works about 50-60% of the time) so don't worry if the fluid stays in the hub.
- 'Walk off' the edge of the bone as described above. If the needle hits bone, then can be inserted deeper when you move it to 'probe' for the space, the needle is in the space!
- Use the 'loss of resistance' technique. This is the most definitive technique for insuring that the needle is in the epidural space!
  - Connect a syringe that has about 2 mls of saline and 0.5-1 ml of AIR (you need an air bubble!) to the needle **(Figure 7-19 H)**.
  - STABILIZE the needle - you don't want to move it out of the space! Luer-lock syringes require more manipulation to connect and may cause the needle to move so we recommend syringes that are not luer-lock.
  - Inject some saline **(Figure 7-19 I)**. Then stop and take your thumb off the syringe plunger.
  - The fluid should continue to flow into the space (which you can tell because the fluid at the bottom of the air bubble will continue to flow).
  - If the plunger goes back up instead of the fluid going down, the tip of the needle is NOT in the space!

- **ASPIRATE** to ensure that you do not have CSF fluid (which means you are in the subarachnoid space which is deeper than the epidural space) or that you do not have blood (which means that the needle is in an epidural vein).
- If CSF fluid is aspirated inject only half of your calculated drug volume. If blood is encountered withdraw the needle 1 to 2 mm, aspirate, and inject if no blood. Keep withdrawing if still getting blood. Some people advocate starting completely over if blood is aspirated.
- Remove the syringe with saline and attach the syringe with the opioid solution carefully so as not to move the needle. **STABILIZE THE NEEDLE!**
- Again leave roughly one ml of air in the syringe to check again for loss of resistance. Also aspirate again before injecting. Inject slowly over about 30 to 60 sec.
- Remove the needle. If local anesthetics were used, consider laying the patient with the leg scheduled for surgery 'down' so that the local anesthetics can spread to those nerves. The true efficacy of this technique is questionable. This technique will not be effective if opioids were used without local anesthetics since the opioids don't work locally but instead must migrate cranially and bind to receptors in the spinal cord.

TIP
Don't be afraid to do epidurals in cats! The technique is the same but the epidurals are actually often easier in cats than in dogs because the landmarks are easy to palpate. If you can palpate landmarks, you can do an epidural! (Figure 7-20 A-D).

NOTE
The spinal cord can extend farther caudally in the cat than in the dog and it is possible to get some CSF fluid. If that happens go ahead with the epidural, but inject only one-half of the calculated volume.

TIP
Epidural analgesia has many uses - not just surgery! Use for treating pain from pancreatitis and to aid in passing urethral catheters to relieve urethral obstruction (see 'sacrococcygeal epidural').

TIP
Epidural catheters are fairly easily placed in larger dogs and can be maintained for several days to allow continuous or intermittent delivery of analgesic drugs.

NOTE
Epidural injections can also be used in non-anesthetized patients but the animal must be heavily sedated.

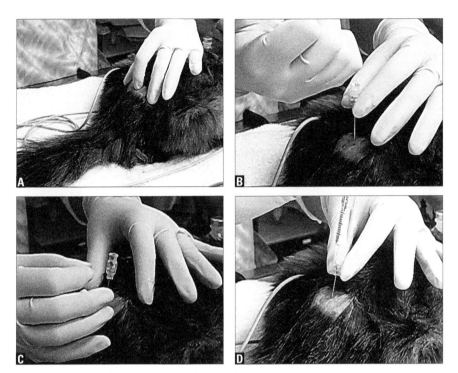

Figure 7-20. Epidural injection in cats: Landmarks for epidurals are the same in cats and dogs **(A)**. The injection technique is also the same but the needle should be moved in very small increments when finding the space. Insert the needle subcutaneously ON MIDLINE, remove the stylet and place a drop of saline in the hub for the hanging drop technique **(B)**. The needle is in the lumbosacral epidural space if the hanging drop disappears **(C)** or can be 'walked off' the edge of the bone. Stabilize the needle and inject the drug **(D)**. In these photos the needle is at a steeper than normal angle but disappearance of the hanging drop indicates proper needle placement.

Contraindications/Precautions
• The epidural space is a bad place to get a hematoma or an abscess so don't use epidural injections in patients with clotting disorders or skin lesions in the LS area.
• Ineffective block is by far the MOST COMMON complication, and it is still rare. If the patient is painful, assume that the block did not work and provide additional analgesia like boluses of opioids or constant rate infusions.
• Opioid epidurals do NOT affect motor function of the rear limb or diaphragm. Local anesthetic drugs can affect motor function but this is rare. Drug volumes that are described here are unlikely to flow far enough cranially to affect the diaphragm so ventilation is unlikely to be impaired.
• Location of the LS space can be difficult in patients with pelvic injuries or abnormal anatomy and other analgesic options (like constant rate infusions) might be a better option for analgesia.
• Don't add local anesthetics if the patient is at risk for hypotension. These are patients that are dehydrated, hypovolemic or in shock. Local anesthetics cause

vasodilation in the area affected by the epidural injection and this can cause or worsen hypotension.

• Urinary retention may occur following an opioid epidural. Express the bladder at the end of the surgery and monitor for urination for the next several hours.

▌IMPORTANT TIP

Have a place on the chart or the cage card that can be checked if a patient-care person sees urine in the cage or litter box or sees the dog urinate when it is taken out for a walk.

▌IMPORTANT POINT

Hair may grow back slowly after clipping anywhere on the dorsum of the patient, including the LS space. This fact needs to be communicated to the clients since it is sometimes blamed on the epidural, but it is just the location of the clipping and has nothing to do with injection of drugs into the LS space. Hair just grows back slowly on the topline of dogs and cats.

Sacrococcygeal or Intracoccygeal Epidural

The injection site for this epidural is the space between the sacral and coccygeal (tail) vertebrae or between the first two coccygeal vertebrae **(Figure 7-21)**. Because we are blocking nerves (just like any other nerve block) and not expecting the drug to migrate forward to bind with analgesic receptors in the spinal cord, local anesthetics are used for this block, although opioids could certainly be added. The block desensitizes the tail, perineum (which is the area under the tail), caudal portion of the urogenital tract, anus, rectum and caudal portion of the colon. It can be done in sedated or anesthetized patients. Because a local anesthetic is used for this block, motor function to the tail will be blocked but motor function to the rear limbs is unlikely to be blocked, unless an excessively large volume of local anesthetic is injected. This block is easier than the lumbosacral epidural, but does not provide analgesia as far cranially as the LS epidural (does not provide analgesia for structures in the abdominal cavity or rear limb).

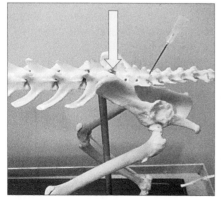

Figure 7-21. Sacrococcygeal epidural:
The Injection site for the sacrococcygeal epidural is the space between the sacral and coccygeal (tail) vertebrae (location in this photo) or between the first two coccygeal vertebrae. For comparison, the arrow indicates where a lumbosacral epidural injection would occur.

WHEN TO USE A SACROCOCCYGEAL EPIDURAL: It can be used for any surgical or trauma pain in the regions desensitized. Examples include: tail amputations, anal sac removal, relief of urethral obstruction ('blocked cat'), insertion of urethral catheter and relief of caudal colon obstruction (constipation). This block is commonly used in standing horses and cows for perineal surgery and delivery of foals or calves.

Technique

- Palpate the sacrococcygeal or intracoccygeal space, which is found by 'pumping' the tail up and down and feeling for the first movable space caudal to the sacrum.
- Clip and scrub the site.
- This is a very shallow site so an epidural needle is not necessary. A regular 22- to 25-gauge 1.0-1.5 inch hypodermic needle is appropriate.
- Insert the needle at a 30 to 45 degree angle to the skin ON MIDLINE at the palpated space. Some people start the needle at a 90 degree angle. It doesn't matter how you start since the needle will be used to probe for the space by 'walking it off' the bone.
- As with the lumbosacral space, slowly insert the needle until the needle enters the space or hits bone. If the needle enters the space, a 'pop' as the needle pierces the ligamentum flavum is common. However, hypodermic needles are sharper than epidural needles and they may penetrate the ligamentum without causing a pop. If the needle hits bone, 'walk off' the bone as described for lumbosacral epidurals. The hanging drop technique may work.
- Slowly inject the drug and remove the needle.
- VOLUME: 0.1 to 0.3 ml total volume of 2% lidocaine or 0.5% bupivacaine for cats and small dogs and up to 1.0-2.0 ml total volume of either of those drugs for medium to large dogs.

IMPORTANT POINT

Do not inject air in this location (air is not contraindicated at the LS site). The drug is being injected into a very small space and there is a theory that the air bubble can alter drug uptake because it will consume a large amount of space.

TIP

Use this block to relieve urethral obstruction in cats (often called a 'blocked cat')! The cat doesn't have to be anesthetized (but should receive systemic opioids +/- sedative drugs), the block provides analgesia and muscle relaxation, which makes the obstruction much easier to relieve and provides analgesia for the cat. Lidocaine onset is 2-5 minutes with a 90 minute duration. We prefer bupivacaine or ropivacaine which have a 5-7 minute onset and a 4 hour duration.

TIP

Use this block for any surgeries on the tail - including tail amputations.

> **TIP**
> Use this block for removal of fecal constipation - works especially well in the cat. This should be done even though the cat is anesthetized since the post-procedure pain relief is important.

Contraindications/Precautions
Do not inject air into the space.

Blocks for the Limbs
Radial/Ulnar/Median (RUM) Nerve Block
This block causes desensitization of the sensory nerves to the structures of the paw but the motor nerves are not blocked **(Figure 7-22 A, B)**.

WHEN TO USE THE RUM BLOCK: Use for any surgery on the paw, including toe amputation, tumor removal, biopsy, foreign body removal (like a migrating grass awn), suturing pad lacerations, etc. **This used to be called the 'declaw block' but it definitely isn't just for declaws!**

Technique for the 3-Point Block
(Figure 7-22 B)

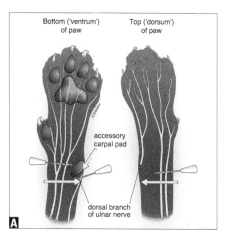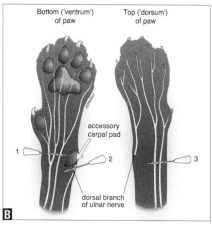

Figure 7-22. Three point and Ring Block Techniques for Radial/Ulnar/Median (RUM) Nerve Block: A ring block desensitizes the same nerves as a three point block. Inject local anesthetic subcutaneously all the way across the top and bottom of the paw to form a ring of anesthetic (injection sites indicated by the horizontal arrows) (A). For the three point block inject local anesthetic subcutaneously across the bottom of the paw at the level of the accessory carpal pad *(needle 1)*, above the accessory carpal pad on the side of the paw *(needle 2)*, and on the top of the paw just above the carpus on the medial side (the side of the paw where digit 1 is located); *needle 3* (B). **(Adapted from Tranquilli WJ, Grimm KA, Lamont AL. Pain Management For The Small Animal Practitioner, Figure 3-4. Teton New Media, 2000).**

- Locate the carpus and the accessory carpal pad, which is the small carpal pad without a nail on the bottom, lateral side ('outside') of the paw.
- Inject 0.1-0.3 mls of local anesthetic <u>subcutaneously</u> at three sites:
  - 1) On the backside of the paw inject from the medial side of the paw (the side with the first digit or 'thumb') to the accessory carpal pad (blocks median nerve and palmar branch of the ulnar nerve; Needle 1 in Figure 7-22 B);
  - 2) On the medial side of the paw immediately above the accessory carpal pad (blocks dorsal branch of the ulnar nerve; needle 2 in Figure 7-22 B); and
  - 3) On the medial side of the front of the paw immediately above the carpus (blocks superficial branches of the radial nerve; needle 3 Figure 7-22 B).
- For each site, aspirate before injecting.

TIP
For cats and small dogs, 0.1ml per injection site is adequate, while 0.1 to 0.3 ml per site is adequate for medium to large dogs. If multiple paws need to be blocked, the total calculated dose of local anesthetic should be drawn up and then can be diluted with saline to increase the total volume, which should be just enough to provide sufficient volume for injection but not enough to create a large fluid 'bleb' in the tissue.

Technique for the 'Ring' Block
The 'ring' block can be used instead of the 3-point block. The landmarks are the same but instead of making 3 separate injections, a line block (meaning a line of local anesthetic) is made subcutaneously all the way across the top of the paw at a level that is just above the accessory carpal pad and a second line block is made at the same level all the way across the bottom of the paw. These two line blocks make a 'ring' around the paw. This technique tends to be a little faster than the 3-point block but also requires a slightly higher volume of local anesthetic (Figure 7-22 A).

TIP
Inserting the needle under the skin and then injecting as the needle is withdrawn is the easiest way to do the ring block. Withdraw the needle slowly so that local anesthetic is evenly distributed over the nerve.

Contraindications/Precautions
There are no contraindications but it is important that you DO NOT use local anesthetics that contain epinephrine since epinephrine causes vasoconstriction, which could compromise blood flow to the paw.

Brachial Plexus Block
This block desensitizes most of the forelimb. Because local anesthetic drugs are used, it also causes loss of forelimb motor function for a short time, but motor function is generally adequate or even normal by the time the patient recovers from anesthesia and is ready to walk. This block provides analgesia for surgeries in or around the elbow and anything below the elbow if the approach described below is used.

WHEN TO USE THE BRACHIAL PLEXUS BLOCK: Use for surgeries at or below the elbow. Examples: elbow arthroscopy or arthrotomy, forelimb amputation and radius/ulna fracture repair.

EQUIPMENT: A 22-gauge needle that is 3-4" long for large dogs or 2 to 3" long for medium dogs (an epidural or spinal needle will work for both of these needle lengths) or a 1½ to 2" hypodermic needle for small dogs and cats; a syringe of adequate size to hold the calculated volume of drug. If a long needle is not available, the metal stylet from an IV catheter will work.

Technique
• Locate the point of the shoulder, which is the part of the humerus (technically the 'greater tubercle of the humerus') that can be felt just below the junction of the scapula (shoulder blade) and the humerus (forelimb; **Figure 7-23 A**). Clip and scrub the area.
• Using sterile technique insert the needle at the point of the shoulder, under the scapula, and keep the needle horizontal (so as not to enter the thoracic cavity) and parallel with the spinal column. The needle may scrape the underside of the scapula.

TIP
It is easier to insert the needle if the leg is rolled so that the scapula is raised up a little.

• Insert the needle to its full length **(Figure 7-23 B)**. Remove the stylet and attach the syringe containing the local anesthetic.
• Aspirate, if you aspirate blood, withdraw the needle a few millimeters and aspirate again.
• Once there is no blood aspirated, slowly inject ⅓ of the calculated dose of the drug, slowly withdraw the needle to the middle of the area to be blocked, aspirate and inject ⅓ of the local anesthetic **(Figure 7-23 C)**.
• Withdraw the needle to a site just before it exits the skin, aspirate and inject the remaining ⅓ of the local anesthetic **(Figure 7-23 D)**.

TIP
Be sure the needle is long enough.

TIP
If blocking both front limbs, split the total dose of the local anesthetic and dilute with saline to increase the volume of the solution to be injected if necessary. Don't exceed the total dose.

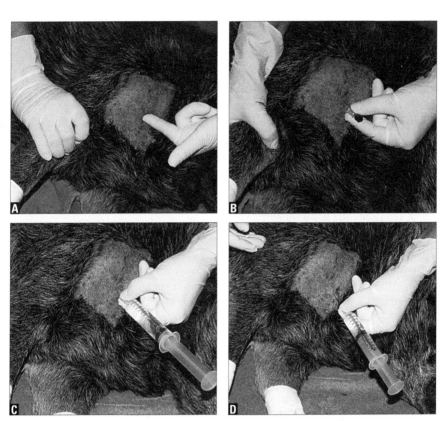

Figure 7-23. Brachial Plexus Block: Roll the leg to raise the scapula and locate the point of the shoulder **(A)**. Insert the needle at the point of the shoulder, under the scapula. Insert the needle to its full length **(B)**. Remove the stylet and attach the syringe containing local anesthetic **(C)**. Aspirate, and inject ⅓ of the local anesthetic. Slowly withdraw the needle, and inject ⅓ of the local anesthetic midway across the brachial plexus **(D)**. Withdraw the needle to a point just before exiting the skin, aspirate and inject the remaining ⅓ of the local anesthetic.

TIP
Accuracy of this block can be improved and dosage of drug decreased by using a nerve finder, but a nerve finder is definitely not required. With a nerve finder, the block can also be done higher up (it is called the 'cervical paravertebral' block), which increases the consistency of the block and provides analgesia all the way up to the shoulder.

Direct Visualization Technique
If the forelimb is being amputated, the surgeon can inject the tissue around the nerves directly during the surgery, thus desensitizing the entire forelimb.

Complications/Precautions
Don't forget that motor function to the leg is blocked so the patient might have difficulty using the leg for a short time postoperatively. However, this rarely occurs

since the motor nerve block is shorter duration than the analgesic block and the patients do not jump up and start trying to walk immediately after surgery.

Intercostal Blocks
This block desensitizes boney and soft tissue structures of the thorax.

WHEN TO USE INTERCOSTAL BLOCKS: Use for any painful lesion or surgery on the thorax. Examples include relief of pain from rib fractures, insertion or removal of chest tubes, removal of tumors, suturing of lacerations and thoracotomies.

EQUIPMENT: You will need a 22 to 25 gauge one-inch needle for cats and small dogs but may need a 1.5 inch needle on big dogs and a 1 to 12 ml syringe to hold the calculated dose and lidocaine or bupivacaine +/- adjunctive drugs.

Technique
• Start at the vertebrae and palpate distally (down towards the sternum) until you can feel the ribs (usually within several centimeters of the vertebrae).
• The nerves run behind each rib so insert the needle off the back side of the rib **(Figure 7-24)**. Sometimes your needle will actually hit the rib so just back it out a little and redirect at an angle so that the needle is 'walked' off the caudal edge of the rib.
• **ASPIRATE.** If you get air, the tip of the needle is in the thorax. Withdraw the needle into the tissue and re-aspirate before you inject. If you get blood, withdraw the needle slightly, redirect, and re-aspirate before you inject.
• Inject local anesthetic as you insert the needle or as you withdraw the needle.
• Repeat the technique in at least 2 intercostal spaces cranial and two spaces caudal to the incision site or fracture because the nerves form a 'network' on the thorax and you want to be sure that you block as many nerves as possible.
• Calculate the total dose, but generally 0.25 to 1 ml of local anesthetic per site is sufficient to cover the area just described.

TIP
The closer to the vertebrae that the drug can be injected, the more consistent the area of analgesia.

TIP
If placing a chest tube, intrapleural analgesia (local anesthesia injected through the chest tube into the intrapleural space) should be used in conjunction with the intercostal block.

Contraindications/Precautions
Be sure to aspirate so that you don't inject local anesthetics into blood vessels or the thorax for this block (they can be injected using the intrapleural technique). The local anesthetics will not likely cause harm, but the skin and deeper tissues at the site of the incision won't be desensitized.

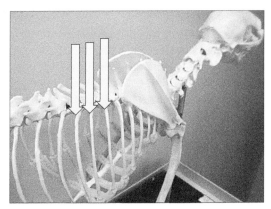

Figure 7-24. Intercostal Blocks: The nerves run on the caudal border (back) of each rib so the needle should be inserted through the skin and into the muscle of the back side of the rib in a location that is as close to the vertebrae (spine) as possible (injection sites are indicated by the arrows).

Summary
Local/regional anesthetic blocks are easy, inexpensive and extremely effective. ALL practices should be incorporating these techniques into their analgesic protocols.

Constant Rate Infusions
Constant rate infusions (CRI) of analgesic drugs are an excellent way to manage pain in both dogs and cats. A CRI of analgesic drugs has several advantages over multiple repeated injections for pain relief:

• A more stable plane of analgesia can be maintained with less incidence of break-through pain (which can be difficult to treat).
• A lower drug dosage can be delivered at any given time, resulting in a lower incidence of dose-related side effects.
• CRIs allow greater control over drug administration (easy to change the dose).
• There is a decreased need for stimulation of resting patients to administer drugs, and a decreased need for painful IM injections.
• CRIs are less expensive (when compared to technician time, needles and syringes required for repeat injections).
• It is possible to use a variety of drugs with continuous infusions - including some that don't work as well for analgesia when administered by other routes.

DRUGS for CRIs
Drugs most commonly used for CRIs include fentanyl, hydromorphone, morphine, methadone, butorphanol, ketamine, lidocaine, dexmedetomidine and a myriad of combinations of these drugs **(See Tables 7-11 & 7-12)**.

Opioids

The opioid class of drugs includes some of the most potent analgesic drugs available and should be considered for any patient experiencing moderate to severe pain. Although opioids are generally sedating in dogs, they can cause excitement in cats. Fortunately, the low dose of opioids delivered in a CRI rarely results in sedation or excitement. However, if excitement does occur, a light dose of a sedative (acepromazine or dexmedetomidine) can be administered to the cat and the CRI rate maintained (if excitement is mild) or reduced (if excitement is moderate). If sedation occurs, the dose of the CRI can be decreased. Fentanyl, hydromorphone, morphine and methadone are potent full agonist opioids that provide profound dose-related analgesia.

> **TIP**
> Morphine is VERY inexpensive and a morphine CRI can be used in all practices, even those with economically challenged clients.

> **TIP**
> Fentanyl is one of the best opioids to use in a CRI. It is extremely potent and is the least likely of the opioids to cause adverse effects. Cats love fentanyl! It is more expensive than morphine, but still not cost prohibitive.

These full agonists are the most commonly used opioids but butorphanol, an agonist-antagonist, has an advantage in that it is more likely to provide sedation than excitement in cats. However, butorphanol provides only moderate analgesia and has a ceiling effect for pain relief (a point is reached where higher dosages result in more sedation but not more analgesia). Thus, butorphanol is only appropriate for short-term mild to moderate pain and should be used as part of a multi-modal protocol rather than as a sole agent, or used as a CRI.

Lidocaine

Lidocaine can be administered systemically to provide analgesia. In addition to pain relief, lidocaine CRIs are anti-inflammatory, antiarrhythmic and improve GI motility. Lidocaine CRIs are commonly used in dogs, especially in dogs with gastro-intestinal pain (e.g., pain from exploratory laparotomy, gastric dilatation-volvulus [GDV], pancreatitis, or parvovirus). Lidocaine CRIs are somewhat controversial in cats because: 1) Cats appear to be more sensitive to the lidocaine-induced adverse effects than other species are, and 2) there is evidence that lidocaine may cause excessive cardiovascular depression in cats (Pypendop & Ilew 2008). Because of the uncertainty of lidocaine adverse effects in cats, some veterinarians feel that a lidocaine CRI is not warranted in the cat at all while others feel that it is an appropriate way to treat pain, especially in patients where other options may be limited. If a lidocaine CRI is chosen for a cat, low-dosages are recommended **(Table 7-12)**.

Ketamine

Painful impulses cause N-methyl-D-aspartate (NMDA) receptors (among others) in the dorsal horn of the spinal cord to depolarize and prolonged depolarization of these receptors can lead to an amplification of the pain stimulus, resulting in central sensitization, which we commonly refer to as 'wind-up' or 'hypersenstization'. When this occurs, the patient may feel more pain than expected (hyperalgesia) or even feel pain in response to a non-painful stimulus (allodynia). By administering drugs that antagonize these receptors (like ketamine), we are able to alleviate this exaggerated response and make the pain easier to control. Ketamine is a NMDA-receptor antagonist that improves analgesia when administered as a low-dose CRI. A single high-dose bolus of ketamine (e.g., like the anesthetic induction dose) can serve as a loading dose for a CRI but is unlikely to improve analgesia when used alone. NMDA receptor antagonists control central sensitization and do not provide true analgesia, thus, these drugs must be administered in conjunction with true analgesic drugs (opioids or NSAIDs). Adverse effects can include dysphoria, although this is rare since the low-dosages administered in the CRI are 'subanesthetic', meaning that they are very low and unlikely to cause dysphoria.

Alpha-2 Agonists

Alpha-2 agonists, including dexmedetomidine and medetomidine, provide both sedation and analgesia and the effects are reversible. Sedation is only minimal when using the CRI, especially at the low end of the dose range, but the light level of sedation or calming makes this CRI excellent for patients that are excited or distressed. The alpha-2 agonists are generally added to an opioid CRI (or any other CRI) at the same dosage as that listed in tables 7-11 and 12. Alpha-2 agonists may cause bradycardia.

Combinations of Opioids, Ketamine, and Lidocaine

CRIs that include multiple drugs are often more effective than CRIs of single drugs because the effects of analgesic drugs from different drug classes are generally additive or synergistic. Combinations include opioids + ketamine, opioids + ketamine + lidocaine or ketamine + lidocaine. However, infusions of a single drug are also effective, especially if the patient is receiving other drugs, like NSAIDs and/or local blocks. So the choice of multiple or single drug infusions is as much personal preference as science. Remember that lidocaine CRIs are controversial in cats.

Calculation of CRI Dosages

Generally, dosing tables or individualized spread sheets (e.g., there are very useful spreadsheets available at multiple websites, including websites for the International Veterinary Academy of Pain Management (**IVAPM.ORG**), Veterinary Anesthesia Support Group (**vasg.org**), Veterinary Information Network (**VIN**) and Veterinary Emergency & Critical Care Society (**VECCS**)), should be used for constant rate infusions. These sheets greatly improve the speed at which CRIs can be initiated (since no one has to take time to do calculations!) and greatly decrease the chance of mathematical errors. However, CRI dosages can also be easily calculated using the formula:

- A = desired dose in microg/kg/min
- B = body wt in kg
- C = Diluent volume in mls
- D = Desired fluid rate in mls/hr
- E = Drug concentration in mg/ml

A x B x C x 60/D x E x 1000 = mls of drug to add to diluent (the fluid bag or syringe)

> ## NOTE
> If the dose at A is in mg/kg/hr, the two conversion factors in the formula (60 in the numerator and 1000 in the denominator) should be removed from the formula and the mg/kg/hr dose be used instead of the microg/kg/min dose.

> ## NOTE
> See numerous ways to calculate infusions at the end of this chapter!

Loading Doses

Administering loading doses of the drugs to be infused is important since the loading dose provides a rapid increase in the serum concentration of the drug **(Figure 7-25)**. The serum concentration of the drug will slowly increase with the infusion, but this may delay time to onset of analgesia. A separate loading dose for opioids may not be necessary if an opioid was used as a premedicant and a separate loading dose for ketamine may not be necessary if ketamine was used as the induction drug. However, if a long delay (> 30 mins) occurred between administration of the opioid and/or ketamine and the start of the infusion, administer the loading dose. The loading dosages are very low and extremely unlikely to cause adverse effects so, if in doubt, administer a loading dose.

When to Start the CRI

- Start as soon as possible! As soon as a painful patient has an IV catheter in place, consider a CRI.
- For patients with pain from trauma (e.g., hit-by-car or attacks from other animals) or medical conditions (e.g., pancreatitis), pain relief is a component of stabilization and infusions can be started immediately after triage.
- For patients undergoing surgery that already have an IV catheter in place, start the infusion prior to anesthesia if possible since pre-emptive analgesia is more effective than analgesia that is administered after pain has started.
- For surgical patients that do not have an IV catheter in place prior to induction, start right after induction or when the patient has been moved into the operating room.
- Infusions can be started postoperatively if the need for an infusion was not recognized until the postoperative period. It is never too late to start! However, infusions

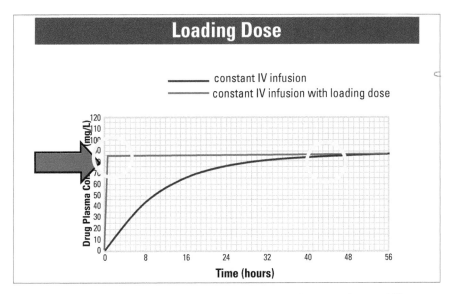

Loading Dose

constant IV infusion
constant IV infusion with loading dose

Figure 7-25. Constant rate infusion loading dose. The loading dose provides a rapid increase in the serum concentration of the drug. In this diagram of a fictional drug, the steep upslope indicates a loading bolus that allows the serum concentration of the drug to rapidly increase to the serum concentration that is needed to provide analgesia in this species. The slow upslope indicates the time required for this drug to reach analgesic concentrations without a loading dose.

should be started pre- or intra-operatively whenever possible so that the patient can benefit from infusion-delivered intraoperative analgesia and infusion-mediated decreases in the dosage of inhalant drugs necessary to maintain anesthesia.

When to Stop the CRI

• The infusion can be stopped at the end of surgery if appropriate on-going analgesia (e.g., NSAIDs, local blocks) has been administered, or the infusion can be continued for several hours, overnight, or even several days. The infusion duration should be based on the continued analgesic needs of the patient.
• Patients with severe medical (e.g., from pancreatitis) or trauma pain often remain on infusions for several days.
• If the analgesic level of the patient is questionable, the infusion can be slowly weaned by cutting the dose in half every 1 to 2 hours and carefully assessing the patient for pain.

How to: Setup and Administer a CRI

See chapter 8

Summary

Constant rate infusions are extremely easy to use and extremely beneficial to the patient. A variety of drugs can be used in the CRI and drug choice should be based not only on what is best for the patient (analgesic potency and safety) but also on what is best for the hospital (comfort level with and availability of drugs). Because calculating CRI dosages can be cumbersome, math is often the only limitation to using these valuable tools. Thus, rather than calculating drug dosages for each CRI, a 'dosing sheet' or computer program is recommended.

Tables
Tips for using Tables 7-11, 7-12, 7-13 and 7-14

The fluid rate in Tables 7-11 and 7-12 was chosen as 1ml/kg/hr but that can easily be doubled (so cut the amount of drug added to the bag in ½ since it will be administered twice as fast), quadrupled, halved, or whatever you need to make the infusion work for the patient. The dosages here may be slightly different than dosages you are currently using because CRIs are administered 'to effect' and some practices see effects at dosages slightly different than dosages used at other practices. However, all dosages are generally within a fairly narrow range. If you are using CRIs and you like your dosages, you don't need to change to our dosages.

References

Abelson AL, McCobb EC, Shaw S, Armitage-Chan E, Wetmore LA, Karas AZ, Blaze C. Use of wound soaker catheters for the administration of local anesthetic for post-operative analgesia: 56 cases. Vet Anesth Analg. 2009; 36(6):597-602.

Barton-Lamb AL, Martin-Flores M, Scrivani PV, Bezuidenhout AJ, Lowe E, Erb HN, Ludders JW. Evaluation of maxillary arterial blood flow in anesthetized cats with the mouth closed and open. Vet J.2013; 196(3):325-31.

Benito J, Monteiro B, Lavoie AM, Beauchamp G, Lascelles BDX, Steagall PV. Analgesic efficacy of intraperitoneal administration of bupivacaine in cats. J Feline Med Surg. 2016;18(11):906-912.

Brummett CM, Williams BA. Additives to local anesthetics for peripheral nerve blockade. Int Anesthesiol Clin. 2011; 49(4): 104-116.

Carpenter RE, Wilson DV, Evans AT. Evaluation of intraperitoneal and incisional lidocaine or bupivacaine for analgesia following ovariohysterectomy in the dog. Vet Anaesth Analg. 2004;31(1):46-52.

Martin-Flores M, Scrivani PV, Loew E, Gleed CA, Ludders JW. Maximal and submaximal mouth opening with mouth gags in cats: implications for maxillary artery blood flow. Vet J. 2014; 200(1): 60-4.

Pypendop BH, Elkiw JE. Assessment of the hemodynamic effects of lidocaine administered IV in isoflurane-anesthetized cats. Am J Vet Res. 2005 Apr; 66(4):661-8.

Scrivani PV, Martin-Flores M, van Hatten R, Bezuidenhout AJ. Structural and functional changes relevant to maxillary arterial flow observed during computed tomography and nonselective digital subtraction angiography in cats with the mouth closed and opened. Vet Radiol Ultrasound. 2014; 55(3):263-71.

Stiles J, Weil AB, Packer RA, Lantz GC. Post-anesthetic cortical blindness in cats: twenty cases. Vet J. 2012; 193 (2):367-73.

Valverde A. Epidural analgesia and anesthesia in dogs and cats. Vet Clin NA Small Ani. 2008; 38:1205-1230.

Zilberstein LF, Moens YP, Leterrier E. The effects of local anesthesia on anesthetic requirements for feline ovariectomy. The Vet J 2008; 178:212-216.

The CSU pain scales are available at http://csu-cvmbs.colostate.edu/vth/diagnostic-and-support/anesthesia-pain-management/Pages/pain-management.aspx

Table 7-11
Dosages Used for Constant Rate Infusions (CRIs) in Dogs

Drug	Loading Dose	CRI Dose	Quick Calculation*	Comments
Morphine (M)	0.5 mg/kg IM (or 0.25 mg/kg SLOWLY IV)	0.12 to 0.3 mg/kg/hr (2.0 mic/kg/min- 5.0 mic/kg/min	Add 60 mg to 500 ml fluid & run at 1 ml/kg/hr for 0.12 mg/kg/hr	MAY cause sedation; can be combined with K &/or L.
Hydromorphone (H)	0.05-0.1 mg/kg IV	0.01 to 0.05 mg/kg/hr	Add 5 to 24 mg to 500 ml fluid & run at 1ml/kg/hr	MAY cause sedation; can be combined with K &/or L.
Fentanyl (F)	0.001 to 0.003 mg/kg IM or IV (1 to 5 mic/kg IV)	**Intraop:** 0.003-0.04 mg/kg/h (0.05-0.7 mic/kg/min; **Postop:** 0.002-0.010 mg/kg/h (0.03-0.2 mic/kg/min)	For 0.005 mg/kg/h, add 2.5 mg to 500 ml fluid & run at 1 ml/kg/hr	2.5 mg =50 ml F, remove 50 ml LRS before adding F; can be combined with K &/or L; **Intra-op dose can be up to 20 to 40 mic/kg/hr.**
Methadone	0.1 to 0.2 mg/kg IV	0.12 mg/kg/hr	Add 60 mg to 500 ml fluid & run at 1 ml/kg/hr	MAY cause sedation; can be combined with K &/or L.
Butorphanol	0.1 mg/kg IV	0.1 to 0.4 mg/kg/hr	Add 50 mg to 500 ml fluid & run at 1 ml/kg/hr for 0.1mg/kg/hr	Only moderately potent & has ceiling effect - use as part of multimodal protocol.
Ketamine (K)	0.25 to 0.5 mg/kg IV	0.12 to 0.6 mg/kg/hr (2 to 10 mic/kg/ min)	Add 60 mg to 500 ml fluid & run at 1 ml/kg/hr for 0.12 mg/kg/hr	Generally combined with opioids; may cause dysphoria; intra-op dose is high end of range.

Drug	Dose	CRI rate	Mixing	Comments
Lidocaine (L)	0.5 to 1.0 mg/kg IV	1.5 to 3.0 mg/kg/hr (25 to 50 mic/kg/min)	Add 750 mg to 500 ml fluid & run at 1ml/kg/hr for 25 mic/kg/min	750 mg = 37.5 ml, remove 37.5ml LRS before adding L; can be combined with opioid &/ or K.
Medetomidine (Med) or Dexmedetomidine(D)	1 to 5 mic/kg Med 1 to 2 mic/kg D Can be IV or IM Preop dose can be loading dose	0.001 to 0.004 mg/kg/hr Med (1 to 4 mic/kg/hr) 0.0005 to 0.002 mg/kg/hr D	Add 500 mic Med or 250 mic D (0.5ml of either) to 500 ml fluid and run 1 to 4 mls/kg/hr	Provides analgesia and light sedation. Excellent addition to opioid CRI, or can be administered as solo drug CRI.
Morphine / Ketamine	M: 0.5 mg/kg IM K: 0.25 to 0.5 mg/kg IV	0.12 mg/kg/hr M & 0.12 mg/kg/hr K	Add 60 mg M & 60 mg K to 500 ml fluid & run at 1 ml/kg/hr	Can be administered up to 3 ml/kg/hr but sedation or dysphoria MAY occur. Can substitute H, F or methadone for M.
Morphine / Ketamine / Lidocaine (MLK)	M: 0.5 mg/kg IM K: 0.25 to 0.5 mg/kg IV L: 0.5 mg/kg IV	0.12 mg/kg/hr M, 0.12 mg/kg/hr K; 1.5 mg/kg/hr L	Add 60 mg of M, 60 mg K and 750 mg L to 500 ml fluid & run at 1 ml/kg/hr	Can substitute H, F or methadone for M. Dr. Muir's dose is 3.3 mic/kg/min M, 50 mic/kg/min L; 10 mic/kg/min K.

*Any of the drug amounts in the bag of fluids can be decreased and the fluids administered at a higher rate if necessary. For example, for morphine, ketamine and morphine/ketamine infusions, 30 mg of morphine & 30 mg of ketamine can be used and the CRI administered at 2 ml/kg/hr if more fluids are needed.

Table 7-12
Dosage for Constant Rate Infusions (CRIs) Used in CATS

Drug	Loading Dose	CRI dose	Quick Calculation*	Comments
Morphine (M)	0.10 mg/kg IM	0.03 mg/kg/hr (0.5 mic/kg/min)	Add 15 mg to 500 ml fluid & run at 1 ml/kg/hr	Cat may need light sedation; can be combined with K & maybe L.
Hydromorphone (H)	0.025 mg/kg IV	0.01 mg/kg/hr	Add 5 mg to 500 ml fluid & run at 1 ml/kg/hr	May cause hyperthermia; can be combined with K &/or L
Fentanyl (F)	0.001 to 0.003 mg/kg IM or IV (1 to 5 mic/kg IV)	**Intraop:** 0.003-0.04 mg/kg/h (0.05-0.7 mic/kg/min); **Postop:** 0.002-0.010 mg/kg/h (0.03-0.2 mic/kg/min)	For 0.005 mg/kg/h, add 2.5 mg to 500 ml fluid & run at 1 ml/kg/hr	2.5 mg=50 ml F, remove 50 ml LRS before adding F; can be combined with K & maybe L. Intra-op dose can be up to 0.02-0.04 mg/kg/hr.
Methadone	0.1 to 0.2 mg/kg IV	0.12 mg/kg/hr	Add 60 mg to 500 ml fluid & run at 1 ml/kg/hr	MAY cause sedation; can be combined with K & maybe L.
Butorphanol	0.1 mg/kg IV	0.1 to 0.2 mg/kg/hr	Add 50mg to 500 ml fluid & run at 1 ml/kg/hr for 0.1 mg/kg/hr	Only moderately potent & has ceiling effect - use as part of multimodal protocol.
Ketamine (K)	0.25 to 0.5 mg/kg IV	0.12 to 0.6 mg/kg/hr (2 to 10 mic/kg/min)	Add 60mg to 500 ml fluid & run at 1 ml/kg/hr for 0.12 mg/kg/hr	Generally combined with opioids; may cause dysphoria. Intra-op dose is high end of range.

Lidocaine (L)	0.25 mg/kg IV	1.5 mg/kg/hr (25 mic/kg/min) Some sources recommend no more than 10 mic/kg/min in cats. Some recommend no lidocaine in cats.	Add 750 mg to 500 ml fluid & run at 1 ml/kg/hr 10 mic/kg/min would be 300 mg lidocaine in 500 ml fluid with a rate of 1 ml/kg/hr	750 mg = 37.5 ml, remove 37.5 ml LRS before adding L; can be combined with opioid &/ or K; **Lidocaine MAY be contra-indicated in the cat due to cardiovascular effects.**
Medetomidine (Med) or Dexmedetomidine(D)	1 to 5 mic/kg Med 1 to 2 mic/kg D Can be IV or IM Preop dose can be loading dose	0.001 to 0.004 mg/kg/hr Med (1 to 4 mic/kg/hr) 0.0005 to 0.002 mg/kg/hr D	Add 500 mic Med or 250 mic D (0.5ml of either) to 500 ml fluid and run 1 to 4 ml/kg/ hr	Provides analgesia and light sedation. Excellent addition to opioid CRI, or can be administered as solo drug CRI.
Morphine/Ketamine	M: 0.10 mg/kg IM K: 0.25 to 0.5 mg/kg IV	0.03 mg/kg/hr M & 0.12 mg/kg/hr K	Add 15 mg M & 60 mg K to 500 ml fluid & run at 1 ml/kg/hr	Can be administered up to 3 ml/kg/hr but dysphoria MAY occur. Can substitute, F, or methadone for M.
Morphine / Ketamine / Lidocaine (MLK)	M: 0.10 mg/kg IM K: 0.25 to 0.5 mg/kg IV L: 0.25 mg/kg IV	0.03 mg/kg/hr M, 0.12 mg/ kg/hr K; 1.5 mg/kg/hr L	Add 15 mg of M, 60 mg K and 750 mg (or 300 mg) L to 500 ml fluid & run at 1 ml/kg/hr	Can substitute H, F or methadone for M. Lidocaine is controversial in cats.

* Any of the drug amounts in the bag of fluids can be decreased and the fluids administered at a higher rate if necessary. For example, for morphine, ketamine and morphine/ketamine infusions, 7.5 mg of morphine & 30 mg of ketamine can be used and the CRI administered at 2 ml/kg/hr if more fluids are needed.

289

Table 7-13
Sample Chart for Adding Analgesic Drugs to IV Fluids for Dogs

(appropriate if you don't think that you will need to change the IV fluid rate - if the patient might need a fluid bolus it is better to have the CRI in a separate fluid bag or syringe).

Amount of **lidocaine** (20 mg/ml) to add to a 1-L fluid bag:

Fluid Rate:*	Maintenance* (50 ml/kg/24hr)	0.5x Maint.	2x Maint.	Surgical (5 to 10 ml/kg/hr)
Lidocaine Dose:				
25 microg /kg/min	36 mls	72 mls	18 mls	15 mls (5 ml/kg/hr) 7.5 mls (10 ml/kg/hr)
50 microg/kg/min	72 mls	144 mls	36 mls	30 mls (5 ml/kg/hr) 15 mls (10 ml/kg/hr)
75 microg/kg/min	108 mls	216 mls	54 mls	45 mls (5 ml/kg/hr) 22.5 mls (10 ml/kg/hr)

Before adding the lidocaine, remove the same volume of LRS as you will be adding of lidocaine. Lower dosages (25 to 50 microg/kg/min) are used for analgesia while all 3 dosages are used for antiarrhythmic therapy.

QUICK CALCULATION: You can easily split the difference between the two analgesic dosages of lidocaine - for 36 mi crog/kg/min of lidocaine add 50 mls of 2% lidocaine to 1-L of LRS and run at 1 ml/POUND/hr (or 0.5 ml/kg/hr).

* Most veterinarians consider maintenance to be 40 to 60 mls/kg/24 hrs in dogs, with the lower end of that rate used in cats. If the infusion rate is halved, the amount of lidocaine in the bag should be doubled to keep the dose constant. We have rounded the volumes slightly up or down to make them clinically useful.

Amount of **morphine** (15 mg/ml) to add to a 1-L fluid bag:

Fluid Rate:*	Maintenance* (50 ml/kg/24hr)	0.5x Maint.	2x Maint.	Surgical (5 to 10 ml/kg/hr)
Morphine Dose:				
0.5 microg /kg/ min (cat dose)	1.0 mls	2.0 mls	0.5 mls	0.40 mls (5 ml/kg/hr) 0.20 mls (10 ml/kg/hr)
1 microg/kg/min	2.0 mls	4.0 mls	1.0 mls	0.80 mls (5 ml/kg/hr) 0.40 mls (10 ml/kg/hr)
2 microg/kg/min	4.0 mls	8.0 mls	2.0 mls	1.60 mls (5 ml/kg/hr) 0.80 mls (10 ml/kg/hr)

QUICK CALCULATION: Ketamine CRI: Add 60 mg (0.6 mls of 100 mg/ml) ketamine to a 1-L bag and run at 2 mls/kg/hr to provide 2 microg/kg/min or at a surgical fluid rate (10 ml/kg/hr) to provide 10 microg/kg/min (intra-op dose).

Table 7-14
Calculating Constant Rate Infusions

(for people that really want to do the math)

For drugs that don't need to be diluted (generally used for drugs in an infusion pump):
• Calculate the TOTAL mgs or microgs needed:
• Dose of infusion in mg/kg/hr or mic/kg/min or whatever (use mg/kg/hr for now) x body weight in kg = total mg/hr needed.

• Divide the calculated mg/hr by the concentration of the drug in mg/ml and now you have the **mls/hour**.
• Divide the number from the calculation above by 60 to get the mls/min:
• Divide by 60 again and to get the mls/second.
• Most drip sets are either 10 drops/ml or 60 drops/ml .
• Calculate the drops/second the patient needs by multiplying the number of drops/ml in the drip set by the number of mls/second.
• Of course if you have a syringe pump, you can stop at mls/min and just program the pump!

• SO, a dog weighs 40 kg and needs a CRI of 2 mg/kg/hr and the drug is 0.2% (2 mg/ml).
• 5 mg/kg/hr x 40 kg = 200 mg/hr divided by 2 mg/ml = 100 ml/hr (program the pump now or move on to drops).

• 100 ml/hr divided by 60 = 1.666, divide by 60 again = 0.027 x 10 drops/ml = 0.2 drops/second or (to make counting easier) 1 drops per every 5 seconds.

For drugs that need to be diluted and administered using a syringe pump:

QUICK TIP from the WSU Technicians: Quick and easy calculation for a 50 ml syringe-pump infusion of lidocaine/ketamine or lidocaine/ketamine/morphine
1. DRAW *42.2 ML SODIUM CHLORIDE INTO A 60 ML SYRINGE.
2. ADD 7.5 ML (150 MG) LIDOCAINE
3. ADD 0.3 ML (30 MG) KETAMINE
4. IF YOU CHOOSE TO ADD MORPHINE, ADD 0.8 ML* (12MG)
*For accuracy, you should subtract another 0.8 mls of saline at the start (so total saline in the syringe would be 41.4 mls so that the total final volume of saline + drugs will be 50 mls. This isn't critical but does increase precision of the concentration of the infusion.
5. ADMINISTERED AT 1 ML/KG/HR, THIS WILL DELIVER LIDOCAINE 50 MCG/KG/MIN; KETAMINE 10 MCG/KG/MIN; MORPHINE 4 MCG/KG/MIN

For drugs that need to be diluted (this is generally for drugs that will be diluted in large volumes, like a bag of fluids)
• Again calculate the number of **mg/hr** that you need.
• Decide the fluid rate you want to deliver in ml/kg/hr.
• Multiply this by the body weight to get the mls/hour.
• We need to deliver 'x' mg/hr of a drug in 'x' mls/hr of a drug so all we need to do is figure out how many mgs we need in each ml. Do this by dividing mg/hr by mls/hr and that gives us mg/ml.

Table 7-14 continued

- Multiply the total number of mls you plan to deliver (e.g., 500 mls, 1-liter, etc.) and that gives you the number of mgs that you need to put in the fluids.
- Finally divide these mgs by the concentration of the drug and you have the number of mls to add to the fluid.
- SO, a dog weighs 20 kg and needs a CRI of 5 mg/kg/hr and a fluid rate of 2 ml/kg/hr and we have 1 liter of fluids and a drug that is 0.5% (5 mg/ml).
- 5 mg/kg/hr x 20 kg = 100 mg/hour. 2 ml/kg/hour x 20 kg = 40 ml/hour. 100 mg/hour / 40 ml/hour = 2.5 mg/ml. 2.5 mg/ml x 1000 mls = 2500 mg. 2500 mg / 5 mg/ml = 500 mls of the drug to add to the 1-L of fluids.
- (For all you math whizzes, you probably see that the kgs could be deleted from this formula and it would still work! Regardless of the wt, you would add 250 mls of the drug to 1000 mls of the fluid and deliver at 2 ml/kg/hr to get 5 mg/kg/hr.)

To make math REALLY easy, use an excel spreadsheet!

Chapter 8
Anesthesia Step-by-Step

Mary Albi, LVT

Shelley Ensign, LVT, CVPP

Janel Holden, LVT, VTS (Anesthesia/Analgesia)

Shona Meyer, BS, LVT, VTS (Anesthesia/Analgesia)

Nicole Valdez, LVT, VTS (Anesthesia/Analgesia)

Introduction

This chapter will quickly get you through all of the anesthesia procedures that you need to do on a routine basis. The other chapters in the book will provide you a more in-depth knowledge of anesthesia but this will most likely be your daily 'go to' chapter. It is organized just like your day should be organized - first get the equipment ready, then choose drugs and calculate dosages, get the patient ready , then go through the 4 phases of anesthesia (preparation/premedication, induction, maintenance, recovery), then clean-up and get ready for the next case! Anesthesia should always proceed in the same order so that nothing is forgotten. Forgetting any step can compromise the patient.

How to Set-Up for Anesthesia

Making sure that EVERYTHING is ready for anesthesia (including all supplies, the anesthetic machine, monitors, drugs and the patient) will greatly improve both the safety and efficiency of the anesthetic episode. There is detailed information about preparing for anesthesia in this chapter and a detailed checklist at the end of the book (pages 466-467). After you read the chapter, use the check-list for every patient. The checklist can be copied and maintained in the anesthesia area.

Anesthesia Phase: Preparation/Premedication

How to Set-up and Pressure-Check the Anesthesia Machine

Please refer to figures 3-37 and 3-38

How to Set-Up the Monitoring Equipment

Make sure that you have all of your monitors ready BEFORE you anesthetize the patient!
1. Turn all of the monitors on (ECG, blood pressure, pulse oximeter, $ETCO_2$, etc.).
2. Choose the correct size blood pressure cuffs.
3. Check the Doppler probe by placing it over your own artery.
4. Set-up the ECG leads, the pulse oximeter probe AND the $ETCO_2$ monitor.
5. Get the esophageal stethoscope ready.
6. Fill out the patient and drug information on the anesthesia record.

How to Prepare the Patient for Anesthesia

Insuring that the patient is healthy and ready to go through anesthesia is one of the most important steps in administering safe anesthesia. Before considering which anesthetic drugs are best for a patient, the following things should be done:
1. Get the patient's history, including any health problems the patient has had and what medications the patient has been on.

2. Understand the patient's diagnosis and the planned surgical procedure.

3. DO A GOOD PHYSICAL EXAM! This is extremely important and should be done prior to administering any medications. If any abnormalities are uncovered, those should be brought to the attention of the attending veterinarian.

   a. Look at the patient for overall signs of health (hair coat, body weight, etc.).

   b. WEIGH THE PATIENT - this is critical for accurate drug dosing. DON'T GUESS THE WEIGHT.

   c. Check the patient's heart rate and respiratory rate (See Chapter 2 for normal values).

   d. Check the patient's body temperature (See Chapter 2 for normal values).

   e. Look at mucous membrane color and capillary refill time (should be pink and < 2 seconds, respectively).

   f. Listen to the heart (both before and after premedications). Understand the impact of premedication drugs on the heart rate. For example, dexmedetomidine will cause bradycardia.

   g. Listen to the lungs.

   h. Obtain a blood work data base. We recommend at least a packed cell volume (PCV) and total protein, even in healthy animals (See Chapter 2).

4. Make sure an anesthesia release form is completed and signed by the owner and that any other forms that your hospital requires are complete. Anesthesia release forms are extremely important! By having the owner sign an anesthesia release form, you know that the risks of anesthesia have been discussed with the owner. You will also have a legal document stating that the owner has given permission for their pet to be anesthetized. This can be very important in the event that something goes wrong.

5. Ideally, the patient's CPR Code should be determined based on the patient's health and the owner's wishes.

6. If patients are sick or geriatric, they may need more assessment prior to anesthesia, which may include:

   a. More complete blood work (CBC, serum chemistry, etc.).

   b. Specific blood tests for specific diseases (e.g., thyroid hormone assay in hyperthyroid cats).

   c. A complete urinalysis.

   d. Assessment of clotting times. May need to cross match & type the patient's blood for a blood transfusion.

   e. Radiographs (e.g., patients with cardiac disease should have a thoracic radiograph) and other imaging like an echocardiogram, if available

   f. Ultrasound (e.g., patients with abdominal disease may need an abdominal ultrasound).

   g. Other tests as needed by the specific patient.

7. If patients are sick, they may also need stabilization prior to anesthesia which may include:

   a. IV fluids.

   b. Additional analgesia.

   c. Supplemental oxygen.

d. Specific drugs (e.g., a patient in heart failure may need furosemide and drugs that improve cardiac function).

e. Body temperature support (warming).

f. Other support specific for the patient.

How to: Calculate Drug Dosages:

1. Weigh the patient.

2. Look up the dose of the drug in milligrams (mgs) per kilogram (kg) or pound (lb or #).

3. Calculate the patient's total drug dosage in mgs:

a. Example, a patient weighs 10 kg (or 20 lbs);

b. The dose of hydromorphone is 0.2 mg/kg (or 0.1 mg/lb);

c. 10 kg x 0.2 mg/kg = 2 mg of hydromorphone for this patient (20 lbs x 0.1 mg/lb = 2 mg).

4. Find the concentration (mg/ml) of the drug on the drug label.

5. Divide the number of mgs calculated above by the concentration of the drug to determine the number of mls the patient needs:

a. Example, hydromorphone is 2 mg/ml;

b. The patient above needs 2 mgs; 2 mgs ÷ 2 mg/ml = 1 ml of hydromorphone.

How to: Administer Premedications:

1. Once the patient has been deemed healthy, or stabilized if unhealthy, premedication for anesthesia should be administered. Drugs to be administered in the premedication period include: sedatives/tranquilizers (e.g., acepromazine, alpha-2 agonists, benzodiazepines, opioids), analgesic drugs (e.g., opioids, alpha-2 agonists, NSAIDs) and any required support drugs (e.g., anticholinergic drugs).

2. Routes of drug administration and their advantages/disadvantages include:

a. Intravenously (IV), intramuscularly (IM) and subcutaneously (SQ).

b. The onset of action is fastest and the degree of effect is most profound (usually 1-5 minutes) and predictable following IV injections but IV injections can be difficult, especially in fractious patients.

c. IM injections are easier to administer and are commonly used for administration of premedicants. Following an IM injection, the onset of action is slightly slower (usually 15-20 minutes) and the degree of sedation is generally not as profound nor as predictable as that following an IV injection. The dosing range for IM injections is generally increased compared to that for IV injections because of the unpredictability of absorption from the tissues.

d. SQ injections provide the least reliable uptake and can significantly impact the speed of onset (often 30 minutes or longer) and predictability of drug effects. This route is not ideal for administration of premedicants. For some drugs, rapid uptake is not necessary (e.g., the NSAIDs) and SQ administration may be appropriate or even recommended.

How to: Administer an IM Injection in the Dog or Cat:

1. First make sure the location you are going to use for the injection will not interfere with any procedures, including imaging.

2. Palpate the muscle you wish to give the injection in. Make sure that the area is not heavily covered with fat ('adipose tissue') since injection into fat will cause very slow absorption, and a very slow onset of action of the drug.

3. Insert the needle with the syringe attached into the muscle using an appropriately sized needle (usually a 25-gauge or 22-guage needle works best for small animals). Keep in mind that you don't always need to insert the needle all the way to the hub into the patient's muscle if the muscle tissue is thin. Just insert the needle in far enough so that the tip of the needle is in the middle of the muscle body.

4. Aspirate to ensure that you are not in a blood vessel. If blood is aspirated, back the needle out slightly and redirect it into muscle again. Aspirate and then inject the drug if there is no blood.

5. Pull the needle and syringe out and discard into a sharps container.

6. Muscles for IM injections in the dog and cat include **(Figure 8-1)**:

    a. Semi-membranous and semi- tendinosis muscles (rear limb);

    b. Biceps femoris (rear limb);

    c. Quadriceps group (rear limb);

    d. Gluteal muscles (rear limb);

    e. Dorsal lumbar muscles or epaxial (over the lumbar area of the back);

    f. Triceps brachii (fore limb);

    g. Latissimus dorsi (over the top of the shoulder);

    h. Pectoral muscles (chest).

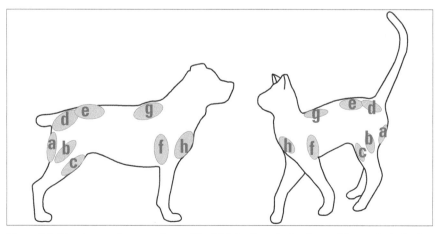

Figure 8-1. Muscles most commonly used for IM injections in the dog and the cat include the: semi-membranous and semi- tendinosis *(a)*, biceps femoris *(b)*, quadriceps group *(c)*, gluteal *(d)*, dorsal lumbar or epaxial *(e)*, triceps brachii *(f)*, latissimus dorsi *(g)*, and pectoral *(h)*.

How to: Administer a Subcutaneous (SQ) Injection in the Dog or Cat:

1. Locate the area you wish to inject. Lift the skin up forming a 'tent'.
2. Insert the needle with syringe attached under the skin at base of the skin tent.
3. Let go of the skin tent.
4. Aspirate and inject if no blood is seen and aspiration is easy.
5. Pull the needle and syringe out and discard them into a sharps container.
6. Sites for SQ injections in the dog and cat include:
    a. Anywhere over the shoulder blades or latissimus dorsi (the thin muscle over the rib cages) where a skin tent can be achieved.

How to: Administer an IV Injection in the Dog or Cat:

1. Identify which vein will be used.
2. Wet the hair with alcohol so that you can see the vein.
3. Clip the hair if the vein is hard to see.
4. Scrub the site if it is really dirty - you don't want to insert dirt into the blood vessel with the needle.
5. Have an assistant occlude the vein or use a tourniquet.
6. Wait for a few seconds (up to a minute) for the vein to fill with blood until you can readily feel and/or see the vessel.
7. Insert the needle through the skin at about a 20° angle from the skin and parallel with the vein. Be assertive getting through the skin - not so assertive that you go through the vein, but don't 'pick at' the skin with the needle.
8. Gently aspirate as you move the needle towards the vein.
9. Once you get blood in the syringe, insert the needle a bit further (about 0.5 to 2 mm, depending on the size of the patient), then aspirate again to be sure that you are still in the vein.
10. Have the assistant release their hold on the vein or release the tourniquet.
11. Inject the drug into the vein.
12. If you are not sure that the needle stayed in the vein, aspirate again at the end of the injection.
13. Remove the syringe and needle, hold off the vein for 10 to 30 seconds.
14. Dispose of the needle in a proper sharps container.
15. Veins for IV injections in the dog and cat include (**Figure 8-2**):
    a. Cephalic vein;
    b. Medial saphenous vein (especially useful in the cat);
    c. Lateral saphenous vein (especially useful in the dog);
    d. Jugular vein;
    e. Dorsal pedal vein.

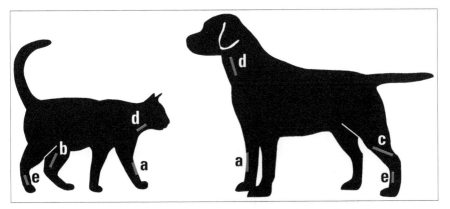

Figure 8-2. Veins that can be used for venipuncture and/or catheterization in dogs and cats include the: cephalic *(a)*, medial saphenous *(b; cat)*, lateral saphenous *(c; dog)*, jugular vein *(d)*, dorsal pedal *(e)*.

What to do with the Premedicated Patient Prior to Induction

After premedicants have been administered IM, the patient should start to show signs of sedation in about 10 to 20 minutes depending on the dose and types of drugs administered. The patient should be placed in a cage in a quiet, dimly lit area to achieve the best sedation. Remove any items in the cage that could cause problems (e.g., water bowls, cat litter, etc.). The patient should be observed frequently to ensure that there are no complications as it becomes sedated. Do not leave any patient that is very old, very young, sick or with respiratory compromise (e.g., brachycephalic dogs or cats) in the cage without continuous observation. Administration of premedicants IV results in almost immediate sedation. The patient should not be placed in a cage but should be gently restrained until sedation is adequate for catheter placement.

Once the patient is sedated:
1. Move the patient from the kennel to the prep table.
2. Start warming, if necessary, using veterinary-approved warmers or warm towels and blankets. Patients that are very small get cold quickly so warming should definitely start now.
3. Place the intravenous (IV) catheter. Remember to pick an appropriate catheter size for the patient. You never know when a routine procedure will lead to a critical situation and the catheter is a tool that you will use to stabilize the patient.
4. Place an oxygen mask (attached to the breathing system of the anesthesia machine) over the muzzle of the patient, turn on the oxygen flow and pre-oxygenate the patient for 3-5 minutes prior to induction. **(Figure 8-3)**
5. Place ECG leads and a blood pressure cuff on the patient and evaluate for any abnormalities. Treat if necessary.

6. Administer IV fluids, if necessary, prior to induction. This can help with perfusion and blood pressure.

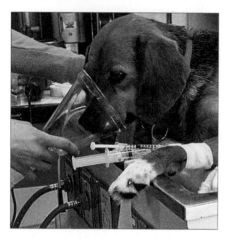

Figure 8-3. Preoxygenating a dog prior to induction.

How to: Place an IV Catheter with Helpful Hints

List of Supplies:
a. Clippers;
b. Tape;
c. T-port or injection cap;
d. Multiple catheters appropriate for patient size;
e. Dry gauze;
f. Scrub and alcohol;
g. Saline or heparinized saline flush;
h. Tourniquet;
i. Bandage material (for covering catheters that will be left in long term).

Veins Commonly Catheterized in Dogs and Cat:
(See Figure 8-2)
a. Cephalic vein/accessory cephalic vein (front leg, used in cats and dogs);
b. Lateral saphenous vein (rear leg, used in dogs);
c. Femoral vein / medial saphenous (rear leg, medial saphenous commonly used in cats).
d. Dorsal pedal vein (rear leg, not commonly used);
e. Jugular vein.

How to: Choose the Correct Catheter Size:

1. Shave the area and evaluate the size of the vein (holding a catheter next to the vein for comparison may help). Remember that it is ideal to select the biggest catheter possible that can be placed in the vein in order to have a good flow of fluids and drugs through the catheter.
2. Catheter sizes are measured by gauges, so the higher the number the smaller the catheter. The commonly used sizes in small animals are 25-gauge, 22-gauge, 20-gauge, and 18-gauge. In large animals commonly used catheter sizes are 10-gauge, 14-guage, and 16-gauge.
3. Keep in mind that if there are two catheters of the same gauge but one is shorter than the other, fluids administered through the shorter catheter will flow faster than fluids through the longer catheter even though they are of the same gauge. However, sometimes longer catheters are better placed in patients that have lots of loose skin due to the fact that movement of the skin (as would occur when the patient is moved) can cause a shorter catheter to be pulled out of the vein. Always consider placing a long catheter when using the lateral saphenous vein in a large dog.

It is Best to Place Two Catheters in a Patient When:

1. The patient is in critical condition;
2. It is possible that the patient will need a blood or plasma transfusion;
3. Multiple types of fluids or drugs will be administered;
4. The current catheter patency is questionable or the size of the catheter is not ideal.

The Best Way to Approach Each Vein:

1. The cephalic and accessory cephalic veins (forelimb):
    a. Remember to start as distal on the limb as possible in case any hematomas form during placement of the catheter. This will allow another attempt higher up the vein.
    b. If the cephalic vein doesn't pop up but the accessory vein of the cephalic does, place the catheter in the accessory vein - it is a good spot to place a catheter.
2. The lateral saphenous vein (rear leg):
    a. This vein is a little harder to catheterize because it tends to move around under the skin.
    b. With this vein it may be easier to start higher up on the leg to get more of a straight line for catheter placement. The straight line may also allow the fluids to flow better.
    c. When the assistant holds off the vein it is often helpful to have them pull the skin tight by slightly pulling the skin towards them. This will help to keep the vein from being so 'bouncy'.
    d. This vein is not useful in cats because it is extremely small.
3. Medial saphenous vein (rear leg):
    a. This vein is commonly used in cats.
    b. Start distal in this vein as well in case any hematomas form during placement of the catheter.
    c. The vein is very shallow and moves around a lot under the skin.

d. When the assistant holds off the vein it is often helpful to have them pull the skin tight by slightly pulling the skin towards them. This will help to keep the vein from being so 'bouncy'.

e. It is very easy to go all the way through this vein so it is best to start at a shallow angle to the skin and to make only small moves with the catheter.

f. This site will work for a surgical catheter but it can be a little hard to keep in place and keep from kinking in an awake and moving animal.

4. Femoral vein (rear leg):

a. Start distal in this vein as well in case any hematomas form during placement of the catheter. Use a long catheter or it is likely to pull out.

b. The vein is fairly deep and can be hard to find in fat animals.

c. Because the vein is deep, the catheter goes through a lot of tissue before it gets to the vein and is usually not deeply seated into the vein. This makes the catheter more difficult to manage since movement of the patient's leg (especially stretching of the leg) can pull the catheter right out of the vein.

d. This site will work for a surgical catheter but it is hard to maintain in a conscious animal for the reason described for the dorsal pedal vein. It must be carefully watched in order to prevent it from being pulled out or kinked.

5. Dorsal pedal vein (rear leg):

c. This site is not commonly used, which may be due to the fact that it is often over looked or may be less preferred. However, this is a great location if all other veins are blown or have all been recently used for catheterization.

d. The only problem with this site may be long term management since once the patient is awake, it will be moving its leg and could cause the catheter to pull out or fail.

6. Jugular vein:

a. This site will require a 'cut down' (small hole through the skin using a small scalpel blade or a large needle) and takes bigger sized catheters than any leg catheter.

b. Jugular catheters are not commonly used unless no other vein is usable or the patient needs a long-term catheter post-operatively.

c. Jugular catheters may also be placed for monitoring central venous.

Placing the Catheter: Step by Step

1. Generously clip the hair from the catheter site. **(Figure 8-4)** This eliminates the potential of contamination from the hair. If the patient has long hair on the back of the leg at the catheter site, it is best to clip hair completely around the leg.

2. Scrub the site with chlorhexidine scrub or iodine scrub, alternating with alcohol wipes. Repeat this step 3 or more times until the alcohol wipes are clean after they have wiped the skin.

3. Flush the catheter with heparinized saline unless blood collection is needed through the catheter for a PCV/TP.

4. Make sure to have an injection port or T-port flushed and readily available.

5. Tear white tape into strips for easy taping of the catheter.

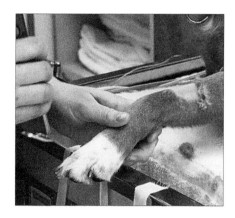

Figure 8-4. Clip and scrub the site for the IV catheter.

6. Have your assistant occlude the vessel, or apply a tourniquet. **(Figure 8-5)**

7. To avoid contamination, do not touch the catheter or the injection site unless you are wearing sterile gloves.

8. Insert the catheter with the bevel side face up towards you into the vein.

9. The catheter is usually at about a 30° angle with the skin to initially get through the skin. Once through the skin, decrease the angle to make it easier to get in the vein without going through it.

10. Hold the catheter so that you can see the hub of the stylet so that you know the instant blood flows into the hub. The hub should be held so that it can be visualized all the time. **(Figure 8-6)**

11. Once blood is seen flowing in the hub of the stylet, decrease the angle of the stylet and catheter and advance both the stylet and catheter a very slight distance (usually 1 mm or so) farther in order to get good placement into the vein. When advancing slightly farther be careful not to push all the way through the vein.

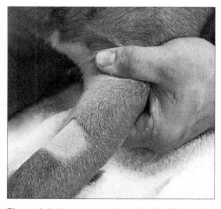

Figure 8-5. Have an assistant hold off the vein.

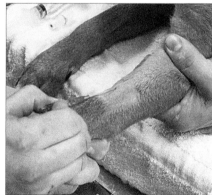

Figure 8-6. Hold the catheter at a 30 degree angle from the skin with your finger and thumb on either side of the hub so that you can see blood as soon as it enters the 'flash' chamber.

TIP

When blood is first seen, the tip of the stylet is in the vein but the catheter might not be in the vein (remember that the stylet is a little longer than the catheter). If this is the case and you try to thread the catheter into the vein, the catheter is not likely to enter the vein and might actually push the vein away (since the catheter is OUTSIDE the vessel wall).

12. Once you have inserted the stylet and catheter a little farther, check to see if blood is still flowing out of the hub of the stylet **(Figure 8-7)**. If so, gently push the catheter off of the stylet and into the vein with one hand while keeping the stylet perfectly still with the other hand.

TIP

Be sure to move the catheter and NOT THE STYLET. If the stylet backs out before the catheter is securely in the vein, the catheter might not thread into the vein.

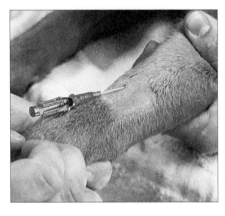

Figure 8-7. After you see blood in the flash chamber, thread the catheter farther into the vein and be sure that blood is still flowing back before removing the stylet.

13. If blood is not flowing, the stylet and catheter probably went all the way through the vein so very slowly back the stylet and catheter out until blood is flowing again, then proceed with step 12.
14. Once the catheter is inserted into the vein, pull the stylet out and see if blood flows out of catheter.
15. If blood is flowing out of the catheter, place the injection cap or T-port on the catheter **(Figure 8-8)**. If blood is not flowing from the catheter, keep the vein held off and squeeze the leg below the catheter. This helps increase blood flow and allows you to see if your catheter is in when the vein is tiny or the patient is dehydrated or hypotensive. You can reinsert the stylet into the catheter (if it is still sterile) and redirect it until blood begins to flow and resume feeding the catheter into the vein. HOWEVER, using this technique can sometimes cause the stylet to cut through the wall of the catheter, so be careful with this. If you are unable to find the vein or to get the catheter to feed into the vein, simply pull the catheter/stylet out and start with a fresh catheter. Choose a new catheterization site either higher up on the same leg or on another leg.

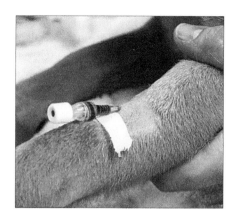

Figure 8-8. Put an injection cap on the catheter.

16. After placing the injection cap or T-port onto the catheter, carefully tape it in place with the white tape that was previously torn **(Figure 8-9)**. Be sure that the catheter stays straight and doesn't kink where it goes through the skin and be sure to tape snugly but not too tightly or the blood flow to/from the paw might be compromised.

TIP
If the paw starts to swell, cut the tape completely through on the back side of the leg to allow blood flow and simply place tape gently over the cut slit of the old tape. Swelling means the tape is too tight! Be sure you watch for this!

17. Flush the catheter with saline or heparinized saline to insure patency. **(Figure 8-10)**
18. Bandage if needed. You can spray with bitter apple or place an E-collar or catheter guard on the patient if they try to chew or lick the catheter.

Catheters and catheter sites should be inspected and monitored several times daily for signs of infection, phlebitis, swelling, soiled bandages, wetness, etc. In addition

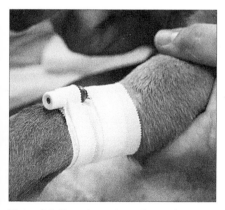

Figure 8-9. Tape the catheter in carefully so that it doesn't accidentally get pulled out of the vein.

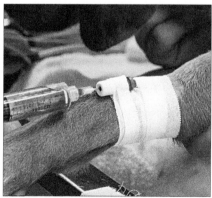

Figure 8-10. Flush the catheter with saline or heparinized saline.

catheters should be flushed for patency, generally every hour. All catheters should be replaced every three days or more often if needed, unless it is a special long-term catheter.

Tips from Technicians for Better Catheter Placement:

1. A bold 'poke' (meaning a fairly aggressive push of the catheter through the skin) usually helps to get a good insertion through the skin and, possibly, straight into the vein. But don't be too aggressive (especially in really small patients) as you might go all the way through the vein!

2. If the patient has tough skin, for example a bulldog or Shar Pei, it is helpful to make a skin nick (or 'cut') with a needle of the same gauge as your catheter. You can make a skin nick by inserting the needle with the bevel facing up right on top of the vein or off to the side, just be careful not to poke the vein! Get the needle tip just under the skin, turn the needle sideways and pull up and out through the skin. This will create a slit in the skin for the catheter placement.

3. When inserting the catheter, pull the skin taught whenever possible. This stabilizes the vein so it doesn't move around as much. This is especially useful when placing a lateral saphenous catheter.

4. Placing the thumb of your non-dominant hand (meaning your left hand if you are right-handed and vice-versa if you are left handed) along the vein will also aid in stabilizing the vein **(Figure 8-11)**.

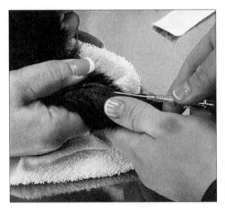

Figure 8-11. A thumb placed alongside the vein will help to stabilize the vein as you are inserting the catheter.

5. Before inserting the catheter into the vein, make sure that it easily comes loose from the stylet (we usually do this as we are flushing the catheter). This makes the catheter easier to 'feed' off the stylet.

6. When flushing the catheter prior to placement in the vein, pull it off of the stylet about half way and then flush with heparinized saline. This technique flushes both the stylet and the catheter and may prevent the catheter from becoming clotted as quickly during a difficult catheterization.

7. When taping in the catheter be sure to overlap the new piece of tape about 50% over the previous piece of tape and wrap the tape going up the leg. This will help keep the catheter from backing out of the vein and allow more skin-to-tape contact.

8. Do not tape over any connection sites where things twist together (like injection caps onto the catheter). These connections may come loose and leak blood. It is difficult to get to those sites to fix them if they are under tape and attempting to get to them may cause you to accidentally pull out the catheter

How to: Choose the Appropriate Endotracheal (ET) Tube

Selection of the appropriate sized endotracheal (ET) tube (both diameter and length) is extremely important for optimizing airway function. The type of material that the tube is made from and the type of cuff are also important. An appropriately sized endotracheal tube will protect the patient's airway and allow for ventilation assistance without causing any trauma to the arytenoids and trachea.

1. Most endotracheal tube sizes are indicated in millimeters (mm) and in French (Fr.) measurements. The size indicates the inside diameter (ID) **(Figure 8-12)**.

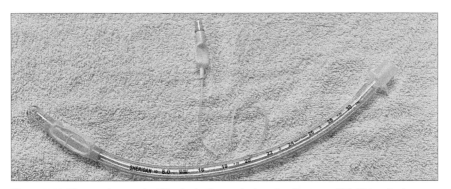

Figure 8-12. The number on the ET tube indicates its interior diameter (ID). This tube is a size 8.0.

2. The diameter of the ET tube should be as close to the diameter of the patient's trachea as possible. Determine the diameter by palpating the trachea and then select 3 tubes: the size that you think best matches the trachea, a tube one half size larger and a tube one half size smaller than the selected tube **(Figure 8-13)**. The diameter is critical!

   a. Breeds with hypoplastic (i.e., smaller than expected for the size of the patient) tracheas, which are primarily brachycephalic breeds like bulldogs and pugs, require endotracheal tubes smaller than expected by their body size.

   b. Hound breeds, including dachshunds, have large tracheas for their body size.
3. An ET tube that is too large will be too tight and may cause irritation/inflammation of the tracheal membrane that can produce clinical problems (e.g., cough, airway stricture). The tube can also cause damage as it passes through the arytenoids (or 'vocal folds') at the larynx to get into the trachea.
4. An ET tube that is too small will make it harder for the patient to breathe.

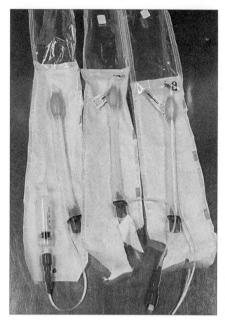

Figure 8-13. A variety of ET tube sizes should be prepared for the patient. In this photo, the cuffs are inflated to check for leaks.

    a. A tube even one size too small increases the work of breathing four fold.

    b. Increased work of breathing means increased muscle activity. Muscles need oxygen to work. Normal muscle oxygen consumption is about 5% with normal breathing but increases greatly with increased work of breathing. This can cause, or add to, hypoxemia.

    c. It can be very hard for patients with 'weak' muscles (geriatric, neonatal or very sick patients) to increase their work of breathing and they are very likely to experience hypoxemia and/or hypercarbia due to respiratory fatigue.

5. An endotracheal tube that is too small may not seal the airway completely and can lead to aspiration pneumonia or breathing of air around the tube cuff, decreasing the amount of inhalant that the patient receives. If the tube does seal the airway, it may require overinflation of the cuff. This may narrow/occlude the airway by constricting the tube, or can cause pressure necrosis in the trachea. The latter is an extremely dangerous condition and the cuff should NEVER be overinflated.

6. The length of the ET tube should reach from the tip of the animal's incisors to the thoracic inlet (the area of the thoracic inlet is approximately located at the tip of the sternum). The tube should be measured against the body of the patient to determine the proper length **(Figure 8-14)**, while keeping the tube sterile or clean.

    a. ET tubes that are too short can potentially come out when the patient is moved.

    b. ET tubes that are too long may go down one of the bronchi instead of staying in the trachea. This causes 'endobronchial intubation' (sometimes called 'one lung intubation') which means that only half of the lung field is participating in gas exchange. This can cause hypoxemia and hypercarbia. This can also cause inadequate concentrations of inhalant to reach the patient and the patient may be hard to maintain at an appropriate anesthetic plane.

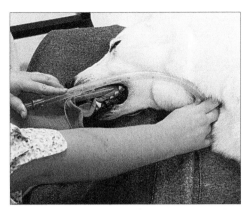

Figure 8-14. The length of the ET tube should reach from the tip of the animals incisors to the thoracic inlet, which is approximately located at the tip of the sternum.

CRITICAL TIP!
If a small patient is hypoxemic or hypercarbic or won't stay asleep in spite of an appropriate setting on the vaporizer and appropriate ventilation, the ET tube might be too long. Try backing it out SLIGHTLY (a few millimeters, maybe up to 1 cm in larger patients). Give the patient 3 to 5 deep breaths (10 to 15 [cat] or 15 to 20 [dog] cm H_2O on the airway pressure manometer) and reassess.

c. Tubes that are too long also increase 'dead space' if they stick out from the incisors too far. Dead space is an area where inhaled gas and exhaled gas mix. This decreases gas exchange efficiency and is likely to result in hypercarbia.
d. Tubes that are too long can be trimmed up to the level of the cuff inflation line ('pilot line'), as needed **(Figure 8-15)**.

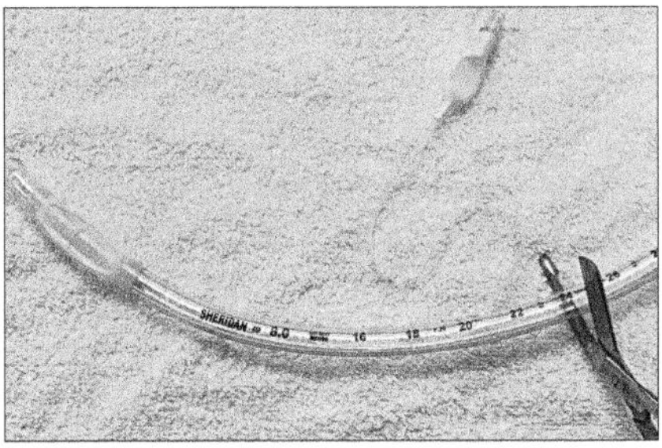

Figure 8-15. To decrease dead-space, the end of the ET tube can be cut off as long as the pilot line to the cuff is still present.

7. Tubes are available with high pressure low volume and high volume low pressure cuffs.
   a. High volume low pressure cuffs are safer because they allow a seal without placing as much pressure on the tracheal wall as high pressure low volume cuffs.
   b. High pressure low volume cuffs can only be used for short periods of time because of the excessive pressure on the tracheal mucosa.
8. The material that the tube is made from is also an important consideration. Tubes

can be made from polyvinyl chloride (PVC) or red rubber. PVC tubes are preferred for the following reasons:

a. Advantages of PVC:
- Relatively inexpensive.
- Not irritating to tissues.
- Less likely than rubber tubes to kink.
- Less likely than rubber tubes to become sticky with age.
- Fairly stiff at intubation which makes them easy to place in the trachea. PVC warms up and becomes softer at body temperature so the tube conforms to the patient's airway shape and is less likely to cause excessive pressure in areas where it contacts the trachea. Rubber tubes do not soften.
- The tube is transparent so that condensation occuring with each breath can be visualized and anything occluding the tube can be easily discovered when cleaning. Rubber tubes are not transparent.

b. Advantages of rubber:
- Can be steam sterilized.

How to: Prepare the Endotracheal Tube (ETT)

Prior to induction, it is necessary to have the endotracheal tube (ETT or ET tube) chosen and prepared.

1. Select the proper size and length of tube for your patient.
2. Have tubes a half size above and below the assumed appropriate size ready to go in case the first tube is not the right size.
3. Inflate the cuff and leave for 10 to 15 minutes to insure that it does not leak (See Figure 8-13).
4. A water soluble sterile lubricant should be used to lightly coat the cuff of the endotracheal tube.
   a. The lube is preferred to water because lubricant helps the cuff to create a lasting seal. Water will dry out and a leak may develop around the cuff.
   b. Use only a very small amount of lube on the tube of cats and small dogs. Excessive amounts of lubricant could occlude the bevel (if the tube is really small) or the Murphy eye (which is the hole near the end of the endotracheal tube that prevents complete obstruction if the tip of the ET tube becomes occluded).
5. Just before induction, deflate the cuff so that the tube is ready for insertion into the trachea.

Anesthesia Phase: Induction

Induction is the process of taking a patient from a state of sedation to a state of unconsciousness. This process can cause some very large physiologic changes (e.g., hypotension and/or hypoventilation are common), requiring that the anesthetist be ready to react if necessary.

How to: Induce the Patient to Anesthesia

1. Before induction it is important to pressure check the anesthesia machine and have monitoring equipment placed on your patient, if tolerated by the patient. If your patient will not tolerate monitoring equipment placement, more sedation may be needed before induction. The monitoring equipment can also be placed immediately after induction of the patient. Preparation is key to a successful and safe induction.

2. It is also beneficial to preoxygenate critically ill patients, patients that are hypoventilating and any patient prone to apnea during induction.

3. Administration of induction drugs should always be preceded by sedative/tranquilizer drugs to decrease the necessary dose, and the dose-dependent adverse effects, of the induction and maintenance drugs.

> **TIP**
> **Proper sedation and pain management will decrease the amount of induction drugs needed to achieve intubation and decrease the amount of inhalant needed to keep the patients asleep. Utilizing multiple sedative/anesthetic drugs is called 'balanced anesthesia' and is imperative for safe anesthesia.**

4. Induction drugs should be titrated 'to effect', which means that the drug should be slowly administered to the point that the patient can be intubated.

6. Titrate the induction drug through the IV catheter or into the vein until the patient is at an anesthetic depth appropriate for intubation. This is determined by muscle relaxation assessed by jaw tone.

a. For propofol and alfaxalone, ⅓ of the calculated dose should be administered and then the patient checked in 20 to 30 seconds for unconsciousness/relaxation.

b. For ketamine/benzodiazepine or Telazol, ½-⅔ of the calculated dose should be administered and the patient checked in 1 to 1.5 minutes for unconsciousness/relaxation.

c. With any of these protocols, more drug (another ⅓ of the propofol or alfaxalone dose or another 10 to 20% of the ketamine or Telazol dose) should be administered until the patient is unconscious and relaxed enough to be easily intubated.

How to: Intubate the Patient

1. If the patient is relaxed and the mouth can be easily opened, the patient can be intubated. If the patient is still conscious, has excess jaw tone, or swallows when the larynx is stimulated, administer more induction drug as described above. DO NOT TRY TO INTUBATE A SEMI-CONSCIOUS PATIENT. This can result in excessive stimulation (making it harder for the patient to go to sleep) and can cause damage of the larynx. Stimulation of the gag reflex, with potential regurgitation/vomiting, can also occur. Excessive coughing and gagging, as can occur when intubating an inadequately anesthetized patient, can increase intracranial and intraocular pressure.

2. Once the patient is relaxed, an assistant should grasp the upper jaw with one hand just behind the canine teeth while retracting the upper lip on either side. The

other hand is used to GENTLY pull the tongue out and down so that the larynx can be visualized by the person intubating. The person helping with intubation should hold the head at a 45 degree angle from the body of the patient **(Figure 8-16)** with the mouth open.

    a. In cats and brachycephalic patients it is useful to grasp the upper jaw behind or just below the cheek bone (zygomatic arch).

    b. Excessive flexion or extension of the head will make it difficult to visualize the larynx.

    c. The holder should not put pressure on the laryngeal area as this can push the structures of the throat into an abnormal position, making it difficult to intubate.

3. A laryngoscope blade should be placed on the base of the tongue just in front of the epiglottis by the person intubating **(Figure 8-17)**.

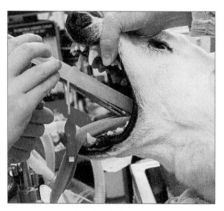 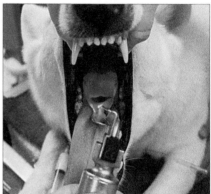

Figure 8-16. The proper technique to hold the mouth open for intubating. One of the holder's hands should be on the maxilla just behind the incisors and the other hand should be gently pulling the tongue out of the mouth.

Figure 8-17. The blade of the laryngoscope should be placed in front of - not on - the epiglottis. The larynx and the opening of the trachea can be clearly visualized in this photo.

4. The tip of the blade can be gently pushed down towards the table (ventrally) to force the base of the tongue down, which will also allow the epiglottis to move down (ventrally).

    a. THE BLADE SHOULD NOT BE PLACED ON THE EPIGLOTTIS BECAUSE THIS CAN EASILY DAMAGE THE EPIGLOTTIS.

    b. If the soft palate is in the way of visualizing the larynx and the arytenoids, use the ET tube to gently push the soft palate up (dorsally).

5. Once the epiglottis has moved ventrally, the arytenoids should be readily visible.

6. If intubating a cat, 1-2 drops of lidocaine (but not cetacaine! Cetacaine is toxic to cats) should be placed on the arytenoids prior to attempting intubation since cats are prone to laryngeal spasm.

    a. Deliver oxygen (1 to 2 liters) through an oxygen mask placed over the cat's nose and mouth for 30 to 60 seconds while waiting for the lidocaine to work.

7. Intubate the patient by placing the tip of the beveled end of the ET tube at the

ventral opening of the trachea and then passing the ET tube through the arytenoids into the trachea.

a. The tube should be PLACED GENTLY. Do not force the tube or push it roughly through the arytenoids and into the trachea.

TIP
The tube should be VISUALIZED PASSING BETWEEN THE ARYTENOIDS. Passage of the tube into the esophagus instead of the trachea delays the delivery time of oxygen and anesthetic gases and may stimulate regurgitation. Regurgitation when the patient cannot swallow (because it is anesthetized) and does not have a protected airway (because the ET tube is in the esophagus) can result in aspiration pneumonia. GET THE PATIENT INTUBATED AS QUICKLY AS POSSIBLE!

8. To help with placement of the tube in cats, a stylet should be placed through the ET tube with the stylet tip just at the end, or barely past the end, of the tube **(Figure 8-18)**. The latter is acceptable ONLY when using a soft stylet or a stylet covered in plastic so that there are no rough or sharp edges. Wire stylets should not pass through the end of the ET tube because the metal can damage the soft tissue of the upper airway and/ or trachea.

a. The soft stylets are often made from a flexible polyethylene (PE) tubing that can pass through the ETT into the trachea prior to insertion of the ETT.

b. PE tubing is beneficial when intubating cats and patients that are having laryngeal spasm. In these patients the stylet generally must be inserted through the arytenoids before the tube can be inserted into the trachea.

c. Once the stylet is through the arytenoids, the ETT is pushed into the trachea using gentle but firm pressure and a rotating motion.

d. Alternatively, the tube can be held ready at the larynx with the stylet through the arytenoids while the anesthetist watches for the patient to breathe. As soon as a breath is taken and the arytenoids open, the ETT tube can be inserted into the trachea. Be ready for that breath!

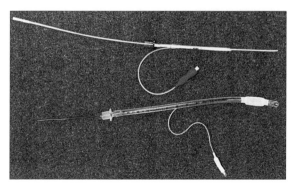

Figure 8-18. Stylets in ET tubes. A soft stylet is at the top and a rigid stylet at the bottom.

9. Methods to confirm proper endotracheal intubation include: feeling air moving in and out of the end of the ETT while the patient is spontaneously breathing, connecting the patient to the breathing system and watching for movement of the rebreathing bag with each breath, watching the ETT 'steam up' with each breath, palpation of only one rigid tubular structure in the cervical (neck) region, placing the laryngoscope blade on top of the ETT and applying downward pressure until you can visualize a the arytenoids on either side of the ETT, and connecting a capnograph to the end of the ETT to measure the production of carbon dioxide.

TIP
ALWAYS confirm proper placement of the ET tube right after it has been inserted into the trachea and any time the patient is moved! If not confirmed at that time, the patient may be in danger by the time the incorrect placement of the tube is noticed.

10. Secure the ETT to the patient's mouth/head with a piece of tape, elastic band, gauze, etc. and connect the ETT to a breathing system **(Figure 8-19)**.
11. If the patient has any trouble breathing or if intubation took a long time, give the patient 2 breaths of pure oxygen (watch the pressure manometer: peak pressure should be 10 to 15 cm H_2O for cats and small dogs; 15 to 20 cm H_2O for medium-large dogs) and assess the patient. Don't turn on the inhalant until the patient's tongue is pink and SpO_2 is 95% or higher.

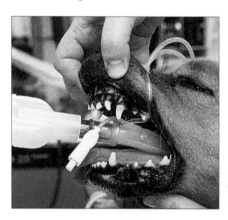

Figure 8-19. The ET tube should be tied to the patient's jaw (maxilla in this photo) and connected to the breathing system.

How to: Pressure Check the Endotracheal Tube Cuff After Intubation
12. THIS IS A CRITICAL STEP!
   a. The cuff should not be under-inflated or there will be a leak in the airway (allowing the patient to breathe room air around the tube which may make the patient light [room air does not contain inhalant gas] or hypoxemic [room air contains only 21% oxygen]). An under-inflated cuff also means that the airway is not 'protected' so if the patient regurgitates or vomits, it could aspirate some

of the regurgitated or vomited fluid into the airway. This can potentially lead to aspiration pneumonia.

    b. Conversely, over-inflating a cuff is just as dangerous since over-inflation creates excess pressure on the tracheal mucosa. This can cause mucosal damage which may lead to airway stricture.

13. Once the tube is in place, the cuff should be CAREFULLY inflated.

    a. Inflate the cuff ONLY to the point where leaks are prevented at a peak inspiratory pressure (PIP) of 20 cm H_2O measured on the pressure manometer **(Figure 8-20)**.

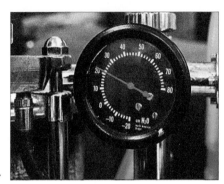

Figure 8-20. A manometer showing 20 cm H_2O, which is the highest pressure that should be used when pressure checking the ET tube cuff.

CRITICAL TIP!

An overinflated cuff can cause tracheal mucosal damage and possible scarring and stricture.

CRITICAL TIP!

To prevent the ETT and the inflated cuff from damaging the trachea, the ETT should be disconnected from the breathing system when the patient is moved or repositioned. Tracheal mucosal tearing, and potentially tracheal rupture, may occur during repositioning while the patient is still connected to the breathing circuit, especially in cats (Hardie et al. 1999; Mitchell et al. 2000). This occurs because the breathing system causes twisting of the tube in the airway and the inflated cuff can catch on, and tear, the tracheal mucosa.

14. Once the cuff is inflated, turn the inhalant on to the desired concentration.

TIP

Do not turn on the inhalant prior to cuff inflation or the inhalant will contaminate the room.

CRITICAL TIP!

Once the patient is intubated and oxygen/inhalant is turned on, don't forget to lubricate the eyes! (Figure 8-21)

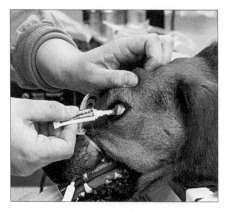

Figure 8-21. Lubricating the eyes immediately after induction.

How to: Handle a Difficult Intubation

CRITICAL TIP!
ALWAYS be prepared for a difficult intubation.

1. If intubation is difficult:
   a. Have the person holding the head reposition so that you can see the larynx better.
   b. Administer another ¼-⅓ dose of induction drug - a relaxed patient is easier to intubate.
   c. Use lidocaine on the arytenoids if they are spasmed closed.
   d. Use a stylet!
   e. Use a smaller tube. It can be replaced with a bigger tube at a later point but getting ANY tube in to start with is critical for safety.
   f. Do all of this QUICKLY. A patient that has not received oxygen for only four minutes is in serious danger. Four minutes passes quickly!
   g. If these techniques do not work, stop trying, put the patient back on oxygen (QUICKLY!) and call for help. The patient may need a tracheostomy or other routes of intubation.

Anesthesia Phase: Maintenance

During the maintenance phase of anesthesia the anesthetic depth should be continuously assessed and the vaporizer percent changed as needed to deliver anesthesia 'to effect'. Analgesia should be reassessed and monitoring and support should be provided as needed for each patient.

How to: Choose an Inhalant

Both isoflurane and sevoflurane will be suitable for all patients. Desflurane is also suitable but rarely used because of the need for special vaporizers. All of the inhalants cause dose-dependent cardiovascular and respiratory depression so more important than the inhalant itself is the dose. Keep it low!

Sevoflurane is faster-acting than isoflurane so if rapid change in anesthetic depth or rapid recovery from anesthesia is necessary/desired, sevoflurane is a better choice.

How to: Assess Anesthetic Depth

Assessing anesthetic depth is one of the most important jobs of the anesthetist. CNS depression is necessary (or otherwise the patient will wake up during surgery!) but unfortunately it is very easy to over-anesthetize the patient ('too deep'). This is very dangerous because it can cause dysfunction of all organ systems and can rapidly lead to death. Monitoring anesthetic depth means monitoring the response of the central nervous system (CNS) to the dose of the anesthetic drugs and to external stimuli, like pain.

CRITICAL TIP!
Even though the CNS is the most important organ system since it controls all of the other organ systems, we have no way of mechanically monitoring its status. Thus, the anesthetist is critical since the seemingly minor but critically important monitoring tools listed below depend on the vigilance of the anesthetist.

a. Assess response to a painful stimulus. This can be as simple as the response to pinching the toe if the patient isn't having surgery (like a patient anesthetized for radiographs) or response to a surgical incision or manipulation of tissues. If the patient responds, provide analgesia or increase the anesthetic depth. If the patient doesn't respond, make sure the patient isn't too deep and consider decreasing the vaporizer setting by 0.25 to 2.0% (depending on patient is depth and specific inhalant).
b. Assess jaw tone by moving the jaw up and down. Muscle relaxation associated with anesthesia should allow the jaw to be easily movable ('loose'). For tight jaw tone, provide analgesia or increase the anesthetic depth. For loose jaw tone, make sure the patient is adequately but not excessively anesthetized.

TIP
Jaw tone in patients with very muscular jaws (like Rottweilers) may always feel a little 'tighter' than in patients with less mandibular muscle.

c. Assess the palpebral reflex by gently stroking the eyelashes or by gently touching the medial canthus (the inner part of the eyelid next to the nose; **(Figure 8-22)**. The patient should have a light 'blink' in response to this stimulus if lightly anesthetized (like for radiographs or other non-painful procedures) but the blink should be very slow or not present for deeper planes of anesthesia.
d. Eye position and pupil size are important but can also be deceiving. The eyes of dogs and cats in a light plane of anesthesia are in a central position (meaning they are staring straight ahead) and the pupils is generally normal size. Animals in a good surgical plane of anesthesia will have eyes in a ventral (downward) position with the white part of the eye [sclera] showing. **(Figure 8-23)** The tricky part is that when an animal becomes too deep their eyes come back to central but in this

instance, the pupils are generally dilated. If you are not sure about depth assess other parameters, e.g. jaw tone, heart rate, respiratory rate, etc....

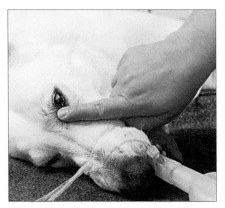

Figure 8-22. Checking the palpebral reflex by gently touching the medial canthus of the eye.

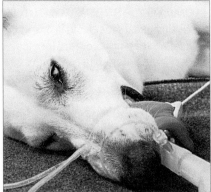

Figure 8-23. The eye rotated down showing the sclera, which indicates a medium plane of anesthesia.

TIP
Many drugs (for example, ketamine, atropine, and high dosages of opioids) can affect eye positioning and pupil constriction/dilation so the anesthetist should also assess signs other than eye position and pupil size to determine depth of anesthesia.

e. Assess cardiovascular (i.e., heart rate and rhythm and blood pressure) and respiratory (i.e., respiratory rate and volume, SpO_2 [oxygen saturation as measured by the pulse oximeter] and end-tidal CO_2 [measured by capnography]). Although anesthesia affects these organ systems directly, depression of the CNS also affects these systems. If there are any abnormalities, be sure to check anesthetic depth.

How to: Calculate Drip Rates for Fluid Administration

Intravenous fluid administration should usually start just before induction so that the fluids can help push the induction drug into the patient's circulation, but starting fluids right after intubation is also acceptable. The IV fluid drip rate for your patients is easy to calculate once you have determined which size drip set to use. Use a 60 drop/ml set for patients under 11 kgs and a 15 drop/ml set for patients over 11 kg. There are other drop/ml sets so be sure to check yours!

a. Determine the weight of your patient in kilograms.

b. Determine the desired fluid volume/kg to be administered.

c. Determine the size drip set to be used.

d. Use the following formula to calculate drops/minute:

e. (Weight (kg) x rate x drip set) ÷ 3600

How to: Choose the Appropriate IV Fluid for your Patient

Mary Albi, LVT

Balanced electrolyte solutions are the right place to start until you can determine acid/base status. Patients with dehydration, anorexia, diarrhea, vomiting from most causes, diabetes, hyperadrenocorticism, renal failure, sepsis, shock, heat stroke and most other conditions can all be started on a balanced electrolyte solution. The majority of these conditions will have potassium loss and, because potassium (K^+) is an anion (+ charged), the patient will present mildly acidotic. The K^+ in the balanced electrolyte solutions is not enough to correct acidosis, but not enough to cause an issue should the patient be hyperkalemic either. Since normal IV fluid K^+ is around 4 mEq/L, the balanced electrolyte solution may actually help to decrease potassium in the body. The balanced electrolyte solutions are also buffers so the acidosis is generally corrected by the buffer even if K^+ is abnormal. Most sick patients, like those described above, are acidotic so this is an important component of the fluids. The buffer in LRS is lactate which requires metabolism by the liver to become a buffer. Thus, Normosol-R or Plasmalyte may be preferred in patients with hepatic disease since the buffer in those fluids is acetate, which does not require metabolism to work. The liver disease would have to be severe for this to be a clinically important concern. RARELY, patients are alkalotic. An example is a patient that has a 'high' obstruction (ie, very near the stomach) and has been vomiting out acidic stomach contents. These patients should receive 0.9%NaCl. Otherwise, most patients should receive balanced electrolytes.

How to: Add Potassium to the IV Fluids
Mary Albi, LVT

Hypokalemia is frequently encountered in sick patients since the main source of K^+ is food and these patients may not be eating. K^+ in the form of potassium chloride (KCl) can be added to the isotonic fluids.
- No more than 60 mEq K^+ should be added to a liter of fluids and the administration rate should never exceed 0.5 mEq/kg/hr.

How to: Add Calcium to the IV Fluids
Mary Albi, LVT

Hypocalcemia is another common electrolyte deficiency and calcium can be added in either the form of calcium gluconate (10% solution=9.3 mg of Ca^{++}/ml) or calcium chloride (10% solution = 27.2 mg of Ca^{++}/ml) at 5-15 mg/kg/hr.

How to: Correct Metabolic Acidosis by Adding Sodium Bicarbonate to the IV Fluids
Mary Albi, LVT

- Correct respiratory acid-base imbalance first (ie, increase ventilation if the patient is anesthetized or on a ventilator).
- Make sure the patient can breathe normally. Sodium bicarbonate administered to hypoventilating patients can increase the acidosis since the patient can't exhale the CO_2 that will be produced by metabolism of the sodium bicarbonate and respiratory acidosis will occur.
- Insure appropriate fluid choice and rate of fluid administration. This alone often corrects metabolic acidosis.
- Once ventilation and fluids are correct, sodium bicarbonate can be administered to treat metabolic acidosis if pH is less than 7.2 and CO_2 is NORMAL. Use the following formula:
  - mEq HCO3- = body weight (kg) x base excess (from blood gas) x 0.4;
  - administer ½ dose over 30 mins & reassess pH.

How to: Use and Trouble-Shoot the Pulse Oximeter

The pulse oximeter measures the percentage of hemoglobin that has oxygen bound to it (designated as SpO_2), as does analysis of an arterial blood gas sample (designated SaO_2). Normal SpO_2 or SaO_2 in patients breathing room air is > 90% while normal in patients breathing 100% oxygen (i.e., anesthetized patients) is > 95%. A SpO_2 reading below 90% is considered hypoxemic, requiring immediate revisions in anesthetic technique and/or analysis of the SpO_2 sensor. The pulse oximeter will also count heart rate.

1. The pulse oximeter probe is normally positioned on the tongue **(Figure 8-24)** because the tongue is easily accessible, generally the right thickness for the pulse oximeter to pass light waves through (that is how oxygen saturation is measured), highly vascularized so the pulse oximeter should be able to detect a pulse fairly easily, and usually not pigmented or at least not entirely pigmented (pigmentation at the probe site will decrease the quality of the signal).

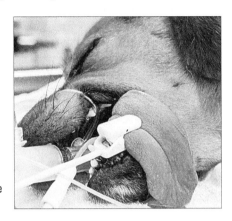

Figure 8-24. The pulse oximeter placed on the tongue.

2. The probe can be positioned in alternate spots if the tongue site interferes with surgery (as in dentistry or oral surgery) or if the probe might be frequently dislodged by the surgeon (as with almost any surgery on the head).
a. Other locations that may work include sites with relatively thin, non-pigmented skin, including the prepuce, vulva, lightly pigmented toes **(Figure 8-25)**, fold of skin at the 'flank' right in front of the stifle **(Figure 8-26)** and rectum. Ears are occasionally used, but they are too thin and often don't give an accurate reading. There is a very useful specialized probe, called a reflectance probe, that can be positioned on the ventral part of the tail or other fairly flat tissue sites.

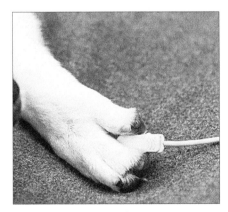

Figure 8-25. The pulse oximeter placed on the toe.

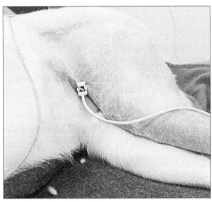

Figure 8-26. The pulse oximeter placed on the flank.

3. If SpO_2 is low, immediately assess the patient for adequate ventilation. Give the patient 1 to 2 breaths and see if the reading changes. If it goes up, hypoventilation is indeed the problem and the anesthetic depth should be decreased (excessive anesthetic depth is the main cause of hypoventilation) and breathing supported until the patient can maintain a normal SpO_2 on its own.

4. If the SpO_2 numbers don't increase, the problem could be that the patient is severely compromised (i.e., close to death). Quickly check other parameters - the patient would also have very weak pulses, very low blood pressure, a prolonged CRT and very pale or blue mucous membranes.

TIP

Using a stethoscope or your fingers on a pulse, check the patient's heart rate and see if that heart rate that you count matches the heart rate given by the pulse oximeter. If so, the pulse oximeter reading is likely correct and you should start breathing for the patient if the SpO_2 is low. If not, the pulse oximeter is probably having difficulty finding a pulse so the reading could be incorrect.

5. The probe might be having a difficult time finding a strong pulse because:

a. The patient is very small so the arteries are also very small. This is a common problem in cats.

b. The patient is indeed severely compromised and blood flow is poor. As above, the patient's blood pressure would be low, CRT prolonged and the mucous membranes might be pale, dusky or blue.

c. The vessels at the site of the probe are constricted ('vasoconstriction'):

   i. Shock (the patient would be extremely pale).
   ii. Hypothermia (take the body temperature!). The tongue can be cold without the entire body temperature being low.
   iii. Alpha-2 agonist (e.g., medetomidine or dexmedetomidine) administration.
   iv. Localized compression of the vessels from prolonged probe pressure at one site.

TIP

Localized vessel compression at the site of the pulse oximeter is a common problem! If the probe is having difficulty locating a pulse, move the probe to a different site nearby or to another location on the body altogether.

TIP

The tip of the tongue can be very difficult to get a reading from in vasoconstricted patients so the probe may need to be moved back to the base of the tongue where the vessels are generally larger or less constricted.

d. The contact is bad because the tongue is really dry.

   i. Moistening the site with water or saline often works to restore the SpO_2 readings.
   ii. The probe may take a moment to stabilize and obtain the SpO_2 reading after moistening the tongue or moving to a new site.

6. If you doubt that your SpO$_2$ monitor is accurate, it is best to draw an arterial blood sample for blood gas analysis, if possible. See Chapter 5 for more information on trouble shooting the SpO$_2$ monitor.

How to: Use and Trouble-Shoot the ECG

The ECG provides information about the electrical impulses through the myocardium (muscle of the heart). The electrical activity is what causes the mechanical activity (i.e., the heart beat) and analysis of the electrical activity is extremely important because some anesthetic drugs and some things that occur under anesthesia (e.g., pain, hypoxemia, and hypercarbia) can cause abnormal electrical rhythm (see Chapters 5 and 10). Correct and routine placement of ECG leads should be part of standard of care for all patients and familiarity with normal ECG tracings will allow rapid recognition of abnormal ECG tracings.

1. There are a myriad of lead numbers and configurations available for diagnosing cardiac disease but a simple three lead configuration (leads I, II, III) is the most commonly used in anesthesia.
    a. The three leads are: white (applied to the right forelimb), red (applied to the left hindlimb), and black (applied to the left forelimb) **(Figure 8-27)**.

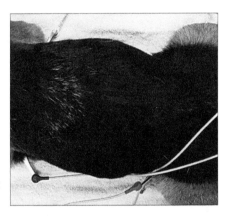

Figure 8-27. The placement of the ECG leads: white lead on right forelimb, black lead on left forelimb, red lead on left rearlimb.

    b. To remember this, use the saying 'white on right; smoke over fire'. The 'smoke' and 'fire' refer to the black and red leads, respectively.
    c. The best sites for lead placement are the triceps for the two forelimb leads and the front of the stifle for the hindlimb lead. Placing the leads on the thorax can create artifacts as the chest moves when the patient breathes.
        i. It is not always possible to put the leads in these locations if they interfere with the surgery site. You may need to be creative with lead placement, but as long as you create a 'triangle' around the heart with the leads, you will get an ECG tracing. Just expect that the ECG might not look normal. But you are monitoring for trends so just watch for changes in the configuration.
2. Use gel or alcohol on the leads to make sure that there is good contact with the skin **(Figure 8-28)**. Gel is often preferred if the surgery will be long or a warm air

blower (like a Bair Hugger) will be used. In both examples, the alcohol is likely to dry out and the leads will stop reading a signal.

3. The different leads (I, II, III) work by combining various configurations of the three lead placement to allow us to look at the myocardial electrical activity in different ways.

a. If one lead is not providing a readable ECG, try another lead. This often occurs in cats because the heart muscle is so small that the electrical activity can be difficult to detect.

b. If an unusual but not diagnostic electrical activity occurs in one lead, switching to another lead may exacerbate or eliminate the activity. If eliminated, assume that it was not a real arrhythmia but instead was an artifact. If exacerbated or unchanged, assume it is a real arrhythmia and start diagnostics and treatment.

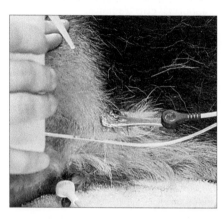

Figure 8-28. Wet the ECG leads with alcohol or gel for better contact with the skin.

4. Pre-anesthesia evaluation of the ECG should always be a part of the pre-anes-thetic protocol, especially in compromised or geriatric patients. The patient should also be evaluated prior to and after induction. There are instances when anesthesia would not proceed because of an abnormal heart rhythm diagnosed by ECG.

5. If the ECG is not working:

a. QUICKLY put your fingers on a pulse or listen to the heart with a stethoscope to make sure that the patient is okay. If the patient is stable, start troubleshooting the equipment. If not, see Chapter 10 for possible causes and treatments.

b. If the problem is the equipment:

i. Check that the leads are still on the patient - they frequently get knocked off. There are also 'dots' which are stick on leads that can be taped to the limbs. These are great for critical patients and procedures where the lead clips may not be accessible.

ii. Check that the cable to the leads is plugged into the monitor.

iii. Reapply alcohol or gel to the site where the leads contact the skin, if this gets dry, the leads can't pick up the electrical activity from the heart.

iv. Switch leads.

v. Increase the amplification of the ECG signal.

vi. Move the leads to locations that are closer to the sites described above.

vii. Remove or turn off anything that could be causing electrical interference, which usually causes very rapid spikes rather than a recognizable ECG tracing. This could be clippers, hot water blankets, cautery, cell phones or anything else that is electrical.

viii. If all of this fails and the problem really is the patient, begin appropriate treatment of the arrhythmia per your clinic protocol. If the problem is the machine, switch to another machine and try to figure out the problem after anesthesia is over. See Chapter 5 for more information on troubleshooting the ECG monitor.

How to: Measure Blood Pressure Using a Doppler

The Doppler is an invaluable monitor for blood pressure, especially in very small patients and in patients with bradycardia or pronounced sinus arrhythmias. In these patients, the oscillometric blood pressure monitor may not be sensitive enough to provide a blood pressure reading (small patients) or may give erroneous blood pressure values (patients with arrhythmias). The audible 'whooshing' sound of blood moving through the arteries is comforting for most, especially for the anesthetist).

Although the Doppler provides only systolic arterial pressure (SAP) values in most patients, the value may be closer to mean arterial pressure (MAP) in cats and, perhaps, toy dogs. Remember, you are monitoring trends over time, and will use the Doppler as an indicator of a blood pressure trend even more than using it to provide an absolute blood pressure number.

1. The Doppler crystal must be placed directly over a palpable artery.

2. It is a good idea to first make sure the crystal is functional prior to taping it on a hairy patient. You can easily do so by placing the crystal on your own artery (applying gel first) and listening for the whooshing sound. Your radial artery, on the inside of your wrist is easily accessed.

3. Common locations for Doppler crystal placement in dogs and cats includes:
   a. Dorsal pedal artery (back leg).
   b. Metacarpal or metatarsal arteries (just above the paw on the front or back leg).
   c. Coccygeal artery (base of tail).

4. Shave off a small area of hair at the site of crystal placement **(Figure 8-29)**.

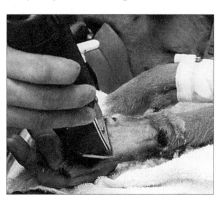

Figure 8-29. Shave the hair over the artery where the Doppler probe will be placed.

5. Apply gel to the crystal **(Figure 8-30)**.

6. It is helpful to tape the crystal in place, then turn on the Doppler **(Figure 8-31)**. By doing so, you eliminate the extremely annoying scratchy sound while taping the crystal securely. Although you may not be directly over your chosen artery, you should be close enough to manipulate the taped crystal to hear the Doppler.

7. The width of the blood pressure cuff to be used should be approximately 40-60% the circumference of the limb or tail being used **(Figure 8-32)**.

8. Wrap the cuff firmly on the leg proximal to (above) the crystal. The cuff should be between the crystal and the patient's body **(Figure 8-33)**.

9. Once the crystal and cuff are in place, attach a sphygmomanometer (pressure bulb) to the cuff. Squeeze the bulb until you no longer hear the sound of blood flow. Slowly release pressure until you can hear blood flowing through the artery.

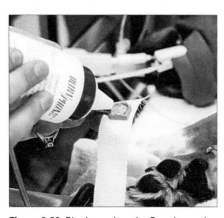

Figure 8-30. Placing gel on the Doppler probe is required for good contact with the skin.

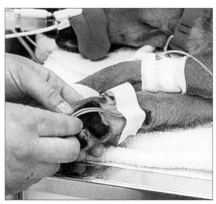

Figure 8-31. Tape the Doppler probe in place before turning on the Doppler speaker to avoid unnecessary noise.

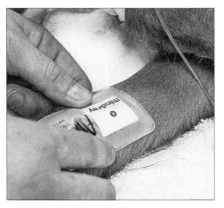

Figure 8-32. Measure the blood pressure cuff. The WIDTH should be approximately 40% of the circumference of the limb on which the cuff will be placed.

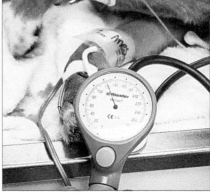

Figure 8-33. Place the cuff above the probe (meaning between the probe and the heart) and measure blood pressure. Systolic blood pressure in this photo is 122 mmHg.

10. When you first hear the sound, this is systolic arterial pressure **(Figure 8-33 and Figure 8-34)**.
11. Release the pressure, repeat the procedure up to three times to ensure an accurate average.

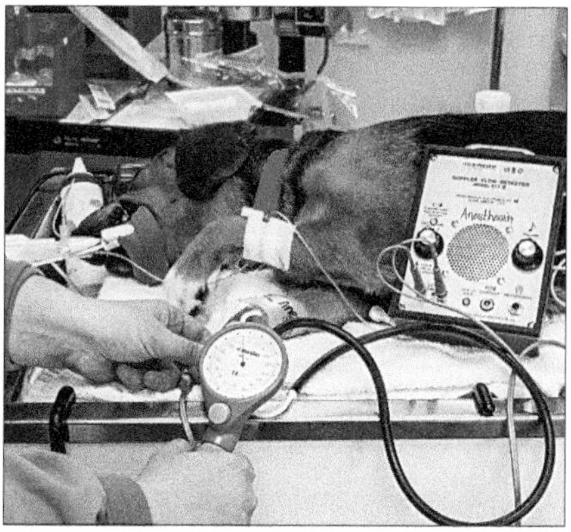

Figure 8-34. Once the Doppler cuff and probe are in place, inflate the cuff by squeezing the bulb attached to the manometer. Inflate until there is no sound coming from the Doppler, then slowly deflate until you hear sound again. The first sound you hear is systolic blood pressure.

12. Be sure to completely release the cuff pressure when your reading is complete, thereby allowing reperfusion of the limb distal to the cuff.
13. It should be noted that there are at least two types of crystals. Small animal crystals are considered "infant". Equine and other large animals use a standard size crystal, which is larger and has a much deeper contact point for gel to be applied.
14. Most Doppler units have a coupler spot to add headphones. Noisy operating rooms are an ideal reason to use headphones, as are faint Doppler sounds. When the headphones are plugged into the Doppler box, there will be no noise other than through the headphones.
15. There are several companies that sell Doppler units, Parks electronics has a specific veterinary Doppler (see their website) and is the Doppler we most commonly use. We recommend leaving the units attached to the charger when not in use, and leaving the crystals plugged in because of fatigue on the points. We also recommend not binding the crystal cords too tightly, but circling them in a relaxed manner. Appropriate care of your Doppler unit will make it last a long time!
16. Other veterinary Dopplers include the Vet-Dop, which works extremely well for smaller patients. Other units can be found using an internet search.

How to : Prevent/Treat Hypothermia
Hypothermia leads not only to delayed recovery but also to impaired immune function, and an increased incidence of arrhythmias, clotting dysfunction and many other adverse effects (see Chapter 6). Hypothermia should be prevented.
1. As soon as the patient is induced to anesthesia, muscle tone is decreased and the thermoregulatory center becomes less effective, both of which lead to a drop in body temperature.
   a. Prevention of hypothermia (which is a lot more effective than treatment of

hypothermia!) should begin at induction. If the patient is small or especially thin, warming can start when the patient is premedicated.

b. Also at this time, minimize the patient's exposure to cold solutions. For instance, scrub the surgical site but don't let scrub solution and alcohol run all over the patient.

2. Core body temperature should be monitored throughout the anesthetic procedure so that changes can be made to keep the patient warm.

3. Active warming devices should be used.

a. Generally, the most effective of these are the forced air warmers like the Baja Breeze (which is a forced air warmer designed specifically for veterinary patients) and Bair Hugger. **(Figure 8-35)**

b. Electrical warming blankets like the HotDog **(Figure 8-36)** and heated surgical tables are also helpful.

c. Although commonly used, circulating hot water blankets are the least effective (but still help). **(Figure 8-37)**

d. Warmed rice bags or hot water bottles near the patient also help, especially if the patient and the warmed devices are then covered by a blanket or surgical drape.

e. Warm towels on the breathing circuit can be helpful, as can use of coaxial breathing circuits.

4. Be sure that only veterinary approved warming devices are used and that towels or blankets are placed between the patient and all warming devices (except for the forced air blankets) so that you don't burn the patient!

CRITICAL TIP!

Placing a towel between the patient and warming device is especially important for patients lying on hot water blankets since the temperature of these is often fairly hot and the weight of the patient on the blanket increases the chance that they will get burned at pressure points (i.e., points where the body is putting the most pressure on the hot water blanket).

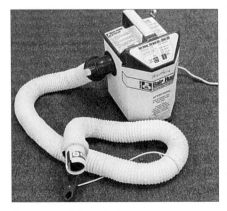

Figure 8-35. A forced air warmer.

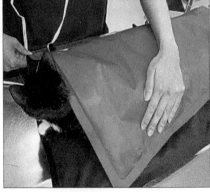

Figure 8-36. A HotDog® electric warmer.

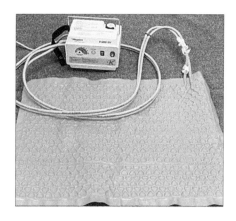

Figure 8-37. A circulating water blanket warmer.

5. Passive warming devices can also be helpful. These are devices that don't add heat, but help the patient to retain heat. This includes gloves or wraps on feet, 'space' type reflective blankets, and 'bubble wrap' or plastic wrap over the patient's body (this is more commonly done in 'pocket pets').
6. Ancillary devices like warmed IV fluids, in-line fluid warmers **(Figure 8-38)** and warmers/humidifiers in the breathing systems can also help. These devices may not add much heat, but they do contribute to slowing down the heat loss.
7. Warming the operating and recovery rooms can make a large difference in patient body temperature.

CRITICAL POINT!
The two most effective measures for preventing hypothermia are:
   a. MINIMIZE SURGERY TIME! Long surgery is directly correlated with lower body temperature.
   b. WARM THE PATIENT'S ENVIRONMENT: Ideally, this means that the surgery room is as warm as can be tolerated by the surgeons.

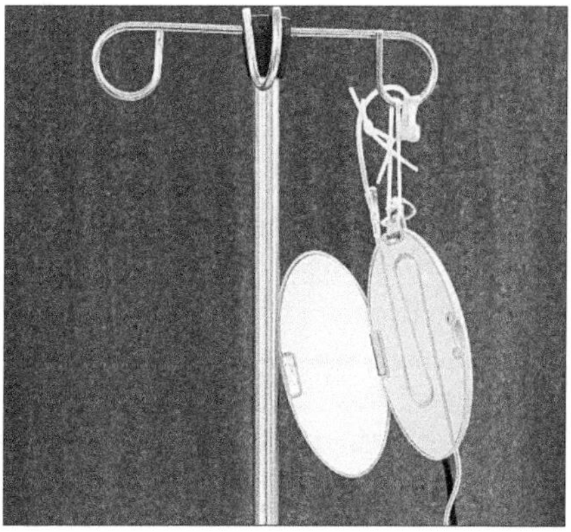

Figure 8-38. An in-line fluid warmer. The warmer should be placed as close to the patient as possible so that the fluid is warmed just before entering the patient.

How to: Measure Blood Pressure Using a Simple Manometer

Shelley Ensign LVT, CVPP

An aneroid manometer can be used to measure the mean arterial blood pressure **(Figure 8-39)**. Supplies needed for set up of a simple manometer: 2 low-volume extension lines, 2 stopcocks, 1 simple manometer, 1 syringe of heparinized saline for flush, 1 22-gauge needle.

First attach the 2 low-volume extension lines together by using a stopcock in between the two.

Place a stopcock to connect to the manometer on the female end of the low-volume extension line.

Attach a 22-gauge needle to the male end of the low-volume extension line. The needle end will be connected to the arterial catheter after the set-up is complete. Attach the heparinized flush syringe to the open port on the stopcock.

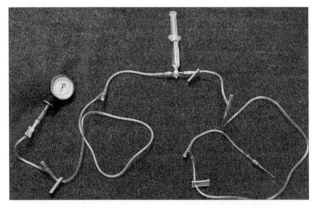

Figure 8-39. The set-up for using a manometer to measure arterial blood pressure. The line on the right ends in the catheter which would be in the patient's artery and the line on the left ends at the manometer. The stopcock in the middle is used to flush the catheter with saline while preventing saline from entering the manometer.

Flush the low-volume extension line on the side that has the needle attached to the end of it. The line can be flushed by turning the stopcock off towards the manometer. Once this line is flushed, it can be attached to the arterial catheter.

The manometer side of the low volume extension line should be flushed until the pressure on the manometer is higher than what the mean arterial pressure is predicted to be. A good pressure to flush to is 150 mmHg. *When flushing towards the manometer, be careful not to get fluid inside of the manometer, this will ruin the manometer. Flush by turning the stopcock off towards the arterial catheter side of the low-volume extension set. The stopcock attached to the flush syringe should be located at the level of the heart for accurate readings.

The manometer itself should be above the level of the heart. Once the pressure of the manometer is set, turn the stopcock off towards the heparinized flush syringe.

The needle on the manometer will begin to bounce when it reaches the mean arterial pressure of the patient.

Once the mean arterial pressure has been recorded, the stopcock that is connected to the manometer should be turned off towards the low-volume extension line between readings. This will prevent flush solution from accidentally being introduced to the manomter.

> ## TIP
> **The simple manometer set-up can be 'mapped'. The components of the set-up appear in this order:**
> > **Heparinized flush syringe**
> > ⬇
> **Manometer < stopcock < low-volume extension line < stopcock > low-volume extension line > needle > artery**

How to: Set up a Constant Rate Infusion (CRI) of Analgesic Drugs

1. Choose the drug (or drugs) that you would like to use (See Chapter 7).
2. Look up the loading dose and the infusion dose of the drug (See Chapter 7).
3. Calculate the loading and infusion dosages.
4. Decide how the infusion will be administered.
   a. Administration of drugs using a syringe pump.
   b. Dilution of the drugs in a small bag of fluids with the small bag 'piggy-backed' into the IV fluid line, which means a needle from the drip set on the small bag is inserted into the injection port of the line on the bag of fluids **(Figure 8-40)** and administered at a slow rate.
   c. Dilution of the drugs in the patient's IV fluids and administered at the regular fluid rate.
5. Set up the infusion as decided above.
6. Administer the loading dose of the drug.
7. Plug the administration line into the accessory port of the IV line.
8. Start the infusion! It's really that easy.

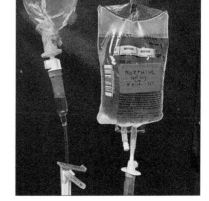

Figure 8-40. A small fluid bag to which analgesic drugs have been added (morphine in this photo) can be 'piggy backed' to the bag of IV fluids for administration of a constant rate infusion (CRI).

How to: Collect Arterial Blood for Blood Gas Analysis

Special syringes with dry lithium heparin are available to use for blood collection **(Figure 8-41)**. These syringes will have a filter attached to the end. Remove the filter and collect the sample. Reattach the filter and remove all excess air from syringe until blood penetrates the filter. Blood can be collected, stored on ice and analyzed within 30 minutes of collection. Be sure to thoroughly blend the sample by rolling it several times before analysis. Sites for collection in small animals include the dorsal pedal **(Figure 8-42)**, femoral, digital and lingual arteries. The transverse facial artery can be used in horses. Arterial catheters can be placed if multiple samples will be needed. Be sure to label the arterial catheter so that nothing is accidentally injected through it! **(Figure 8-43)**

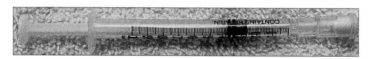

Figure 8-41. A specialized syringe with a filter for collecting arterial blood for blood gas analysis.

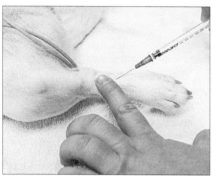

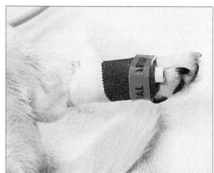

Figure 8-42. Collection of arterial blood from the dorsal pedal artery.

Figure 8-43. An arterial catheter. Note that it is clearly labeled so that it cannot be mistaken for the venous catheter.

How to: Set-Up and Use a Mechanical Ventilator

Please refer to (Figure 3-52).

Anesthesia Phase: Recovery

The recovery phase is just as, or sometimes even more, important as the other phases of anesthesia. Unfortunately, most anesthetic deaths occur in recovery (Brodbelt 2009) so we must continue monitoring and supporting our patients as long as they need extra care. Of course, young healthy patients that had uncomplicated surgeries and did well under anesthesia usually recover without complications. But older, sicker patients, patients that have undergone complicated surgeries, or patients that had adverse events during the other phases of anesthesia, may have complications in recovery and should be watched very carefully.

What to do with the Recovering Patient

1. As soon as the procedure is finished, or as it is finishing, turn off the vaporizer.
2. Squeeze the contents of the rebreathing bag out through the scavenging system so that the patient isn't still breathing anesthetic gases and fill the bag with pure oxygen by increasing the flow of oxygen through the oxygen flow meter. If rapid filling is desired, disconnect the patient from the breathing system and use the oxygen flush valve. Remember, this should not be done when the patient is connected to the machine or the rapid rise in pressure could cause barotrauma.
3. Give the patient a few breaths to help clear the lungs of the inhalant gas. Patients that have been on a ventilator may need to be given a few breaths until they start breathing on their own.
4. Leave the patient on oxygen for 5 to 10 minutes.
   a. This lets the patient wake up a little and start breathing more normally before you switch it from 100% oxygen to 21% oxygen (room air).
   b. This lets the inhalant anesthetics be exhaled into the scavenging system instead of into the room where the staff is exposed to them.
5. Leave the patient on oxygen longer if it needs it. Examples of patients that might need prolonged oxygen therapy include:
   a. Critically sick patients.
   b. Patients that did not oxygenate well during anesthesia.
   c. Patients that aren't breathing adequately.
   d. Patients that have cardiac or pulmonary disease/insufficiency.
   e. Brachycephalic patients may need flow-by oxygen supplementation or even time in an oxygen cage post-extubation.
6. Deflate the endotracheal tube cuff and loosen the tube tie.
7. Check body temperature and start warming if < 98°F. Warm to 100°F - don't overheat the patient.
8. Continue monitoring and support as needed.
   a. Young, healthy patients anesthetized for short, elective procedures are unlikely to need monitoring and support beyond the end of the anesthetic episode.
   b. Other patients might need prolonged monitoring and/or support. Examples include:
      i. Critically ill patients that might need continued fluid administration and measurement of blood pressure.
      ii. Patients with arrhythmias that might need continued ECG monitoring.
      iii. Patients with renal failure that might need continued fluid administration.
      iv. Any patient that had an adverse event during anesthesia or who did not do as well under anesthesia as expected.
9. Keep the patient in a warm, quiet area where you can observe the patient until it starts regaining consciousness (even on the floor of the surgery room wrapped in a warm towel while you are preparing for the next case will work).

10. As the patient regains consciousness, 'challenge' its ability to swallow by gently moving the ET tube a few centimeters in and out. Also check jaw tone and tongue tone (pull on the tongue and see if the patient pulls back). Some animals won't swallow and these techniques can be used to determine the timing of extubation.

CRITICAL TIP!
DO NOT over stimulate the patient by moving the endotracheal tube aggressively, speaking loudly, rubbing aggressively, or moving the patient from side to side. It is possible to wake the patient enough by doing this to extubate but it DOES NOT mean that the patient is really conscious enough to be extubated. This may lead to anesthetic death because the anesthetist may think the patient is recovering and stop monitoring when, in reality, the patient isn't breathing adequately.

11. Once the patient swallows or you have determined that it is time for extubation, gently remove the tube and hold your hand in front of the nose and mouth to make sure that you feel air moving when the patient breathes and watch for chest movement.

CRITICAL TIPS!
• Extubation of brachycephalic breeds should be delayed as long as possible. A roll of tape can be placed in the mouth to prevent them from chewing the tube.
• Prolonged intubation of healthy cats can cause laryngeal spasms, so cats should be extubated at the first signs of swallowing or return of jaw/tongue tone.
• If fluid is suspected to be in the trachea, like after a dentistry or if a patient has regurgitated, the ET tube cuff can be left partially inflated and the patient positioned with the head slightly down (hanging off the table) to facilitate drainage of the fluid. Flush the mouth and throat with water and/or use suction to clear the throat and airway before extubating.

12. If the patient has a bad (or 'rough') recovery, follow the steps in the next section to determine if the patient has dysphoria or is in pain.

13. If the patient has an excessively long recovery, follow these steps:
   a. Determine whether the patient is really having prolonged anesthesia or is just sleeping because it is comfortable. The better you get at pain management, the more you might see patients recovering quietly and sleeping. You can easily tell the difference - a patient that is still anesthetized won't respond to calling its name and petting it, but a patient that is just comfortable and sleeping will respond. If the patient is just sleeping comfortably, leave it alone! It is safe, happy and recovering like you would want to if you just had surgery!
   b. Determine whether or not the prolonged recovery is normal for the situation or the patient. Long anesthesia period = long recovery, there is nothing you can do about it. Also, sick or old patients just recover more slowly. There is nothing you can do about that either.
   c. Take the body temperature. The number one cause of slow recovery is

hypothermia. Warm the patient if that is the problem.

d. If the patient is a pediatric or neonatal patient, a patient with liver disease or a patient that has been on insulin, check the serum glucose. Hypoglycemia can cause long recoveries and this is a critical situation that needs to be diagnosed and treated.

e. If the patient has received reversible drugs like alpha-2 agonists or opioids, consider whether or not they should be reversed. If the patient is in trouble, the answer is yes. If the patient is safe and just slow, the answer may be no. Remember that reversing the sedative effects of these drugs will also reverse the analgesia. Using a lower dose of a reversal drug MAY reverse only a portion of the effects ('partial reversal') but this can't be guaranteed. This is because even a low dose of reversal drug could reverse all of the alpha-2 agonist still in the patient since some of the alpha-2 agonist will have been metabolized. Provide analgesia regardless of the dose of reversal drug used.

f. Placing the patient in sternal recumbency can often promote awakening.

Pain or Dysphoria? How to: Differentiate and Treat

1. Usually we can't tell for sure if the patient is experiencing pain or dysphoria
2. To be humane, assume that it is pain. Ask yourself:

a. How painful was the procedure?

b. How long ago did we administer analgesic drugs and what is the expected duration of that drug?

c. What was the dose of the drug and was it appropriate for this patient?

d. If the time since the last administration of the analgesic drug is approaching or has exceeded the expected duration of that drug, or if the initial dose of the drug was low, administer analgesics!

i. Boluses of opioids or alpha-2 agonists are great choices because they have a rapid onset of action.

3. If you think analgesia is adequate, assume that the patient is dysphoric and administer a sedative.

a. Alpha-2 agonists are ideal because they have a rapid onset of action, provide both sedation AND analgesia in case pain is indeed part of the problem and they are reversible so you can reverse the effects if the patient is too sleepy when it is time for it to go home.

b. Acepromazine is fine when combined with an opioid but it has a slow onset of action, provides no analgesia and is not reversible.

c. In addition, consider patient factors that might cause discomfort but not pain. For instance, after a long anesthesia, the patient may need to have its bladder emptied. A full bladder can be very uncomfortable.

How to: Extubate a Patient with Upper Respiratory Compromise

1. Patients in this category include brachycephalic dogs and cats and patients with laryngeal dysfunction.

2. For these patients, this is the most critical part of the entire anesthetic period.

3. Keep the patient on oxygen as long as possible.

4. Make sure the patient is fully awake but calm and that pain is alleviated prior to extubation.

5. Leave the ET tube in as long as possible.

6. Use the pulse oximeter before and after extubation to be sure that the patient is oxygenating.

TIP

Take a pulse oximeter reading before any drugs are administered in the preanesthesia period if possible. Often patients with airway dysfunction are normally slightly hypoxic.

7. Stretch out the neck and pull out the tongue to help open the airway post-extubation.

8. Administer steroids if the upper airway inflammation is moderate to severe (usually seen at intubation as a really red and swollen airway) or if intubation was difficult.

9. If the patient will tolerate it, prop the mouth open with a roll of tape or syringe case post-extubation if the patient has mild difficulty breathing or a slight drop in SpO_2.

10. If the patient is still having mild difficulty breathing and maintaining normal SpO_2, consider putting the patient in an oxygen cage for several hours. This often allows the patient to fully recover and maintain normal SpO_2.

11. Be prepared to reanesthetize and reintubate if the patient really can't breathe. Have a dose of induction drug (e.g., propofol) and a laryngoscope ready.

12. The patient might need a tracheotomy if the upper airway dysfunction is severe.

How to: Provide Supplemental Inhaled Oxygen

1. First check to see if the patient needs supplemental oxygen by using the pulse oximeter.

2. A face mask with oxygen flowing from the anesthesia machine can be used between the time the patient is extubated and the time that it needs to go into the cage.

3. If the patient still needs oxygen when it is ready to go into the cage, it should be placed in an oxygen cage.

4. If an oxygen cage is not available, one or two red rubber tubes can be placed and secured in the nostrils. Measure from the medial canthus of the eye to the tip of the nose, this is how far the red rubber is placed in the nasal passages. Attach the red rubber by suture or staple to the nostril (alar fold), bend the catheter over the top of the nose and up to the forehead. Attach it here with suture or staples. Oxygen insufflation lines can be attached to the red rubber tubes by various means, including Christmas tree connectors or cut-off syringes.

TIP

Proparacaine or lidocaine gel on the tip of the catheter can help decrease the discomfort of the catheters in the nasal passage.

How to: Handle Complications

Unfortunately, many complications can occur in recovery. Before anesthetizing patients, it would be good to read Chapter 10 so that you can rapidly respond to any situation that occurs.

How to: Assess Pain Once the Patient is Conscious

1. The best way to know for sure whether or not a patient is in pain is to use a pain scoring system (See Chapter 7).
2. Animals HIDE pain and you have to look for it.
3. Ideally, the same person will evaluate the patient before and after the painful stimulus. Changes in behavior are the best indication of pain but the person scoring needs to know the pre-pain behavior.
4. Check the heart and respiratory rates and blood pressure. If they are above the baseline for this particular patient, it may indicate that the patient is in pain.
5. Watch the patient's behavior. Abnormal behavior (like hissing and growling or hiding in a patient that was previously friendly and interactive) is the most accurate indicator that a patient might be in pain.
6. Interact with the patient (open the cage door and handle the patient) and palpate the incision or other painful area (be gentle and respectful! You are checking for a painful response, which might not be that comfortable for the patient!).
7. If in doubt, treat changes in HR, RR, behavior and response to palpation of potentially painful areas as if the patient is indeed in pain and administer analgesic drugs (opioids, alpha-2 agonists, NSAIDs or local anesthetics). REASSESS the patient in 10 to 30 minutes. Just as a change in behavior can be an indication of pain, it can also be an indication of the RELIEF of pain.
8. If your clinic isn't currently using scoring systems, we recommend that you implement one. You can't identify pain unless you look for it (See Chapter 7).

How to: Get Ready for the Next Case

1. Be absolutely sure that the patient that you are finishing with is comfortable and safely awake. As a veterinary nurse or technician, you are the patient's 'voice' so speak up if you need more time with the patient!
2. If the patient isn't ready to be left unobserved but you must proceed to the next case, put the patient where you can see it. In a recovery cage with another technician watching is ideal but if not possible, put the patient at your feet (or the receptionist's feet!) on a warm towel (appropriate for large patients) or in a laundry basket full of warm towels (appropriate for small patients).
3. Put the ET tube in the sink to be washed.
4. Clean the table in the induction and surgery areas.
5. Check your patient again.
6. Start back through the check list in Table 8-1.

CRITICAL TIP!
Treat every patient like the first patient of the day and check all of the equipment, including the inhalant level in the vaporizer, the oxygen level in the tanks, adequacy of the CO_2 absorbent, the position of the pop-off valve (OPEN!), etc. Also pressure check the machine again since machine and breathing system components can get dislodged at any time.

References

Brodbelt D. Perioperative mortality in small animal anesthesia: Vet J. 2009; 182: 152-161.

Chapter 9
Anesthesia/Analgesia
Protocols for Specific Cases

Introduction

Commonly used anesthesia and analgesia protocols and suggestions for patient management are presented in this chapter. Of course, these are guidelines and the final protocol should depend on the health status and demeanor of the patient, the drugs available in your practice and the complexity/duration/pain level of the procedure that the patient is anesthetized for. In order to fully utilize the information in this chapter, refer to other chapters in this book, including chapters that cover normal physiologic parameters, drug dosages, patient monitoring & support and treatment of complications.

General Protocols
Sample Protocols for Anesthesia & Analgesia for Healthy Dogs (ASA I-II)
Preanesthesia

Analgesia for moderate to severe pain: 0.1-0.2 mg/kg hydromorphone OR 0.5-1.0 mg/kg morphine OR 0.3-0.5 mg/kg methadone or 0.1-0.3 mg/kg oxymorphone IM or IV (use the lower end of the dosing range for IV; if administering morphine IV, administer SLOWLY). Analgesia for mild pain: 0.02-0.03 mg/kg buprenorphine IM or IV. Butorphanol should be used as a sedative but not an analgesic unless the pain is predicted to be VERY brief (< 60 minutes in the dog), the butorphanol dose will be repeated, or a longer lasting opioid will be administered after the butorphanol. If the latter solution is chosen, remember that butorphanol will reverse some of the effects of the more potent opioid. Sedation: Add to the opioid 0.002-0.010 mg/kg dexmedetomidine OR 0.01-0.03 mg/kg acepromazine IM or IV (use the lower end of the dosing range for IV). Start NSAIDs now if appropriate.

Induction

Any of the injectable induction drugs.

Maintenance

Administer Isoflurane, sevoflurane or desflurane to effect.

- Monitoring & Support: Use all of the monitors available. Suggested monitors include blood pressure, pulse oximeter, ECG, and end-tidal CO_2, along with a person checking mucous membrane color, capillary refill time, pulse strength, heart rate, respiratory rate and depth of anesthesia. Routine support should include IV fluids and support of blood pressure, ventilation and normothermia.
- Analgesia: Provide analgesia appropriate for the procedure (opioid/alpha-2 agonist boluses, local/regional blocks, constant rate infusions [CRI]).

Recovery

Provide sedation and analgesia as indicated by the procedure and patient. The most common protocol is to administer another bolus of the opioid that was used for premedication +/- sedation if the patient is dysphoric or excited. Half of the dexmedetomidine dose that was used for premedication is very useful since it provides both sedation and analgesia, thereby providing the appropriate treatment no matter if the stress/excitement is due to dysphoria or pain. The effects of the dexmedetomidine can be antagonized with atipamezole later, if necessary. Start or continue NSAIDs and other postoperative/discharge drugs.

Sample Protocols for Anesthesia & Analgesia for Healthy Cats (ASA I-II): Inhalant Drug Based Protocol
Preanesthesia
Analgesia for moderate to severe pain: 0.1 mg/kg hydromorphone OR 0.2-0.3 mg/kg morphine OR 0.3-0.5 mg/kg methadone or 0.05-0.1 mg/kg oxymorphone IM or IV (use the lower end of the dosing range for IV; if administering morphine IV, administer SLOWLY). Analgesia for mild pain: 0.02-0.03 mg/kg buprenorphine IM or IV. Butorphanol should be used as a sedative but not an analgesic unless the pain is predicted to be VERY brief (< 90 minutes in the cat), the butorphanol dose will be repeated, or a longer lasting opioid will be administered after the butorphanol. If the latter solution is chosen, remember that butorphanol will reverse some of the effects of the more potent opioid. Sedation: Add to the opioid 0.005-0.015 mg/kg dexmedetomidine OR 0.03-0.05 mg/kg acepromazine IM or IV (use the lower end of the dosing range for IV). Start NSAIDs now if appropriate.

Induction
Any of the injectable induction drugs.

Maintenance
Administer Isoflurane, sevoflurane or desflurane to effect.

- Monitoring & Support: Use all of the monitors available. Suggested monitors include blood pressure, pulse oximeter, ECG, and end-tidal CO_2, along with a person checking mucous membrane color, capillary refill time, pulse strength, heart rate, respiratory rate and depth of anesthesia. Routine support should include IV fluids and support of blood pressure, ventilation and normothermia.
- Analgesia: Provide analgesia appropriate for the procedure (opioid/alpha-2 agonist boluses, local/regional blocks, constant rate infusions [CRI]).

Recovery
Provide sedation and analgesia as indicated by the procedure and patient. The most common protocol is to administer another bolus of the opioid that was used for premedication +/- sedation if the patient is dysphoric or excited. Half of the dexmedetomidine dose that was used for premedication is very useful since it

provides both sedation and analgesia, thereby providing the appropriate treatment no matter if the stress/excitement is due to dysphoria or pain. The effects of the dexmedetomidine can be antagonized with atipamezole later, if necessary. Start or continue NSAIDs and other postoperative/discharge drugs.

Sample Protocols for Anesthesia & Analgesia for Healthy Cats (ASA I-II): Injectable Drug Based Protocol

Preanesthesia
For injectable based protocols, the drugs are usually administered IM, which allows the drugs to be injected with only minimal restraint compared to the restraint needed for IV injections. However, IV injection is also acceptable. Choose an opioid/opioid dose from the list presented in the inhalant based protocol and add 10-15 microg/kg dexmedetomidine PLUS 5-10 mg/kg ketamine OR 5-10 mg/kg Telazol all combined in the same syringe and administered IM. Start NSAIDs now if appropriate.

Induction
The ketamine (or Telazol) in the combination listed above is the induction drug, if the patient is deeply sedated but not asleep, a bolus of any of the injectable drugs or more of the drug combination used for premedication can be administered. If this is necessary, IV administration is recommended, just for speed of onset of drug effects.

Maintenance
The ketamine (or Telazol) in the combination listed above can be the maintenance drug for SHORT (e.g., castration) procedures. If the anesthesia is inadequate or the procedure is prolonged, more ketamine (or Telazol) can be administered IM or IV or an inhalant can be used.

- Monitoring & Support: Even though the patient isn't receiving inhalant anesthetic drugs, this is general anesthesia! Use all of the monitors available. Suggested monitors include blood pressure, pulse oximeter, ECG, and end-tidal CO_2, along with a person checking mucous membrane color, capillary refill time, pulse strength, heart rate, respiratory rate and depth of anesthesia. Routine support should include IV fluids and support of blood pressure, ventilation and normothermia. Supplemental oxygen should be administered to ALL anesthetized patients.
- Analgesia: Provide analgesia appropriate for the procedure (opioid/alpha-2 agonist boluses, local/regional blocks, constant rate infusions [CRI]).

Recovery
Same as for recovery in patients that received an inhalant based protocol.

CLINICAL TIP

Total injectable protocols also work for dogs but total IM protocols are limited to small dogs to keep the volume of injected drugs from getting too large to be practical. For medium to large dogs, sedation can be administered IM and maintenance drugs can be administered IV. Repeat boluses or an infusion of the drug can be administered as needed.

CLINICAL TIP

A very common injectable protocol in cats (often called 'kitty magic') is a combination of an opioid (commonly buprenorphine), dexmedetomidine and ketamine. The drugs are dosed at 0.1 mL of EACH drug per 4.5 kgs (10 lbs) of body weight for deep sedation (so 0.3 mls total volume) and 0.2 mL of each drug per 4.5 kgs (10 lbs) of body weight for true anesthesia (so 0.6 mls total volume). The drugs should be combined in the same syringe and administered IM. Adjust the volume up or down if the cat is larger or smaller than 4.5 kgs. Onset of sedation/anesthesia is 5-10 minutes and duration of sedation/anesthesia is usually 20-45 minutes. If deeper or longer anesthesia is needed, a an additional ¼-½ dose of the combination can be administered IM or IV. Alternatively, a small dose of propofol, ketamine or alfaxalone can be administered IV. This combination can also be used as a premedication, followed by patient intubation and maintenance on low-dose inhalant (if necessary) for the duration of the procedure.

Anesthesia and Analgesia for Patients with Specific Diseases or Conditions
(in alphabetical order)

Brachycephalic Airway Disease (BAS) or Other Upper Respiratory Dysfunction
(e.g., laryngeal paralysis or high collapsing trachea)

Patient Signalment and History
Puggles is a 6-year old male neutered pug who has blood in his urine, which is the presenting complaint. Puggles is panting and makes a lot of respiratory noise (stridor). The owner reports that Puggles struggles to breathe if the weather is really hot or if Puggles plays too much. But the owner isn't interested in fixing the airway, just the blood in the urine. (NOTE: Although these conditions occur less commonly in cats, if the patient were a cat the protocol would be the same but the drug dosages might change slightly.)

Physical Exam
No abnormalities except panting and fairly profound respiratory noise.

Serum Chemistry and CBC
No abnormalities.

Other Diagnostic Tests Recommended
Abdominal radiographs focusing on the area of the bladder. Urinalysis (UA) with focus on the presence of indicators of infection and on type of stones if not going to surgery for stone removal. A laryngeal exam should be done at induction (more information below).

Procedure
Abdominal surgery for removal of bladder stones.

Concerns and Plan
ASA Status III-IV. ASA depends on degree of respiratory distress rather than on presence of bladder stones. If bladder stones were the only problem, the patient would likely be assigned an ASA status of II. Some brachycephalic patients breathe normally and would be an ASA I-II. Puggles has moderate respiratory distress so is a III-IV. If the patient were having extreme difficulty it might be an ASA IV-V and that patient would likely need to have a low dose of a tranquilizer and be placed in an oxygen cage or might need an emergency anesthetic induction with intubation or an emergency tracheotomy.

Successful anesthesia for patients with upper airway dysfunction depends more on patient management than on drug choice. Intubation can be difficult, extubation can be very 'scary' for the anesthetist and dangerous for the patient. Almost any drugs will work but the most appropriate drugs are those that are fast acting (for rapid intubation) and reversible (for quick return to consciousness and, hopefully, to normal breathing), but low-dose acepromazine is also a good option since it provides long-term calming that lasts into recovery. Brachycephalic patients often have: 1) a hypoplastic trachea so be prepared with a smaller endotracheal tube than you would expect based on body size; 2) a small epiglottis that does not adequately cover the laryngeal opening so aspiration is a concern if the patient vomits; 3) other upper airway abnormalities including everted saccules, elongated soft palates and upper airway inflammation, all of which might complicate intubation; and 4) a profound vagal response with the potential for bradycardia during intubation.

Drug Contraindications
None but avoid deep sedation unless prepared to quickly induce and intubate if sedation causes respiratory difficulty. Drugs that might cause prolonged recoveries (e.g., high dosage of Telazol) are not ideal. Drugs that cause vomiting are not recommended unless maropitant has been administered. These drugs can be administered after induction, when they won't cause vomiting, if necessary.

Anesthetic Plan

Preanesthesia/premedication: Keep the patient calm, excitement can cause rapid and/or deep breathing, which can cause/exacerbate airway collapse. PREOX-YGENATE! Administer maropitant at least 1 hour before induction to prevent vomiting, which could lead to aspiration pneumonia. Premedication: Opioid based on pain level (moderate to high in this case: morphine, hydromorphone, methadone, oxymorphone) at dosages listed for healthy patients + low-dose acepromazine (0.01-0.02 mg/kg) IM or IV. An alpha-2 agonist (e.g., dexmedetomidine) at 25-50% of the dosages listed for healthy (ASA I-II) patients or a benzodiazepine (e.g., midazolam) at the same dosages as those listed for healthy patients could be used instead of or along with the acepromazine. An anticholinergic could be included because of the possibility of a strong vagal response at intubation. If this occurs, an alpha-2 agonist should not be administered.

Induction: Administer propofol or alfaxalone rapidly and INTUBATE as quickly as possible! Ketamine is also acceptable. **DO NOT MASK INDUCE** -this is too slow to obtain an airway quickly. In order to intubate with as little trauma as possible and to have an idea of how dangerous extubation will be, the larynx should be visualized using a laryngoscope or light. A stylet placed through the endotracheal (ET) tube is often useful to help with intubation.

Maintenance: LOW DOSE inhalants. A patient that is too deep during the maintenance phase will have a slow recovery. We want these patients to wake up quickly (but smoothly!) with no residual respiratory depression from the inhalants.

Monitoring & Support: Once intubated, utilize standard monitoring and support as described for ASA I-II patients.

Analgesia: Good analgesia during the maintenance phase will 1) allow a lower dose of inhalant to be used and 2) provide postoperative analgesia. The former is important for rapid recovery, the latter is important for excitement-free recovery. Opioid boluses and CRIs are appropriate. Focus on non-sedating techniques that won't prolong recovery like regional/local blocks. In this patient, use an opioid + local anesthetic lumbosacral epidural.

Recovery: Recovery is the most critical phase & preparation for recovery is crucial. Leave the patient intubated for as long as it will tolerate the ET tube. Often the patient will be totally awake and still tolerating the tube **(Figure 9-1)**.

If the patient isn't breathing well after extubation, extend the neck, & gently pull the tongue out to open the airway. Administer oxygen by mask or flow-by. Be ready to reinduce and reintubate if the patient is not breathing at all or is not moving any air from the trachea. The patient should be kept calm, pain-free & warm for optimal recovery. Excitement, pain and shivering can all be detrimental. Pain & excitement can increased work of breathing which can lead to airway collapse. Shivering increases oxygen consumption, which may not be met by oxygen delivery if the patient can't breathe and oxygen debt (not enough oxygen to the tissues) may occur. Drugs for recovery would include acepromazine if calming is required and non-sedating analgesic drugs like NSAIDs and buprenorphine. For brachycephalic dogs that breathe more normally than Puggles, recovery drugs and dosages include all those listed for healthy dogs.

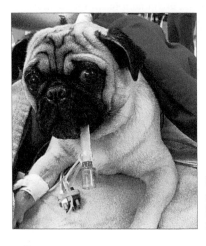

Figure 9-1. A brachycephalic dog recovering from anesthesia. The dog is completely conscious but is not objecting to the endotracheal tube in the airway.

Castration

Patient Signalment and History
Mayson is a 1-year old male intact Brittany Spaniel. (NOTE: This could also be a cat and the protocol - including the intratesticular injection of local anesthetic - would be the same but the drug dosages might change slightly.)

Physical Exam
No abnormalities.

Serum Chemistry and CBC
No abnormalities.

Other Diagnostic Tests Recommended
None.

Procedure
Castration

Concerns and Plan
ASA Status I so no undue concerns based on health of the patient. Castrations are called 'routine' because the surgery is easy - but that does not mean that a

skin incision and a crushing injury of the spermatic cord is 'routine' to the patient. Sounds pretty painful!

Drug Contraindications
None.

Anesthetic Plan
Preanesthesia/premedication: Any of the options in the ASA I-II protocol. A common choice is either morphine or hydromorphone PLUS dexmedetomidine or acepromazine.

Induction: Any of the injectable induction drugs.

Maintenance: Inhalants.

Monitoring & Support: Standard monitoring and support as described for ASA I-II dogs.

Analgesia: Testicular injection of local anesthetic drugs **(Figures 9-2 and 9-3)**.

Recovery: Same as described for recovery of ASA I-II patients.

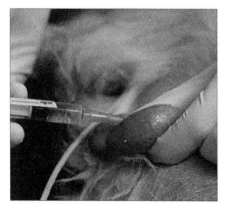

Figure 9-2. Testicular injection of local anesthetic drugs in a dog.

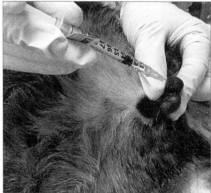

Figure 9-3. Testicular injection of local anesthetic drugs in a cat.

Cesarean Section ('C-Section')
Patient Signalment and History
Rita, a 4-yr old female Chihuahua that has been in Stage II labor, which is the active contraction phase, for several hours without delivering any puppies. (NOTE: This could also be a cat and the protocol would be the same but the drug dosages might change slightly.)

Physical Exam
Obviously stressed, tachycardic and panting, MM & CRT normal.

Serum Chemistry and CBC
Surgery will proceed without bloodwork. This is an emergency cesarean section but the dog is otherwise healthy so no abnormalities suspected.

Procedure
Cesarean section.

Other Tests Recommended
None required but a radiograph of the abdomen is often useful **(Figure 9-4)**.

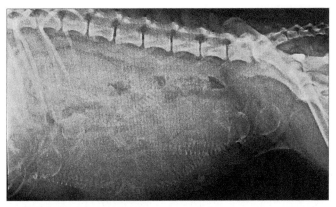

Figure 9-4. Lateral radiograph of a dog being prepared for cesarean section. Note the skulls and spinal columns of the fetuses.

Concerns and Plan
ASA Status III-IV Depending on Health of Mother. These are tough because there are TWO patients - the mother who needs anesthesia/analgesia AND the fetuses who don't need - and could even potentially be harmed by - anesthesia/analgesia. Any drug that crosses the blood brain barrier to produce anesthesia will cross the placental barrier and sedate or anesthetize the neonates. Anesthetic drugs can cause neonatal depression but time in Stage II labor has a bigger impact on fetal demise than any anesthetic drug so the owners should be educated about getting the patient into the clinic quickly if she is having any difficulty delivering the pups or kittens.

The factor that will have the biggest impact on fetal survival that is in our control is oxygen delivery. Support of oxygen delivery is even more important than the actual anesthetic drug choice. We can support oxygen delivery by supporting both blood pressure and ventilation - but this will take more work than it does in a nonpregnant patient. The pressure from the gravid ('full') uterus on the diaphragm can make it difficult for the patient to breathe and placing the patient in dorsal recumbency causes the uterus to place even more pressure on the diaphragm. Expect the patient to have difficulty maintaining normal breathing and gas exchange, especially in dorsal recumbency (on its back). There are many fluid shifts that occur during a C-section, primarily at induction due to vasodilation caused by the anesthetic drugs and when the uterus is lifted from the abdomen to remove the fetuses. Expect the patient to become hypotensive at these times. Dorsal recumbency will also contribute to hypotension since the uterus may put pressure on the venae cava, which will compromise the amount of blood returning to the heart. Pregnant patients are often nauseous and may regurgitate at induction.

Premedication, induction, provision of analgesia and preparation for surgery need to happen quickly because the fetuses need to be delivered quickly, but don't work so rapidly that the patient isn't appropriately prepared to be as stable as possible during anesthesia.

Drug Contraindications

None, but want to choose drugs that have a short duration of action and that are cleared rapidly, or whose effects are reversible. This choice is made not so much for the mother but for rapid recovery of the neonates.

Anesthetic plan

Preanesthesia/premedication: Remember to focus on oxygen delivery. PREOXY-GENATE! Start IV fluids at 10ml/kg/hr. Start monitoring if possible. If blood pressure is already low, increase the fluid rate or give a 5-10 ml/kg crystalloid or 2 ml/kg colloid fluid bolus over 5-10 minutes. Consider a dose of maropitant 1mg/kg IV. This should be administered IV or SQ as early as possible to allow time for onset. Try to place the mother in lateral recumbency (on her side) and clip and scrub the surgery site and do a local block at the site of the incision. If she resists this recumbency and struggles, administer a mu opioid agonist (morphine, hydromorphone, methadone, oxymorphone, fentanyl) at full or ½ dose listed for healthy patients IV. IM is okay, but a catheter should be in with fluids running through it and IV administration will speed the onset of effect of the drug so you can proceed more quickly. If using morphine IV, inject slowly. Don't be afraid of the opioid - this will allow a lower dose of inhalant anesthetic and the opioid effects are reversible by placing a drop of naloxone under the puppy's or kitten's tongue after it is delivered, if necessary. Fentanyl is commonly used because it has a short duration and will likely be cleared before the pups or kittens are delivered. If the mother is still struggling, induce anesthesia and intubate but still clip and scrub as much as possible in lateral recumbency.

Induction: Propofol (alfaxalone is also likely acceptable) +/- a benzodiazepine should be administered and the patient intubated as quickly as possible to prevent aspiration if the patient regurgitates. The anesthetist should give the patient a few breaths immediately after induction. DO NOT MASK INDUCE. The time to induction and placement of an endotracheal tube is prolonged, increasing the chance that the mother will vomit and aspirate. Also, the high dose of inhalant required for induction will cause hypotension and hypoventilation in the mother, which will decrease oxygen delivery to the fetuses.

Maintenance: Use low-dose inhalants - as low as possible since the inhalants will contribute to the hypotension and hypoventilation already occurring. Some people prefer sevoflurane since the patient will wake up more quickly from that gas - as will the puppies or kittens if they are experiencing any effects from the inhalants when they are delivered. Once all of the puppies or kittens are delivered, another dose of opioid can be administered IV to the mother and the inhalant dose can be increased, if needed.

Analgesia: Inject morphine into the lumbosacral epidural space immediately after induction. Morphine will provide analgesia for up to 24 hours postoperatively with little to no systemic uptake of the drug - so it is unlikely that drug will be delivered to the pups or kittens in the milk. After the epidural is complete, place the patient in dorsal recumbency and quickly do an incisional block if one wasn't done in the preanesthetic period. **Local anesthesia should be administered at the incision site whether or not an epidural was done.** The skin is highly innervated and pain from the incision is a big part of the overall pain experienced by the mother. Providing local analgesia decreases the pain experienced intra-operatively (allowing the inhalant dose to be lower) and postoperatively (allowing the mother to let the pups/kittens nurse without experiencing pain at the incision site). After the epidural and incisional block, finish the scrub and proceed with surgery. Once the pups or kittens have been delivered, administer the other ½ dose of the opioid used as a premedication. If fentanyl was used, administer a full dose of one of the longer lasting opioids (e.g., morphine, hydromorphone, methadone).

Monitoring & Support: Monitoring blood pressure and respiratory function (pulse oximetry and end-tidal CO_2) is critical! Cardiovascular Support: Administer IV fluids to compensate for fluid loss during surgery. A large bolus of fluids (5-10 ml/kg crystalloids or 2 ml/kg colloids) might be required just before or after exteriorization of the uterus if the patient is hypovolemic (low circulating blood volume) and/or hypotensive. Respiratory Support: The mother will have difficulty breathing until the abdomen is open and the pressure from the gravid uterus is removed from the diaphragm. Start support of ventilation immediately after induction by administering two-four breaths/minute - or as many as required to keep the SpO_2 and $ETCO_2$ in the normal range. Other support: Maintain normothermia.

Recovery: The epidural can be done post-operatively if there was no time pre-operatively. IV or IM opioids can also be administered since opioids have minimal to no uptake in the milk. Consider administering another dose of full mu opioid agonists, or administer buprenorphine since it causes minimal to no sedation (depending on the dose) and lasts 4-6 hours. Continue to keep both pups and mother warm.

After delivery, if the pups/kittens are lethargic and the opioid is suspected, put a drop of naloxone under the tongue of the pup/kitten. Absorption is very rapid from this site.

Diabetes

Patient Signalment and History
BatMan, a 10-yr old male neutered domestic shorthair (DSH) cat who was diagnosed with diabetes several months ago is presented for advanced dental disease, which is causing anorexia, weight loss and pain. The diabetes is currently controlled with daily insulin. (NOTE: This could also be a dog and the protocol would be the same but the drug dosages might change slightly.)

Physical Exam
No abnormalities except the teeth have excessive tartar buildup and palpation of the maxilla and mandible elicits oral pain.

Serum Chemistry and CBC
Normal except for a glucose of 180 mg/dL. This is not surprising since the last insulin dose was 6 hours prior to admission and because the cat is stressed, which can cause hyperglycemia even in non-diabetics.

Other Diagnostic Tests Recommended
Depending on how stable the diabetes is, a urinalysis (UA) might be useful.

Procedure
Dental prophylaxis with extractions.

Concerns and Plan
ASA Status III. Successful anesthesia for diabetic patients depends more on patient management than on drug choice. Management goals for anesthesia include minimal disruption of food intake with return to eating as soon as possible postoperatively, maintenance of intraoperative glucose around 150 mg/dL and minimization of patient stress in order to decrease the degree of disruption of insulin control. Patient stress can be minimized by limiting the time in the hospital, keeping the patient calm and utilizing effective analgesic techniques.

Even with stable diabetes, diabetic patients are likely to be dehydrated (because of osmotic diuresis caused by the hyperglycemia) and to suffer swings in their serum glucose concentrations, which can be dangerous (especially hypoglycemia). Diabetics may also be more prone to infection than non-diabetic patients. Thin patients (as some diabetic patients may be) are more likely to get hypothermic and may get painful areas or burns over boney points if they are placed on hard surfaces or directly on heating pads with no cover. Fat patients (as many diabetics are) may have difficulty breathing and may need ventilatory support.

Diabetic ketoacidosis occurs when insulin is not provided or the patient is insulin resistant and the body burns fat for fuel instead of burning glucose. This produces ketones which causes acidosis. This disease can be severely life threatening and a cat with diabetic ketoacidosis should not be anesthetized unless there is no other choice. This cat would be an ASA IV-V.

Drug Contraindications

None, but should choose drugs with short duration of action and/or reversible effects so that the patient recovers quickly and starts normal meal consumption as soon as possible. Drugs that might delay recovery and prolong time to eating (e.g., high dosages of acepromazine or Telazol) are not ideal.

Anesthetic plan

Preanesthesia/premedication: Fast the patient only briefly (4 hours) and don't remove water (not from this patient or any other patient). Do surgery first thing in the morning so that you have all day to make sure that the patient is awake and eating. Administer ½ the regular dose of insulin on the morning of the procedure. Consider maropitant since dogs have been shown to return to normal feeding more quickly if they have had maropitant - this is probably true for cats too. Recommended protocol: Maropitant one hour prior to premedication. Premedicate with the opioid of choice based on the pain of the procedure and use the dosages listed for ASA I-II patients. Buprenorphine, because of its long duration of action and minimal sedative properties, is often a good choice for mild to moderate pain, especially in cats. However, buprenorphine alone is not potent enough for severe pain so multimodal analgesia is imperative. Add dexmedetomidine if the cat is fairly healthy and active or midazolam if the cat is sick. Alpha-2 agonists are controversial because they cause transient hyperglycemia but this is generally clinically insignificant - and safer than hypoglycemia.

Induction: Any induction drug will be appropriate but propofol and alfaxalone would be the least likely to contribute to prolonged recovery.

Maintenance: LOW DOSE inhalant. The deeper the patient is during the maintenance phase of anesthesia the longer recovery will take.

Monitoring & Support: Standard anesthetic monitoring as listed for ASA I-II patients PLUS glucose. Check the glucose prior to anesthesia, once per hour throughout the surgery and in recovery. Administer 5% dextrose IV fluids if the blood glucose drops below 150 mg/dL. If glucose can't be measured in your practice, administer 5% dextrose solution throughout the procedure. Make sure that body temperature is monitored and supported. Position the patient carefully and pad well. Be sure to use aseptic technique where required to decrease the chance of infection.

Analgesia: <u>Local anesthetic blocks</u> allow lower inhalant concentration which will allow quicker recovery. Use oral/dental blocks in this patient.

Recovery: Keep the patient warm with blankets and external heating sources **(Figure 9-5)**, may need to continue to monitor glucose if the patient had fairly low glucose during anesthesia. If recovery is unexpectedly prolonged, definitely check glucose. Start NSAIDs if appropriate.

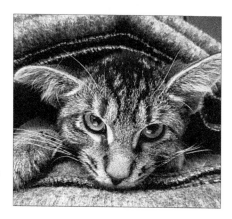

Figure 9-5. A cat recovering from anesthesia with warm blankets for support of body temperature.

Heart Disease
Patient Signalment and History
Sissy, a 9-yr old female spayed Cocker Spaniel, was diagnosed with mitral insufficiency and congestive heart failure 6 months previously. Her disease is being controlled with medications but she still has exercise intolerance and often coughs. Her teeth are covered with tartar and the gingiva is red and inflamed. (NOTE: This could also be a cat and the protocol would be the same but the drug dosages might change slightly.)

Physical Exam
No abnormalities except an audible murmur, tachycardia and panting.

Serum Chemistry and CBC
No abnormalities.

Other Diagnostic Tests Recommended
Repeat thoracic radiographs **(Figure 9-6)**, and preoperative ECG.

Procedure
Dental prophylaxis with extractions.

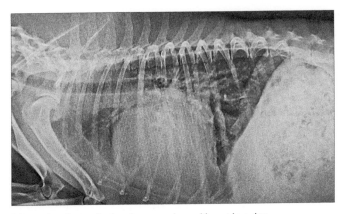

Figure 9-6. A lateral radiograph showing an enlarged heart in a dog.

Concerns and Plan

ASA Status III-IV. Sissy has cardiac disease that is controlled, but of course can't be cured, and still has some signs of disease (coughing, exercise intolerance), which contributes to a higher ASA status. Extractions are painful and will require moderate to profound analgesia. Appropriate analgesia will also contribute to anesthetic safety by preventing the need for maintenance at an excessively deep plane of anesthesia, which is very dangerous since the inhalants cause a dose-dependent cardiovascular depression. Hypotension is likely and will need to be treated with positive inotropic drugs (dopamine or dobutamine) that improve cardiac contractility. The volume of fluids administered to the patient should be limited since a failing heart will have difficulty pumping excessive fluids. The procedure is likely to be long and long-duration procedures contribute to risk of anesthesia-related morbidity or mortality. In all patients, and especially in patients with heart disease, the dentist should work efficiently and try to minimize anesthesia time. Hypothermia can cause arrhythmias and decreased cardiac contractility so aggressive warming may be necessary.

Drug Contraindications

Alpha-2 agonists are generally contraindicated in patients with most types of cardiac disease. The presence of a minor abnormality, like a murmur with no other signs of cardiac disease, may not exclude the use of an alpha-2 agonist if one is needed for appropriate sedation. This patient is very calm and does not need an alpha-2 agonist.

Anesthetic Plan

Preanesthesia/premedication: Opioid based on pain level (high: morphine, hydromorphone, methadone, oxymorphone) at dosages that are 100%, or slightly reduced to 75%, of the dosages administered to healthy patients, IM or IV. The opioid alone may provide sufficient calming for the patient. If not, a low dose of acepromazine (0.01 mg/kg) can be added IM or IV. Acepromazine may improve cardiac function because it allows decreased cardiac work secondary to slight vasodilation. A high dose of acepromazine (0.03 mg/kg or higher) should be avoided as it may contribute to hypotension in patients with cardiac disease. Alternatively, 0.2 mg/kg midazolam (IV or IM) or diazepam (IV only) can be administered along with the opioid in patients that are fairly sick and/or calm. Benzodiazepines won't be calming if used in excited patients and can cause paradoxical excitement in patients that are healthy or have only mild disease.

Induction: Etomidate is the drug of choice for moderate to profound cardiac disease but in this stabilized patient, any of the injectable induction drugs would be appropriate as long as the dose is kept as low as possible - which means that good premedication is critical. If the patient isn't very sedate from the premedications, administer a bolus of midazolam or diazepam (0.2 mg/kg) or fentanyl (0.002-0.005 mg/kg) just before administering the induction drug.

Maintenance: LOW DOSE inhalants. Inhalants contribute more to hypotension, hypoventilation and hypothermia than any other drug we use. But the contribution is dose-dependent so keep the dose low by relying on analgesia to keep the patient from responding to pain.

Monitoring & Support: Blood pressure should be monitored starting at induction and continuing into recovery. Expect hypotension and start treatment with dopamine or dobutamine immediately if turning down the vaporizer and administering a small bolus of crystalloids (2 ml/kg) or colloids (1 ml/kg) doesn't return the patient to normotension. **Judicious** volumes of fluids (2-5 ml/kg/hr) can be administered throughout the procedure. There is detailed information on treating hypotension in Chapter 10. **KEEP WARM!**

Analgesia: Analgesia improves anesthetic safety by allowing the vaporizer to be turned down and decreases the chance for pain-induced adverse cardiovascular effects like arrhythmias and tachycardia. Use opioids and **local blocks**.

Recovery: Keep the patient quiet and warm, continue to monitor cardiac function and support as necessary. Shivering can cause increased oxygen demand which, if not met by oxygen delivery, can cause myocardial ischemia (damage from decreased oxygen) which can also cause decreased myocardial contractility and arrhythmias. Start NSAIDs if appropriate.

Hepatic Disease/Dysfunction
Patient Signalment and History
Rylie, a 10-yr old male neutered Beagle dog with a history of elevated hepatic enzymes and bile acids, is being treated with SAMe (S-Adenosyl methionine) and prescription liver diet. Rylie was seen eating a bone and is now vomiting and anorexic. (NOTE: This could also be a cat and the protocol would be the same but the drug dosages might change slightly.)

Physical Exam
HR 80; RR 16; body condition score 4/5; Slightly lethargic and dehydrated, no other abnormalities.

Serum Chemistry and CBC
Elevated hepatic enzymes (ALT 180, ALP 300 [normal in our lab ALT 0-113; ALP 4-113]); no other abnormalities.

Other Diagnostic Tests Recommended
Abdominal radiographs to determine presence/absence of an intestinal foreign body. This patient's liver function is stable and mildly elevated liver enzymes occur fairly commonly in older dogs so no other tests are needed. If concerned, a bile acids test can be used to determine the degree of liver dysfunction after recovery from the surgery. Since the liver makes clotting factors and proteins, tests for patients with severe liver disease might include prothrombin time (PT), partial thromboplastin time (PTT) and/or buccal mucosal bleeding time (BMBT) to determine clotting function and albumin/total protein to determine the concentration of serum protein.

Procedure
Abdominal exploratory to remove an intestinal foreign body.

Concerns and Plan
ASA Status III. Support oxygen delivery to the liver by supporting both blood pressure and oxygenation. Decreased oxygen delivery can be more detrimental to impaired organs than for healthy organs. Be prepared for a prolonged recovery since many anesthetic drugs are metabolized by the liver. Hypothermia will further delay metabolism of drugs and prolong recovery time. Patients with hepatic disease are often more likely to vomit/regurgitate.

If the hepatic dysfunction was severe enough to cause protein and clotting abnormalities, the patient should not be anesthetized unless anesthesia is required for an emergency procedure. If this is the case, the patient might need to be treated with plasma.

Drug Contraindications
No drugs are truly contraindicated but, as mentioned, drugs that rely primarily on hepatic metabolism for elimination are best avoided. This includes acepromazine, ketamine, Telazol and the NSAIDs. Opioids and alpha-2 agonists are also metabolized by the liver but their effects are reversible. Propofol is metabolized in part by the liver but has other routes of clearance. Drugs of choice include reversible or short duration sedative, analgesic and anesthetic drugs.

Anesthetic Plan

Preanesthesia/premedication: Maropitant should be administered SQ or IV approximately one hour prior to surgery for both decreased vomiting/regurgitation and for provision of abdominal analgesia. Choose an opioid based on pain level (moderate to profound in this case) + dexmedetomidine at dosages for, or at 75% of, those for healthy patients, both administered IM or IV. In many patients with hepatic disease, the opioid alone may provide adequate sedation.

Induction: Propofol is the least dependent on hepatic metabolism. Alfaxalone metabolism is likely similar to that of propofol.

Maintenance: Low-dose inhalants.

Monitoring & Support: Standard monitoring and support as described for ASA I-II patients and KEEP WARM!

Analgesia: Injection of morphine +/- local anesthetic in the epidural space at the lumbosacral junction if clotting is normal **(Figure 9-7)**.

Recovery: Keep warm and be prepared for a slightly prolonged recovery. The effects of the dexmedetomidine could be reversed with atipamezole, if necessary.

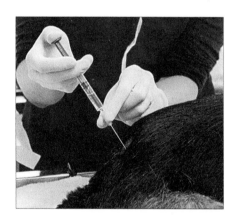

Figure 9-7. Epidural injection of morphine/ bupivacaine in the lumbosacral space of a dog anesthetized for abdominal surgery.

Ovariohysterectomy (OHE or 'Spay')
Patient Signalment and History
Blue is a 1-year old female intact Blue Heeler. (NOTE: This could also be a cat and the protocol - including the mesovarian ligament injection or abdominal lavage of local anesthetic - would be the same but the drug dosages might change slightly.)

Physical Exam
No abnormalities.

Serum Chemistry and CBC
No abnormalities.

Other Diagnostic Tests Recommended
None.

Procedure
Ovariohysterectomy (OHE or 'spay')

Concerns and Plan
ASA Status I so no additional anesthetic concerns based on patient health. Ovario-hysterectomies are called 'routine' because the surgery is easy - but that does not mean that a skin incision, stretching/tearing the mesovarian ligaments and clamping/crushing of the uterine body is 'routine' to the patient. Sounds pretty painful!

Drug Contraindications
None.

Anesthetic plan
Preanesthesia/premedication: Any of the options in the ASA I-II protocol. A common choice is an opioid based on pain level (in this case moderate to high: morphine, hydromorphone, methadone, oxymorphone) + dexmedetomidine, both administered at dosages for healthy patients and delivered IM or IV.

Induction: Any of the injectable induction drugs.

Maintenance: Inhalants.

Monitoring & Support: Standard monitoring and support as described for ASA I-II patients.

Analgesia: Local block at the incision site **(Figure 9-8)** before surgery. Lavage of local anesthetic drugs into the abdomen prior to closure (Chapter 7).

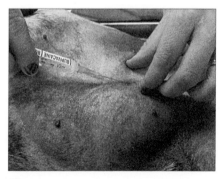

Figure 9-8. Local block of the incision site for an OHE.

Recovery: Same as described for recovery of ASA I-II patients.

Renal Disease/Insufficiency

Patient Signalment and History

Nikita, a 14-yr old female spayed Domestic short hair cat **(Figure 9-9)** returned home from a visit outdoors with multiple bite wounds, presumably from a fight with another cat. She also has chronic kidney disease that is currently stabilized with a prescription renal diet and intermittent administration of subcutaneous fluids by her owner. She is also on maropitant to control nausea/vomiting. (NOTE: This could also be a dog and the protocol would be the same but the drug dosages might change slightly.)

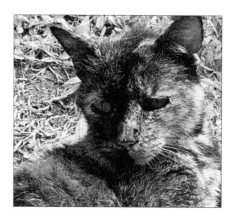

Figure 9-9. A cat with chronic renal failure. Note the thin body condition

Physical Exam

No abnormalities other than the bite wounds, some of them are fairly deep, low body condition score and slight dehydration.

Serum Chemistry and CBC

BUN 60mg/dL and creatinine 3.5mg/dL (normal in our lab 14-36 mg/dL and 0.6-2.4 mg/dL, respectively). The PCV is slightly low, as commonly occurs with chronic kidney disease. No other abnormalities.

Other Diagnostic Tests Recommended

A urinalysis (UA) might be useful if renal function is changing, but her condition is stable so probably not necessary at this time.

Procedure

Wound debridement and cleaning.

Concerns and Plan

ASA Status III since her renal disease is currently stable. Hypovolemia could decrease renal blood flow (RBF) so start IV crystalloid fluid administration prior to anesthesia, if possible. In Nikita's case, fluids for 1-2 hours would probably be sufficient. With more severe and/or unstabilized renal disease, IV fluids may need to be administered overnight prior to anesthesia. Support oxygen delivery to the kidneys by supporting both blood pressure and oxygenation. Decreased oxygen delivery can be more detrimental to impaired organs than to healthy organs.

Drug Contraindications: In cats, ketamine and Telazol should not be used or should be used at the lowest dosages possible. Ketamine is partially excreted by the kidney without having undergone hepatic metabolism. This means that active ketamine could continue to circulate in patients with renal disease, thus delaying recovery. The tiletamine in Telazol is likely to have the same excretion/metabolism. In general, avoid nephrotoxic drugs like NSAIDs and aminoglycoside antibiotics.

Anesthetic plan

Preanesthesia/premedication: Continue maropitant. Choose an opioid based on pain level (moderate in this patient, full mu agonists would be appropriate, as would buprenorphine) at dosages for, or 25-50% lower than, those administered to healthy patients. A benzodiazepine (midazolam or diazepam) can also be administered as part of the premedications. Alpha-2 agonists are commonly used since their effects are reversible and not dependent on metabolism or clearance. However they are somewhat controversial since they MAY constrict renal vessels and decrease renal blood flow. Acepromazine may dilate renal vessels and improve renal blood flow. The effects of both drugs on the renal vessels are probably clinically irrelevant in most patients. Pad and position carefully and keep warm.

Induction: Propofol or alfaxalone.

Maintenance: Low dose inhalants.

Monitoring & Support: Standard monitoring and support as described for ASA I-II patients. Fluids at slightly higher rate in most patients (10-20 ml/kg/hr). MAINTAIN NORMAL BLOOD PRESSURE! Administer dopamine or dobutamine if hypotension occurs and is unresolved by decreasing the inhalant dose and administering IV fluids. Thin patients (as some chronic kidney patients may be) are more likely to get hypothermic and may get painful areas or burns over boney points if they are placed on hard surfaces or directly on heating pads with no cover (which should NEVER happen!).

Analgesia: Important because pain can stimulate the sympathetic nervous system, which can potentially lead to vasoconstriction, which can cause a decrease in renal blood flow. Opioid boluses or infusions can be used. Use local anesthetic blocks wherever possible. In this patient inject local anesthetic into or around all of the bite wounds.

Recovery: Opioids. The long lasting buprenorphine (Simbadol®) would be a good choice.

Seizures

Patient Signalment and History

Fuzzy is an 8-yr old female spayed Pomeranian. She has a history of seizures which are now controlled with medication and she has not seized in several months. Her owner noticed a large lump on her right forelimb about a month ago and is bringing her in now because she won't use the leg. (NOTE: This could also be a cat and the protocol would be the same but the drug dosages might change slightly.)

Physical Exam

Fuzzy is extremely nervous and doesn't want to be touched at all but especially not on the leg with the mass. The owner said that she used to be friendly but has increasingly become 'snappy'. Radiographically, osteosarcoma is diagnosed. It is likely that her behavior changes are due to allodynia (pain induced by non-painful stimuli like touch) and hyperalgesia (exaggerated pain response to mildly painful stimuli like gently palpating the tumor) secondary to central sensitization (or 'wind-up'). She is tachycardic and panting, both probably from anxiety and pain, but no other abnormalities. The owner understands that this is an incurable disease and that a forelimb amputation is the best option for Fuzzy's quality of life.

Serum Chemistry and CBC

No abnormalities.

Other Tests Recommended

Radiograph the thorax to be sure that there is no metastasis of the tumor. Because she also has had previous seizures, take a careful history with a focus on seizure presentation and/or any abnormal mentation.

Procedure

Forelimb amputation.

Concerns and Plan

ASA Status II-III. The main concern is profound and prolonged pain since the patient is very painful and that impacts our anesthetic drug choices and management. Be very aggressive with pain management - surgical pain will exacerbate the existing pain from the tumor. Once the leg is removed the dog's pain should eventually decrease, but not for several days-weeks postoperatively. The pain may not fully resolve since pain of central sensitization AND neuropathic pain, which can both be hard to treat, are major components of this patient's discomfort. See more information in Chapter 7. The patient is currently not seizing but anesthesia-induced changes in the nervous system could potentially precipitate a seizure - unlikely, but potentially. Use drugs that decrease the incidence of seizures. Keep pain & excitement at a minimum as they also could potentially precipitate seizures.

Drug Contraindications

Ketamine and Telazol MAY increase incidence of seizures, although this concern is overrated. Ketamine administered as an infusion is the treatment of choice for central sensitization pain. Fortunately, the low-dose administered in the infusion is safe, even in a patient with seizures. Contrary to popular belief, acepromazine does NOT cause seizures and is not contraindicated.

Anesthetic plan

Preanesthesia/premedication: Choose an opioid based on pain level (in this case very high: morphine, hydromorphone, methadone, oxymorphone) + dexmedetomidine at dosages for healthy patients, either IM or IV. Start NSAIDs now if possible, or immediately postoperatively if that is the preferred protocol in the hospital. Start gabapentin for postoperative control of neuropathic pain.

Induction: Midazolam or diazepam (0.2 mg/kg) plus propofol to effect. All of these drugs decrease seizures. Alfaxalone is likely also acceptable but there is no data on the impact of alfaxalone on seizures.

Maintenance: Inhalants + aggressive analgesia

Monitoring & Support: Standard monitoring and support as described for ASA I-II patients. If moderate to excessive hemorrhage occurs, check the PCV and TP intraoperatively and postoperatively.

Analgesia: Intraoperatively administer a CRI and perform a brachial plexus local anesthetic block with either regular bupivacaine or Nocita®, which is liposome-encapsulated bupivacaine that provides analgesia for up to 72 hours. The best choice for a CRI would be a multimodal infusion like morphine (or fentanyl, hydromorphone, oxymorphone or methadone) plus lidocaine plus ketamine. The ketamine is crucial in this patient because it treats the pain of central sensitization. During closure of the incision, insert a wound or 'soaker' catheter **(Figure 9-10)** or inject Nocita® into the tissue layers of the incision (Chapter 7).

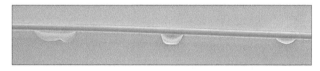

Figure 9-10. A wound infusion or 'soaker' catheter. Note the fluid flowing out of the small holes in the catheter.

Recovery: Keep pain & excitement at a minimum, monitor for seizures. If postoperative seizures occur, treat with benzodiazepines. Continue the CRIs at full dose for at least 1-2 hours and potentially up to 24 hours. Ideally, the full-dose CRI administration should be followed by ½ dose for several hours before discontinuing. The opioid infusions may be stopped postoperatively if Nocita® or a wound infusion catheter has been used. However, the ketamine infusion should continue to treat the pain of central sensitization. Infuse a dose of bupivacaine (1-2 mg/kg) through the wound catheter as soon as it is sutured in place and administer the second dose 4 hours after the first dose. Generally, the dosing interval can be increased to every 6-8 hours after 3-4 dosages. To decide whether or not the dosing interval can be extended, gently palpate the incision at the time when the next dose is due. If the patient is comfortable, extend the dosing interval. If not, dose now. Be careful! If the patient is painful they may resent having the incision touched and may bite. Leave the wound catheter in for 2-5 days, depending on the pain level **(Figure 9-11)**. The Nocita® does not need to be re-dosed since the duration is 72 hours. However, if the patient is painful after the drug wears off, it can be re-dosed (off-label). Continue NSAIDs for at least 1-2 weeks and an aggressive dose of gabapentin (≥ 10 mg/kg TID-QID) for at least 4 weeks.

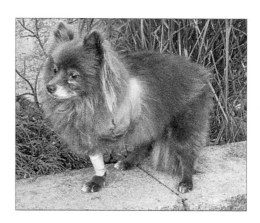

Figure 9-11. A patient after a forelimb amputation.

Trauma

Patient Signalment and History

Two patients: Meteor a 2-yr old intact male Domestic Short Hair (DSH) cat and his buddy Pluto a 1-yr old intact male mixed breed dog were hit by a car 15 minutes prior to presentation to the hospital.

Physical Exam

Both patients are very obviously distressed. Meteor, who is normally very friendly and loves people, is trying to hide under a towel and is growling and hissing when touched. Pluto, who is usually a very friendly dog who likes to be petted, is trying to bite anyone who touches him. Both patients are alert and have no signs of head trauma. Both patients are tachycardic and tachypneic with pale mucous membranes and a slightly prolonged CRT and both have obvious fractures (Meteor femur fracture; Pluto radius/ulna fracture) but no other obvious injuries except for scrapes and a few minor lacerations.

Serum Chemistry and CBC
Important, but not as important as stabilizing the patient. Proceed without it. It will be available before surgery to fix the fractures - which won't be until tomorrow.

Other Tests Recommended
After analgesia and potentially sedation, complete radiographs and other diagnostic tests as required based on the location of the injuries (e.g., may need to do an abdominal ultrasound, radiograph or abdominocentesis if the abdomen was injured; may need a neurologic exam and radiographs of the skull if head trauma is expected, etc.). ECG! Arrhythmias are common with trauma - especially if the thorax was traumatized. PCV and TP to assess blood loss.

CRITICAL TIP!
Do NOT proceed without analgesia. Opioids can be administered at low dosages if necessary but they should not be omitted!

Procedure
Stabilize both patients. Even if these patients need surgery, it would be dangerous to rush them into surgery before stabilization.

Concerns and Plan
ASA Status III or IV for both: It is difficult to decide if they are a III or IV until a more thorough exam can be performed. Start stabilization as described below and continue patient evaluation.

Drug Contraindications
Probably none but more diagnostics are required to be certain. Definitely opioids are NOT contraindicated and should be administered NOW.

Stabilization Plan
Fluids and analgesia! The fluid type will most likely be a balanced electrolyte solution like LRS or PlasmaLyte and the rate will depend on the patient's needs. Remember that cats have a smaller blood volume than dogs so the volume of IV fluids administered should be lower in the cat. Analgesia is a critical part of stabilization. Some people are afraid of giving analgesia at this point because it 'might mask something' but pain can actually contribute to shock and make the patient worse. Alleviating the pain - and the contribution of pain to shock - will make the patient more hemodynamically stable. The heart rate will come down, the mucous membranes will become more pink, the CRT will normalize and the breathing will slow and become deeper. If these things don't happen, now you know that pain is

not the problem so keep doing diagnostics and find the problem!

Opioids are the best choice for analgesia during stabilization. They are rapidly acting, provide profound analgesia and cause minimal to no adverse physiologic effects. Opioid effects are reversible if they are concerning, but that is unlikely to happen in patients with this much pain. A bolus of morphine, hydromorphone, oxymorphone or methadone should be administered as soon as possible. In extremely frantic patients, a bolus of an alpha-2 agonist should also be adminis-tered. The best thing for the patient is to decrease the pain and stress. Overnight care should/could include repeated boluses of opioids or, better, a constant rate infusion (CRI) that includes an opioid and might also include lidocaine and/ or ketamine (Chapter 7). Lidocaine CRIs are controversial in cats but an opioid/ ketamine infusion would definitely be appropriate. Local blocks are appropriate if there are wounds or other painful sites that can be blocked.

Anesthetic Plan
Now that the patients have been stabilized - at least for several hours but probably best overnight - we can proceed with anesthesia.

Preanesthesia/premedication: Choose an opioid based on pain level (high in both patients: morphine, hydromorphone, methadone, oxymorphone) + dexmedeto-midine at dosages for healthy patients, both IM or IV. Even if opioids were admin-istered as an infusion, a bolus of opioids as a premedication is still appropriate to ensure that the serum opioid concentration is high enough to prevent/treat surgical pain, but a ¼-½ dose is generally sufficient. Remember that cats require higher dosages of alpha-2 agonists like dexmedetomidine than dogs require. Preoperative NSAIDs may be appropriate in stabilized patients.

Induction: Any of the induction drugs would be appropriate for both patients.

Maintenance: LOW DOSE inhalants.

Monitoring & Support: Standard monitoring and support as described for ASA I-II patients. Arrhythmias, hypotension and hypoventilation are common in patients with traumatic injuries. May need to monitor PCV/TP if hemorrhage occurs.

Analgesia: Local/regional blocks! An epidural in the case of Meteor **(Figure 9-12)** and a brachial plexus block **(Figure 9-13)** in the case of Pluto. The epidural should contain morphine +/- a local anesthetic. The brachial plexus block can be done with regular bupivacaine or with Nocita®.

Recovery: Continue analgesia. May need to continue monitoring and support depending on what is happening with the patient (e.g., arrhythmias, low SpO$_2$ because of pulmonary trauma, etc.). If not started preoperatively, NSAIDs may be appropriate for many patients at this time.

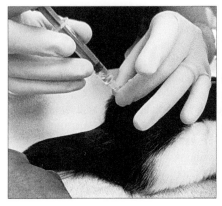 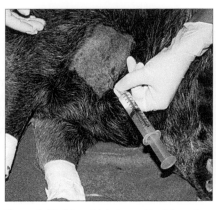

Figure 9-12. Epidural injection of morphine/bupivacaine in the lumbosacral space of a cat.

Figure 9-13. A brachial plexus block in a dog.

Case Examples: Anesthesia Complications
Shona Meyer BS, LVT, VTS (Anesthesia/Anaglesia)

CASE 1
Postoperative Respiratory and/or Cardiac Arrest

Patient Signalment and History
Blizzard is a 2-year old intact female Siberian husky mix.

Physical Exam
No abnormalities. Body weight 23 kg, HR 80 bpm, RR panting, body condition score 3/5, body temperature 101.2°F.

Serum Chemistry and CBC
No abnormalities.

Other Diagnostic Tests Recommended
None needed.

Procedure
Ovariohysterectomy (OHE or 'spay')

Concerns and Plan
ASA status I. Although there is always risk involved in anesthesia even in the healthiest of patients, there are no additional anesthesia-related concerns for this patient.

Drug Contraindications
None

Anesthetic Plan
Preanesthesia/premedication: Standard protocol example: Administer 0.1-0.2 mg/kg hydromorphone or 0.5 mg/kg morphine or 0.4 mg/kg methadone + 0.02 mg/kg acepromazine or 0.005 mg/kg dexmedetomidine IM. When the dog is sedate, place a 20G IV catheter in either cephalic vein, preoxygenate, place oscillometric blood pressure cuff and ECG leads. Start NSAIDs.

Induction: 1 mg/kg propofol bolus, followed by propofol to effect until the patient can be intubated (expect to administer another 2-3 mg/kg).

Maintenance: Isoflurane in 100% oxygen delivered through a rebreathing circuit with a fresh gas flow of 20 ml/kg/min with a minimum flow of 500 ml/min (Chapter 3).

Monitoring and Support: Continuously monitor the ECG, non-invasive blood pressure, pulse oximeter, end tidal capnograph, and esophageal temperature. Administer crystalloid fluids IV at 5-10 ml/kg/hr, maintain body temperature with a circulating hot water blanket.

Analgesia: Administer boluses of opioids, if needed. Use local anesthetics in the incision and in the abdomen (intraperitoneal lavage, Chapter 7). Consider a morphine +/- bupivacaine or lidocaine epidural block. Although epidurals aren't commonly administered for OHE, maybe they should be! They provide effective analgesia for most abdominal procedures, including OHE.

Recovery: Keep quiet and warm, monitor pulse oximeter after removing from 100% oxygen, pain score immediately following anesthesia and 2-4 hours post-operatively.

Problem
After an uneventful anesthesia, Blizzard is moved to a quiet area to recover and administered 100% oxygen with the intent to switch to breathing room air after 5 minutes **(Figure 9-14)**. Three minutes into the recovery process she is observed to become apneic and cyanotic (blue mucous membranes). How do you proceed?

Solution
The fact that the patient is apneic and cyanotic means this is an emergency. Cyanosis is a sign of profound hypoxemia. Start breathing for the patient IMMEDI-ATELY and quickly check the pulse. If there is a pulse, this is likely respiratory arrest and the guidelines for treating hypoventilation/hypoxemia presented in Chapter 10 should be immediately instituted. If there is no pulse, this is likely cardiac arrest and the steps in Figure 10-14 (CPR flow chart) should be instituted IMMEDIATELY.

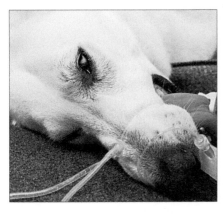

Figure 9-14. A dog recovering from anesthesia just before it went into respiratory arrest.

CASE 2:
Intraoperative Hypotension

Patient Signalment and History
Odie is a 6-year old castrated male Basset Hound who has been anorexic and vomiting for 24 hours. He was seen playing with a sock and now the sock is missing.

Physical Exam
Weight 26 kg, HR 120 bpm, RR panting, body condition score 3.5/5, body temperature 101.5°F, 7% dehydration as determined by skin tenting and dry mucous membranes. Mucous membranes are slightly pale and CRT is slightly prolonged, probably due to dehydration.

Serum Chemistry and CBC
Increased PCV, TP (both likely due to dehydration) and hypokalemia (likely due to not eating).

Other Diagnostic Tests Recommended
Abdominal radiographs to determine presence of an intestinal foreign body. ECG prior to anesthesia since patients with abdominal abnormalities often have arrhythmias. Noninvasive blood pressure measurement prior to anesthesia to determine the impact of the dehydration on blood pressure.

Procedure
Laparotomy to remove foreign body.

Concerns and Plan
ASA III. The dehydration and electrolyte abnormalities should be corrected prior to anesthesia. This patient's surgical procedure is urgent but not an emergency so stabilization can be the priority. When anesthesia commences, rapid airway

protection will be crucial since this patient is already vomiting, which increases the risk of regurgitation/vomiting at induction.

Drug Contraindications: None. Drugs that are less likely to cause vomiting or that prevent vomiting are preferred.

Anesthetic Plan

Preanesthesia/premedication: Place a 20G IV catheter in either cephalic vein and start on IV fluids prior to anesthesia. The patient is dehydrated so administer 10-20 ml/kg for one hour and reassess. Administer 1mg/kg maropitant IV (or SQ but the drug stings so if the catheter is already placed, administer the drug through the catheter) as soon as possible. When it is time for anesthesia, administer 0.1 mg/kg of hydromorphone or 0.2-0.5 mg/kg morphine (slowly!) or 0.2-0.3 mg/kg methadone through the catheter. For calm or very sick patients, no extra sedative is needed for premedication. If the patient is fairly alert or anxious, 0.01mg/kg acepromazine or 0.002 mg/kg dexmedetomidine could be added to the opioid. Preoxygenate, place oscillometric blood pressure cuff and ECG leads.

Induction: 1 mg/kg propofol bolus, followed by propofol to effect until the patient can be intubated (expect to administer another 1-2 mg/kg). If sedatives were not used in the premedication phase, diazepam or midazolam at 0.2 mg/kg should be injected IV immediately prior to or along with the propofol. This decreases the propofol dose needed for induction, which improves anesthetic safety.

Maintenance: Isoflurane in 100% oxygen delivered through a rebreathing circuit with a fresh gas flow of 20 ml/kg/min, with a minimum flow of 500 ml/min (Chapter 3).

Monitoring and Support: Continuously monitor the ECG, non-invasive blood pressure, pulse oximeter, end tidal capnograph, and esophageal temperature. Administer crystalloid fluids at 5-20ml/kg/hr depending on how quickly the initial dehydration is corrected and how much volume is continually lost through evaporation from the open abdomen, hemorrhage, etc…. Maintain normothermia with circulating hot water blanket or forced warm air (eg, Bair Hugger, Baja Breeze).

Analgesia: Administer 0.1 mg/kg morphine +/- local anesthetics in the lumbosacral epidural space. Constant rate infusions can be used if epidurals are not done in your practice or if added analgesia is needed. Regardless of whether or not an epidural injection occurs, an infusion of lidocaine should be administered since lidocaine infusions provide analgesia, improve GI motility (probably secondary to analgesia), decrease endotoxemia effects (endotoxins often leak from compromised bowel) and treat/prevent arrhythmias that often occur in patients with abdominal abnormalities.

Recovery: Keep quiet and warm, monitor pulse oximeter after removing from 100% oxygen. Continue the lidocaine CRI. May need to continue IV fluids as, or in addition to, the lidocaine CRI. Pain score immediately following anesthesia and 2-4 hours post-operatively.

Problem
One hour into the procedure Odie becomes hypotensive. How do you proceed?

Solution
There are many causes of anesthesia-related hypotension including excessive anesthetic depth, hypovolemia, vasodilation and decreased myocardial contraction. Immediately turn down the inhalant dose and start a treatment plan (See Chapter 10, Figure 10-7). The treatment plan will include identification and treatment of the cause of hypotension. Hypovolemia will require administration of crystalloids, colloids and perhaps whole blood. Decreased myocardial contractility will require a positive inotrope (eg, dopamine, dobutamine) infusion. Profound vasodilation will require a vasopressor (eg, norepinephrine, epinephrine, vasopressin).

CASE 3:
Hyperkalemia

Patient Signalment and History
Max is a 3-year old castrated male domestic long hair cat that has been straining to urinate and is now fairly lethargic and dehydrated.

Physical Exam
Weight 5.3 kg, HR 220 bpm; RR 40; body condition score 3/5, body temperature 102.2°F, distended urinary bladder. The presumptive diagnosis is a stone in the urethra.

Serum Chemistry and CBC
Increased PCV, TP and glucose. Potassium 6.8 mEq/L (normal 3.8-5.3 mEq/L in our lab).

Other Diagnostic Tests Recommended
ECG. Patients with hyperkalemia are often bradycardic, and have ECG abnormalities including 'tented' T waves and absent P waves. When the patient is stabilized, radiographs of the bladder/urethra are appropriate but not important right now. This patient is in bad shape!

Procedure
STABILIZE THE CAT, then relieve the urethral obstruction and place a urinary catheter while providing analgesia.

Problem

At presentation Max has the ECG changes described above. How do you proceed? **(Figure 9-15)**

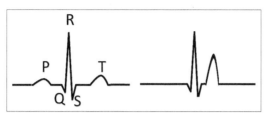

Figure 9-15. Normal ECG on the left, ECG from patient with hyperkalemia on the right. Note the absence of P waves and the 'tented' or enlarged T waves.

Concerns and Plan

Don't proceed without treatment! Uncontrolled hyperkalemia is life threatening and is a much bigger concern than the distended bladder. The potassium should be decreased to 6.0 mEq/L or less and the ECG abnormalities should be resolved prior to anesthetizing this cat. Use the flow chart **Figure 9-16** for treatment. In the meantime, the cat can be lightly sedated with buprenorphine or butorphanol for passing a catheter to relieve the obstruction. Pain contributes to the obstruction by causing muscle spasm at the site of the stone so analgesia will make moving the stone easier. In addition to the systemic opioids, use lidocaine mixed with gel to aid in decreasing the pain of urethral catheter placement. Also consider a sacro-coccygeal (sometimes called intracoccygeal) epidural injection of lidocaine, which will provide both analgesia and urethral muscle relaxation. But remember, stabilize the patient first! The distended bladder will not result in death of the cat, but the hyperkalemia is potentially lethal.

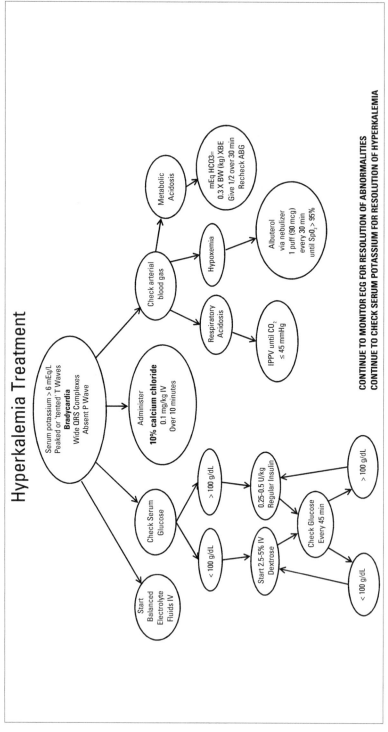

Figure 9-16. Flow chart for treating hyperkalemia. Abbreviations: ABG=arterial blood gas; BE=base excess; BW=body weight; HCO3=bicarbonate; IPPV=intermittent positive pressure ventilation or mechanical ventilation; mEq=milli-equivalents. A good reference for treating hyperkalemia can be found in the Veterinary Emergency and Critical Care Manual 3rd Edition, edited by Karol Mathews, published by Life Learn 2017.

Chapter 10
Treating Complications and Emergencies

Shona Meyer, BS, LVT, VTS (Anesthesia/Analgesia)

Introduction

Complications and emergencies sometimes occur in spite of appropriate anesthetic protocols and diligent patient monitoring and support but, ideally, the anesthetist should be able to identify and treat complications before they become emergencies. Complications and emergencies occurring in the central nervous (CNS), cardiovascular and respiratory systems can become immediately life-threatening. Monitoring and support are focused on these organ systems. Anesthesia-induced changes in other organ systems (e.g., slowing of hepatic metabolism, decreased renal function) are not generally immediately life-threatening, although they can create postoperative complications. Fortunately, support of the CNS, cardiovascular and respiratory systems provides support for other organ systems by promoting adequate oxygen delivery.

CNS Complications and Emergencies

Complications of the CNS include excessive and inadequate anesthetic depth. The main emergency is profound anesthetic depth causing the patient to be near death.

Excessive Anesthetic Depth

This is the most commonly occurring anesthetic complication but, unfortunately, is the least recognized complication. Excessive anesthetic depth can precipitate all of the other potential complications and can rapidly become an emergency rather than a complication. Excessive anesthetic depth is a leading cause of anesthesia-related death. Appropriate patient monitoring - and response to each patient as an individual - are imperative for prevention of this complication. Excessive anesthetic depth is MUCH easier to prevent than to treat!

Most Common Causes

The most common cause of excessive anesthetic depth is a true over-dose of anesthetic drugs as would occur from a dosage miscalculation or an excessively high vaporizer setting. But a relative overdose (the dose is correct but not for that patient or that situation) can occur due to the age and health status of the patient (neonates, geriatric and compromised patients often require a lower dosage of anesthetic drugs), duration of surgery (the dose can be cumulative over time), and/or hypothermia (which causes a decreased need for anesthetic drugs).

Treatment

Decrease anesthetic depth IMMEDIATELY. If necessary, turn the vaporizer completely off, fill the rebreathing bag with oxygen and ventilate for the patient to increase the rate at which the inhalant gases are removed from the patient's lungs. If necessary, antagonists can be administered for those drugs with reversible effects (e.g., atipamezole can be administered to reverse the effects of xylazine, medetomidine and dexmedetomidine). (See Chapter 4).

Inadequate Anesthetic Depth

This complication is less common and more easily fixed than excessive anesthetic depth. Prevention through diligent monitoring and appropriate use of analgesic drugs are the keys to success.

Treatment

Insure that the patient really is at an inadequate anesthetic depth and not just responding to pain. If in pain, provide analgesia. If truly too lightly anesthetized, turn up the inhalant or give a low-dose bolus of the induction drug. The latter is preferable if the patient is excessively light since the injectable drug will work faster than the inhalant.

TIP
Be sure to hold the patient's mouth gently closed around the endotracheal tube if the head is moving so that the patient doesn't pull the tube out of the trachea or bite through the tube.

CRITICAL POINT!
Hypoxemia and hypercarbia can cause physiologic changes (tachycardia, tachypnea) that make the patient seem to be too lightly anesthetized. However, in these situations, the changes are occurring in an attempt to improve oxygenation and/or to eliminate carbon dioxide. This state can generally be differentiated from a light plane of anesthesia by 1) recognition that the vaporizer setting is too high, 2) identification of low blood pressure (blood pressure is usually normal to high with inadequate anesthesia) and 3) evaluation of other reflexes that might indicate the patient's plane of anesthesia (including movement, palpebral reflex, jaw tone). If there is a chance that the patient is actually too deep, don't increase the vaporizer setting! Doing this will blunt or abolish the changes needed to improve tissue oxygen delivery and carbon dioxide elimination, which can lead to adverse events including death.

Cardiovascular System Complications and Emergencies

Complications of the cardiovascular system include abnormal heart rate, arrhythmias with minor impact on blood pressure, mild hypotension or hypertension and mild anemia or hypoproteinemia (low protein). Emergencies include arrhythmias that can be fatal, arrhythmias that have a major impact on blood pressure, profound hypotension from any cause and severe blood loss.

Abnormal Heart Rate

Abnormal heart rate is defined as rates that are too low (bradycardia) or too high (tachycardia) for the species and size of the patient.

Normal Ranges for Heart Rate (beats/min) in Anesthetized Dogs & Cats

Dogs   Small 80-120   **Cats** 120-180
           Medium 60-80
           Large 40-60

Sinus Tachycardia

The heart rate is higher than normal for the patient but the ECG tracing is normal, i.e., the electrical impulse starts at the sinus or 'SA' node [hence the name 'sinus' tachycardia] and generates a normal looking P wave which generates normal QRS and T waves. Sinus tachycardia is depicted in **Figure 10-1**, bottom tracing. Tachycardia is important because an excessively fast heart rate can cause decreases in blood pressure secondary to decreased time for the ventricles to fill with blood and can predispose the patient to other arrhythmias.

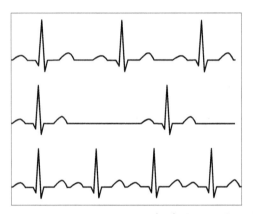

Figure 10-1. ECG tracing depicting normal heart rate (top), sinus bradycardia (middle) and sinus tachycardia (bottom). Regardless of the rate, the ECG tracing has a normal configuration, indicating that the electrical impulse originated at the sinus node (hence the name 'sinus' bradycardia and tachycardia) and followed the normal electrical pathway through the heart (depicted in Chapter 5).

Most Common Causes of Sinus Tachycardia: Excessively fast heart rate is generally due to an underlying cause and it is important to identify and treat the problem since the underlying cause itself may contribute to patient morbidity or even mortality. Causes include:

• Any condition or drug that triggers an increased release of endogenous catecholamines, which are 'excitatory' neurotransmitters like epinephrine. Examples include pain and an excessively light anesthetic plane.
• Exogenous catecholamine administration (e.g., dopamine, dobutamine), especially if the patient is hypovolemic.

IMPORTANT TIP
Administration of dopamine or dobutamine to a patient that is hypovolemic will almost always lead to tachycardia. Assess hydration if this occurs.

- Any drug or condition that blocks vagal tone, like anticholinergics (atropine, glycopyrrolate).
- Any condition that causes hypoxemia, decreased tissue oxygen delivery, dehydration, anemia, hemorrhage, hypercarbia, or an excessively deep anesthetic plane (tachycardia only occurs in the very early phases of excessive anesthetic depth, followed rapidly by bradycardia).
- Primary cardiac disease - which should be identified and treated prior to anesthesia if at all possible.

When/How to: Treat Sinus Tachycardia: Treat if the patient is both tachycardic AND hypotensive. A rule of thumb is to consider treatment if the heart rate is ≥ 20-30% higher than the heart rate obtained on the physical exam immediately prior to anesthesia or ≥ 20-30% higher than the normal upper limit heart rate for the size and species of patient. The treatment depends on the underlying cause **(Table 10-1)**.

Table 10-1
Causes and Treatment of Sinus Tachycardia

Cause	Treatment/Comments (HR = Heart Rate)
Anesthetic drugs: ketamine, Telazol	No treatment necessary, HR is usually high normal to slightly tachycardic and does not generally create adverse effects.
Anesthetic support drugs that stimulate the sympathetic nervous system: dopamine, dobutamine, norepinephrine, epinephrine, ephedrine	All drugs except for ephedrine are administered as an infusion so stop the infusion. No treatment for ephedrine, just wait for the rate to decrease (usually 5 to 15 mins). **IMPORTANT TIP: Also assess hydration because using these drugs to improve blood pressure in a patient that is hypovolemic will almost always lead to tachycardia.**
Anticholinergic drugs: atropine, glycopyrrolate	No treatment available, just wait for the rate to decrease (usually 5 to 15 mins). Administering these drugs IM results in a lower peak HR so try to anticipate the need for an anticholinergic and administer the drug IM, if possible. Use IV administration in emergencies. Glycopyrrolate causes a lower peak HR than atropine.
Pain	Very common cause of tachycardia. Administer analgesic drugs: opioids, alpha-2 agonists, local anesthetic drugs, NSAIDs (although the slow onset of NSAIDs is not ideal for treatment of intra-operative tachycardia).

Table 10-1 continued

Excessively light plane of anesthesia	Not as common as we think - more likely to be due to pain, so treat pain first! If the patient is really too light, turn up the inhalant or give a bolus of injectable anesthetic drug (e.g., propofol, ketamine, etc.).
Excessively deep plane of anesthesia	**CRITICAL TIP: Patients that are too deep and hypovolemic, hypoxemic or hypercarbic can also be tachycardic - SO BE SURE THAT THE PATIENT IS REALLY TOO LIGHT BEFORE YOU ADMINISTER MORE ANESTHETIC DRUGS!** If the increase in HR is blocked by increasing the anesthetic depth, the patient is critically deep and likely close to death. If the patient is too deep, turn down - or turn off - the inhalant anesthetic and breathe for the patient to increase the rate of inhalant elimination from the patient's lungs.
Hypotension	Blood pressure is tightly regulated by the body and low blood pressure will cause an increase in heart rate in an attempt to increase blood pressure. Use techniques to increase blood pressure: decrease the inhalant dose, administer IV fluids, administer colloids, inotropes and vasopressors as needed.
Hypovolemia, dehydration, vasodilation, decreased cardiac contractility	All of these contribute to hypotension with subsequent tachycardia. Treatments: Hypovolemia, dehydration - administer crystalloids, colloids, or blood; Vasodilation - may need to administer vasopressors; Decreased cardiac contractility - administer positive inotropic drugs (e.g., dopamine & dobutamine).
Hypoxemia/hypoxia, hypercarbia/hypercapnia, respiratory acidosis	Oxygen delivery and acid/base status are tightly controlled by the body and will cause an increase in heart rate to increase cardiac output. This will allow more oxygen delivery to the tissues and more blood returned to the lungs so that the excess CO_2 can be exhaled and the pH can be maintained in a normal range. Treatment: Supplement oxygen if the patient isn't already on oxygen, breathe for the patient, decrease anesthetic depth, look for reasons for hypoventilation (more information later in this chapter).
Anemia	Can result in decreased oxygen delivery, which will cause a reflex increase in heart rate in a physiologic attempt to increase cardiac output, and subsequent oxygen delivery, to the tissues. Treatment: TRANSFUSION!
Hyperthermia	If the body temperature is high enough to cause tachycardia, start active cooling including fans, cool water baths, cooled IV fluids.

Sinus Bradycardia

The heart rate is lower than normal for the patient but the ECG tracing is normal (i.e., the electrical impulse starts at the sinus node or 'SA' node [hence the name 'sinus' bradycardia] and generates a normal looking P wave, which generates normal QRS and T waves). Sinus bradycardia is depicted in **Figure 10-1, middle tracing**. Bradycardia is important because it can contribute to hypotension. Profound bradycardia may indicate that cardiac arrest is about to happen.

Most Common Causes of Sinus Bradycardia:

• Anesthetic drugs, primarily opioids, propofol and alpha-2 agonists.
• Anesthetic support drugs that cause hypertension and reflex bradycardia, like phenylephrine, norepinephrine, vasopressin, and sometimes dobutamine and even dopamine (although less common with the latter drug).
• Inherent high vagal tone since the vagus nerve has a profound influence on heart rate. This is often seen in very athletic dogs like many hound dogs.
• Vagal stimulation that occurs when organs with extensive vagal innervation such as the larynx, neck, viscera, urinary bladder (especially when full) and eye are stimulated.
• Hypothermia, hyperkalemia, hypertension, hypothyroidism, hypoglycemia, hyper-calcemia.
• The use of rate slowing drugs for cardiac disease (beta agonists and calcium channel blockers).
• Local anesthetic toxicity.

When and How to: Treat Sinus Bradycardia: Treat if the patient is both bradycardic AND hypotensive. In general, DO NOT TREAT if blood pressure is normal. A rule of thumb is to consider treatment if the heart rate is ≥ 20-30% lower than the heart rate obtained on the physical exam immediately prior to anesthesia or ≥ 20-30% lower than the normal lowest limit heart rate for the size and species of patient. Treatment depends on the cause **(Table 10-2)**. In general, the use of anticholinergic drugs, treatment of underlying causes and cessation of stimulation of areas with extensive vagal innervation will fix the problem.

ADVANCED TIP

If the low heart rate is contributing to hypotension and the anticholinergic drugs are ineffective, consider an infusion of sympathomimetic drugs (drugs that stimulate the sympathetic nervous system) like dopamine or epinephrine. If the patient is extremely cold, neither anticholinergic drugs nor sympathomimetic drugs will increase the heart rate and the patient is in a very dangerous situation. Start warming immediately.

Table 10-2
Causes and Treatment of Sinus Bradycardia

Cause	Treatment/Comments (HR = Heart Rate)
Anesthetic drugs: opioids, propofol, alpha-2 agonists	Treatment is not necessary if the patient is bradycardic but the blood pressure is normal. If HR and blood pressure are low, anticholinergics are usually the best option. If low HR is caused by a reversible drug, reversing the drug MAY be an option, but reversing opioids in a painful patient can cause other problems which can be more difficult to treat than the slow heart rate. In this instance, instead of reversing the opioid, administration of an anticholinergic would be more appropriate. If alpha-2 agonists are reversed in an anesthetized patient, be ready to increase the inhalant dose or administer a bolus of an injectable anesthetic since the patient is highly likely to wake up. Although anticholinergics should not be used with alpha-2 agonists if the blood pressure is normal, anticholinergics CAN BE USED if the patient is bradycardic AND hypotensive. For propofol, the bradycardia is of short duration and will dissipate on its own, but anticholinergics can be used if necessary.
Anesthetic support drugs that stimulate the sympathetic nervous system: dopamine, dobutamine, norepinephrine, epinephrine, ephedrine	These drugs traditionally cause tachycardia but may cause reflex bradycardia, especially if they cause hypertension. Most of the drugs in this category are administered by infusion so decrease the rate of, or stop, the infusion.
High vagal tone (common in very athletic patients, certain breeds and manipulation of some organ systems - like traction on intestinal viscera)	Anticholinergic drugs are usually the best option. They can be used to prevent bradycardia in patients that are highly likely to have decreased heart rate (e.g., highly athletic dogs like Greyhounds or some brachycephalic dogs like Bulldogs) or can be used to treat bradycardia once it occurs. If surgical manipulation is the cause of the bradycardia, have the surgeon STOP MANIPULATING until the anticholinergic drugs take effect. This is commonly seen in surgeries of the neck, abdominal viscera and eye. If anticholinergics don't work, try sympathomimetic drugs like dopamine or epinephrine.

Hypothermia	Start active warming immediately. If the patient is so cold that its heart rate is low, it is dangerously cold. CRITICAL POINT: If patients are profoundly hypothermic, neither anticholinergic nor sympathomimetic drugs will work to treat bradycardia. Only rewarming the patient will return the heart rate to normal. A patient that is so cold that it is bradycardic is a high risk patient and should be closely monitored.
Hyperkalemia, hypercalcemia	Start treatment to decrease the potassium or calcium, including IV fluids.
Hypertension	Determine the cause of the hypertension and treat if necessary (see more information later).
Hypothyroidism	Would likely have been diagnosed and treated preoperatively. If bradycardia occurs intraoperatively, treat with anticholinergic or sympathomimetic drugs.
Hypoglycemia	Treat with IV dextrose or dextrose containing fluids. Most common in neonates and some small breed dogs that have been anorexic. May occur in dogs that have had recent excessive physical exertion.
Drugs that directly slow the heart rate, ie, drugs used in patients with cardiac disease (beta-blocking drugs, calcium channel blocking drugs, etc.)	IF POSSIBLE, discontinue these drugs the morning of the surgery. Can try treating with anticholinergic and/or sympathomimetic drugs but this is often only marginally effective. Keep anesthesia time as short as possible.
Local anesthetic toxicity	EMERGENCY! Discontinue any local anesthetic CRIs and treat with anticholinergics and vasopressors (e.g., norepinephrine, epinephrine, vasopressin). Use special lipid emulsion ('intralipid') if available.

Abnormal Heart Rhythm (Arrhythmias)

Abnormal heart rhythm is defined as a rhythm that occurs in an irregular pattern; has irregular transmission through the AV node (e.g., second degree AV block); or is initiated by the atria (e.g., atrial premature contractions), ventricles (e.g., ventricular premature contractions, ventricular tachycardia, and ventricular escape beats) instead of the sinus node. Of course, many abnormal rhythms can occur, especially in patients with heart disease, but the rhythms covered here are those that are most likely to develop in anesthetized patients. Heart rhythms are diagnosed by evaluating the ECG tracing. A normal rhythm as depicted by a normal ECG tracing appears in **Figure 10-1, top tracing**.

2nd Degree Atrial-Ventricular (AV) Block

Is identified as P waves occurring intermittently without a subsequent QRS complex. Second degree AV block is depicted in **Figure 10-2**. If the AV block is frequent and/or the patient is also hypotensive treat by increasing the heart rate or by correcting the underlying cause of the bradycardia as described in **Table 10-2**. This is a commonly occurring normal rhythm in the horse and does not require treatment.

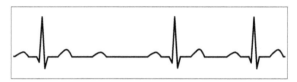

Figure 10-2. ECG tracing depicting 2nd degree AV block. Note that the second P wave from the left does not have an accompanying QRS complex or T wave.

Ventricular Premature Contractions (VPCs)

Occur when the electrical impulse originates in the ventricles, instead of the sinus node. These are intermittent early beats (meaning that they occur earlier than the next normal, sinus node generated beat would have occurred and there is a very short interval between the last normal beat and the VPC) and the associated complexes are wider and 'bizarre' (meaning not normal configuration) in comparison to a normal complex. They do not have a P wave associated with the QRST wave. The VPC is usually a single beat typically followed by a compensatory pause (meaning that the next beat will not occur at its normal time, instead there will be a long pause before the next beat occurs). A VPC is depicted in **Figure 10-3**. Intermittent VPCs themselves are generally not important unless they are occurring frequently enough to alter blood pressure. However, the underlying cause of the arrhythmia (e.g., pain, hypoxia, hypercarbia, electrolyte imbalances) should be investigated since treatment of the cause may be necessary.

NOTE
The term VPC is interchangeable with the term PVC (Premature Ventricular Contraction). Both terms are correct.

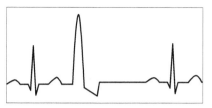

Figure 10-3. ECG tracing depicting ventricular premature contraction (VPC). VPCs occur when the electrical impulse originates in the ventricles instead of the sinus node. Note that the beat occurs early (meaning before the next normal beat would have occurred); that the complex has no P wave, a very large and abnormally configured QRS complex and a large inverted [upside down] T wave; and that there is a long pause before the next normal beat. The overall heart rate with this rhythm is usually normal.

Most Common Causes of VPCs: This arrhythmia is usually due to an underlying cause: hypotension, hypoxia/hypoxemia, hypercarbia/hypercapnia, electrolyte imbalance, excessively deep plane of anesthesia, pain or an excessively light plane of anesthesia. Cardiac disease can also cause VPCs and should be diagnosed and stabilized prior to anesthesia. A low number of VPCs may occur in geriatric patients due to age-related changes.

When and How to: Treat VPCs: Treatment may not be needed if the VPCs are infrequent and are not altering blood pressure.
- Treat the arrhythmia itself if:
  - The VPC does not create a pulse (keep your fingers on an artery while looking at the ECG). This means that there is electrical activity but no cardiac output.
  - Ten or more VPCs occur in a row.
  - The number of VPCs exceeds 20% of the total ventricular rate (count VPCs and normal QRS complexes for a total ventricular rate).
  - The VPCs rate is high (which is actually ventricular tachycardia - see next section).
  - The R wave of the QRS overlaps with the T wave ('R on T').
- Treatment
  - **First try to identify and treat the underlying cause.** The causes and their treatment are generally similar to those for sinus tachycardia (See Table10-1).
  - Lidocaine is the first choice for treatment of the arrhythmia itself.
    - NOTE THAT THE DOSE FOR CATS IS LOWER THAN THE DOSE FOR DOGS.
  - Procainamide can be used to treat refractory (i.e., hard to treat) VPCs. Procainamide causes profound negative inotropic (i.e., decreased contractility) effects and should not be administered to patients with impaired contractility. Arterial blood pressure should be monitored during the administration of procainamide. Again, the dose is lower for cats than dogs.

NOTE
Procainamide is not commonly available in most practices but, fortunately, it is rarely needed.

Ventricular Tachycardia

An excessively high ventricular rate (generally defined as > 160-180 bpm in medium to large dogs and > 220 bpm in cats and small dogs) which can cause hypotension (because the ventricles don't have time to fill with blood) and can lead to ventricular fibrillation and death. Ventricular tachycardia is depicted in **Figure 10-4**.

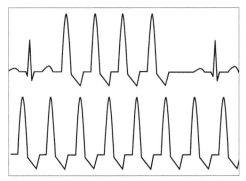

Figure 10-4. ECG tracing depicting ventricular tachycardia. Note that the complexes look like rapidly occurring VPCs. They can be intermittent *(top tracing)* or continuous *(bottom tracing)*.

When and How to: Treat Ventricular Tachycardia: Causes and treatment are generally the same as for VPCs, except that ventricular tachycardia is likely to impair blood pressure so instead of first treating the underlying cause and then treating the arrhythmia if necessary, the arrhythmia is generally treated (with lidocaine) and then the underlying cause identified and treated, if possible.

CRITICAL POINT!
If ventricular tachycardia is sustained (meaning it doesn't quit), immediate treatment is necessary as blood pressure is likely to decrease.

Ventricular Escape Beats

These are generally caused by excessively slow heart rates. The beat looks like a VPC but it is 'late' (meaning that it occurs later than the normal beat should have occurred - there is a long pause between the normal beat and the escape beat). Ventricular escape beats are depicted in **Figure 10-5**.

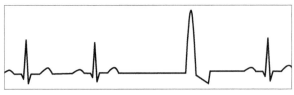

Figure 10-5. ECG tracing depicting ventricular escape beat: Note that the complex looks like a VPC but the beat occurs late (meaning after the next normal beat would have occurred). The overall heart rate with this rhythm is usually slow.

When and How to: Treat Ventricular Escape Beats: Treat if the escape beats are frequent and/or the patient is also hypotensive. Treat by directly increasing the heart rate (e.g., administer atropine or glycopyrrolate) or by correcting the underlying cause of the bradycardia as described in **Table 10-2**.

CRITICAL POINT!

DO NOT TREAT THIS ARRHYTHMIA WITH LIDOCAINE. It is CRITICAL to distinguish escape beats from premature ventricular contractions. Escape beats occur after a long pause from the previous QRS complex (so are called 'late' beats) and are associated with bradycardia. VPCs occur very soon after the previous QRS complex (so are called 'early' or 'premature' beats) and are associated with tachycardia. Escape beats keep the heart rate fast enough to support perfusion, lidocaine will abolish escape beats (just as it abolishes VPCs) and can cause asystole (cardiac arrest).

Ventricular Fibrillation

This arrhythmia occurs when there is absolutely no coordinated myocardial electrical activity or myocardial contraction, and no cardiac output. It is fatal if not treated immediately. START CPR - this is basically cardiac arrest. The definitive treatment is electrical conversion of the arrhythmia with a defibrillator. In the absence of a defibrillator, a 'precordial thump' (single, hard blow to the patient's thorax in the area of the heart) MIGHT restart the normal heart rhythm. Ventricular fibrillation is depicted in **Figure 10-6**.

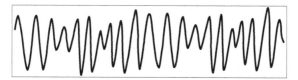

Figure 10-6. ECG tracing depicting ventricular fibrillation. Note that the complexes are differing sizes and erratic.

Abnormal Arterial Blood Pressure

Abnormal arterial blood pressure is defined as pressure that is too low (hypotension) or too high (hypertension).

Normal Ranges for Arterial Blood Pressure

For dogs and cats the normal range is: Systolic 80 to 120 mmHg, Diastolic 40 to 80 mmHg, and Mean 60 to 100 mmHg.

Hypotension

In anesthetized small animal patients hypotension is defined as mean arterial blood pressure (MAP) < 60 mmHg, and the systolic arterial blood pressure (SAP) < 90 mmHg. In horses, the definition of hypotension is the same but MAP should be kept at > 70 mmHg to prevent myopathies and neuropathies (see Chapter 11).

IMPORTANT POINT
Hypotension is the third most common complication that occurs during anesthesia (excessive anesthetic depth is the first, hypoventilation is the second), so a fair number of your patients might be hypotensive!

CRITICAL POINT!
Hypotension is important because: Hypotension = decreased blood flow = decreased oxygen delivery to tissues. Tissues need oxygen to function normally.

Most Common Causes of Hypotension: There are numerous causes of hypotension:
- Excessive anesthetic depth (the most common cause).
- Hypovolemia, dehydration, and excessive hemorrhage.
- Low heart rate or extremely high heart rate.
- Poor cardiac muscle ('myocardium') contractility.
- Vasodilation (dilated blood vessels).

When to Treat Hypotension: Hypotension often occurs briefly right after induction. A brief period is normal but treatment should begin anytime that MAP is < 60 mmHg for > 5-10 minutes in adult animals. Neonates/pediatrics normally have slightly lower blood pressure and a MAP as low as 50 mmHg (but no lower) is normal and does not require treatment.

How to: Treat Hypotension (Figure 10-7): Make sure that the patient is as stable as possible - meaning address all underlying disease conditions.
- Decrease the dose of inhalant (meaning, TURN DOWN THE VAPORIZER). Inhalants cause profound vasodilation and can decrease myocardial contractility, both of which contribute to hypotension.
  - Don't forget to empty the rebreathing (or 'reservoir') bag since it will be filled with the higher concentration of inhalant.
  - Add analgesia if the patient keeps waking up at the lower concentration of inhalant.
- Check the heart rate and if it is too fast or too slow, treat as described in Tables 10-1 and 10-2, respectively.
- Administer a bolus of crystalloid fluids (e.g., Lactated Ringer's solution [LRS], PlasmaLyte, 0.9% saline) of 5 to 10 mls/kg IV (dog) 3 to 8 mls/kg (cat) (See Chapter 6).
  - If the patient is dehydrated, continue to administer crystalloids.
  - If the patient is already hydrated, continuing to administer large volumes of crystalloids is unlikely to improve blood pressure so move on to the next step. OR, if the patient does not respond to the crystalloid bolus move on to the next step.

CRITICAL TIP!
If the patient has cardiac disease, excessive IV fluid administration can be very dangerous since the heart cannot pump the extra fluid and edema will result. In these patients go straight to a colloid bolus or, better yet, straight to dopamine or dobutamine to treat hypotension.

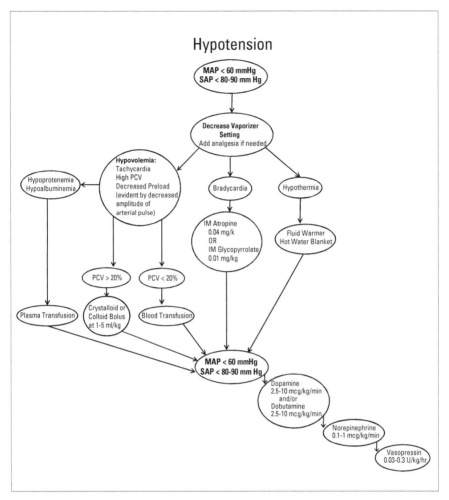

Figure 10-7. Flow Chart for treating hypotension.

- Administer a colloid fluid bolus (e.g., VetStarch) of 2-3 (up to 5) mls/kg IV (dog) or 1-2 (up to 3) mls/kg IV (cat) OR if the patient is anemic, start a blood transfusion OR if the albumin is low administer plasma.
  - This should increase blood pressure if circulating volume is low.
  - Move on to the next step if there is no increase in blood pressure. Administration of excess volume could be detrimental (e.g., can cause edema).
- Administer a positive inotropic drug (e.g., dopamine, dobutamine, ephedrine; dosages Table 10-6) to increase myocardial contractility.
  - Even if the patient does not have cardiac disease, myocardial contractility may be decreased by age, underlying diseases, and/or the anesthetic drugs themselves (especially the inhalant drugs).
- If the patient does not respond to any of these treatments or if the diastolic

pressure is really low, administration of a vasoconstrictive drug or 'vasopressor' (e.g., epinephrine, norepinephrine, vasopressin; Dosages Table 10-6) may be necessary.

- Excessive vasodilation is common in patients in shock or with sepsis.
- Determine if excessive vasodilation is the problem by checking for a very low diastolic blood pressure and mucous membrane color that is red instead of pink (remember that other things can cause red mucous membranes so don't go by this alone).
- Constricting the vessels increases cardiac work (because it is harder for the heart to pump blood into constricted vessels than into dilated vessels) so this is often the last choice for treatment. However, if vasodilation is causing hypotension, it must be treated.
- If treatment does not seem to be improving the blood pressure, determine that the low blood pressure is real by putting your fingers on the patient's pulse, checking the mucous membrane color and the CRT. If the patient seems fine but the blood pressure reading on the monitor is low, trouble shoot the monitor as described in Chapter 5.

Hypertension

Is not as clearly defined as hypotension but the general consensus is SAP > 150 mmHg; MAP > 115 mmHg; DAP > 95 mmHg in anesthetized patients.

Most Common Causes of Hypertension: Hypertension is uncommon in anesthetized patients, and is usually a sign of an underlying problem, which can be pain, inadequate anesthetic depth, drugs that affect heart rate (e.g., anticholinergics such as atropine and glycopyrrolate), drugs that affect cardiac contractility (e.g., positive inotropic drugs such as dopamine, dobutamine and ephedrine), and drugs that cause vasoconstriction (e.g., alpha-2 agonists, epinephrine, norepinephrine and vasopressin).

When to Treat Hypertension: If the hypertension is sustained for > 15 minutes, the underlying cause should be identified and treated, if necessary and/or possible. Rarely is the hypertension itself treated. Mild hypertension is often normal following administration of certain drug classes (like alpha-2 agonists) and treatment is not necessary. Treatment of hypertension appears to be less critical in animals than in humans as animals do not seem to have the same magnitude of adverse events from brief hypertension.

How to Treat Hypertension: Administer an analgesic drug. A bolus of opioids is a good choice because opioids are potent and fast-acting.
- Increase the depth of anesthesia if the patient is too light.
- Discontinue drugs that might cause hypertension (e.g., dopamine, dobutamine).
- Administer vasodilating drugs if the patient is extremely hypertensive. Turning up the vaporizer will cause vasodilation. Acepromazine will cause vasodilation. Beta-agonists (e.g., propranolol and esomolol) are sometimes used for extreme hypertensive emergencies. Both the availability of the drugs and the situation described are very rare in most practices.
- If treatment does not seem to be improving the blood pressure, determine

that the high blood pressure is real by palpating the pulse and checking mucous membrane color/CRT. If the problem does not seem to be the patient trouble shoot the blood pressure monitor as described in Chapter 5.

Low Packed Cell Volume (PCV) or Total Protein (TP)

The cardiovascular system is composed not only of the heart and blood vessels, but also blood and plasma.

• Normal packed cell volume (PCV; which is a measure of the volume of red blood cells) is 36 to 56% in the dog and 30 to 46% in the cat. This range can vary slightly depending on the normal values from the laboratory used by your clinic.
• IMPORTANCE: Low PCV = decreased red blood cells to carry oxygen to the tissues, which means that the tissues may suffer from ischemia (injury from low oxygen).
• If the PCV drops to < 18% (cat) or < 22% (dog) in a patient with chronic anemia or < 20% (cat) or < 25% (dog) in a patient with acute anemia, the patient is in danger of suffering ischemia and should receive a blood transfusion. Loss of 20-25% of the patients blood volume (blood volume in liters is roughly 10% of the patient's body weight in kgs) is another way to determine the need for a transfusion.
• Normal total protein (TP) is 5.5 to 7.5 g/dL in dogs and 6.2 to 8.5 g/dL in cats. This range can vary slightly depending on the normal values from the laboratory used by your clinic.
• IMPORTANCE: Low TP = decreased protein to support oncotic pressure (see Chapter 5), which can lead to edema. If the TP is low, the patient should receive plasma.

How to: Transfuse Blood

Volume to be transfused: When active hemorrhaging is occurring, blood replacement volume should equal the volume lost. When a patient presents with post-hemorrhage or with anemia from other causes, the volume of blood transfused is determined by the formula:

Mls of donor blood = [2.2 x recipient wt in kg x 40 (dog) or 30 (cat)] x [(PCV desired - PCV recipient)/PCV of donor blood]

Blood should be warmed to 37°C and transfused through a filter. The initial transfusion rate should be approximately 5 ml/kg/hr for 10-15 minutes. If no adverse events occur, the rate can be increased. The rate in a hypovolemic patient can be as high as 20 ml/kg/hr but lower rates (eg, 5 ml/kg/hr) reduce the risk of volume overload. Patients with cardiac disease should always receive transfusion at rates ≤ 5 ml/kg/hr. If patients are to receive concurrent crystalloids, 0.9% NaCl or Normosol-R are the most appropriate choices (LRS contains Ca^{2+}, which promotes clotting; hypotonic solutions promote hemolysis). During the transfusion the patient should be observed carefully for any signs of volume overload or hypersensitivity (eg, panting, increased lung sounds, tachycardia, distress, excessively red [ie, hyperemic] mucous membranes, hives).

Respiratory System Complications and Emergencies

Complications of the respiratory system include mild hypoventilation (i.e., decreased respiratory rate, tidal volume or both), hypoxemia and hypercarbia. Emergencies include profound hypoventilation or apnea, profound hypoxemia or hypercarbia and respiratory arrest.

Hypoventilation

Defined as alveolar ventilation (meaning the amount of air that moves in and out of the alveoli over time) that is too low to maintain adequate gas exchange (gas exchange = oxygen into and carbon dioxide out of the lungs). Hypoventilation can be caused by an excessively slow respiratory rate or small tidal volume, or both. Tidal volume is the amount of air moved in and out of the lungs with each breath.

Normal Ranges for Respiratory Rate and Tidal Volume in Anesthetized Dogs and Cats

Respiratory rate: 5-10 (medium to large dogs) or 10-20 breaths per minute (small dogs & cats)

Tidal volume: 10-15 ml/kg/breath.

> **IMPORTANT POINT**
>
> Hypoventilation is the second most common anesthetic complication and can result in hypercarbia (excess carbon dioxide), and potentially, hypoxemia (inadequate oxygen), and low oxygen saturation.

> **IMPORTANT POINT**
>
> The respiratory rate (RR) can be very high but hypoventilation might still occur if the tidal volume (TV) is low. This often happens in patients that are panting because most of the air just moves in and out of the trachea and doesn't reach the alveoli. It is important to evaluate both RR and TV.

Most Common Causes of Hypoventilation

Hypoventilation is often due to underlying causes and it is important to identify and treat those causes since they may contribute to patient morbidity or even mortality (**Table 10-3**).

The primary cause of hypoventilation is EXCESSIVE ANESTHETIC DEPTH. However, patients that are very old, very young or very sick may not respond to increasing CO_2 and may hypoventilate even if at an appropriate plane of anesthesia. This is also true of patients with head trauma or cranial pathology, like brain tumors.

Table 10-3
Causes and Treatment of Hypoventilation

Cause	Treatment/Comments (RR = Respiratory Rate; TV = Tidal Volume)
Excessively deep plane of anesthesia with any drug	**CRITICAL TIP: This is the most common cause of hypoventilation. If the patient is too deep, turn down - or turn off - the inhalant anesthetic and breathe for the patient to increase the rate of inhalant elimination from the patient's lungs.**
Specific anesthetic drugs that directly cause hypoventilation: opioids, propofol, alfaxalone, INHALANTS	DECREASE the drug dose if possible (especially with inhalants) and breathe for the patient if necessary. Hypoventilation can be normal right after induction, you can breathe for the patient but don't breathe more than 1-3 times/minute or the patient won't build up enough CO_2 to stimulate breathing on its own.
Pulmonary disease: pneumonia, pulmonary contusions, pulmonary edema, lung tumors, asthma, etc.	Can decrease the efficiency of gas exchange in the lungs. When possible, wait until pulmonary disease is resolved before anesthetizing the patient.
Upper airway disease: brachycephalic airway syndrome, laryngeal paralysis, collapsing trachea, airway occlusions, etc.	Can cause limited air flow to the lungs. Intubate! See 'extubating the brachycephalic patient' in Chapt 8 for tips on how to extubate safely when anesthesia is done. **Also remember that an occlusion or kink in the endotracheal tube will cause the same problem.**
Anything that limits movement of the lungs: pneumothorax, hemothorax, pyothorax, etc.	Will decrease TV and can lead to atelectasis. When possible, wait until the condition is stable. Remove as much of the air or fluid out of the chest cavity as possible before anesthetizing. May need to maintain chest tubes throughout surgery and into recovery.
Anything that limits movement of the thorax: ties/ropes that cross the thorax, legs tied too tightly across the thorax, surgeon leaning on the thorax, fractured ribs, etc.	Will decrease TV and can lead to atelectasis. Don't let this happen! Always position the patient carefully and don't allow anything to put pressure on the thorax during anesthesia.
Anything that limits movement of the diaphragm: ascites, distended abdomen, distended stomach [like in a gastric dilatation-volvulus], obesity, pregnancy, diaphragmatic hernia, etc.	Will decrease TV and can lead to atelectasis. When possible, wait until disease or condition is resolved before anesthetizing the patient. If immediate anesthesia is necessary, be prepared to breathe for the patient beginning immediately after induction. Spontaneous breathing may recur once the pressure is removed from the diaphragm.

Table 10-3 continued

Anything that causes thoracic pain: fractured ribs, contusions, etc.	May make the patient unwilling to breathe normally. Use analgesics!!! Local anesthetic blockade is ideal since this won't contribute to hypoventilation. Opioids titrated to effect or administered as an infusion, ketamine &/or lidocaine CRIs and NSAIDs (in appropriate patients) are other good choices.
Hypothermia	Mild hypothermia causes hyperventilation, moderate to severe hypothermia causes hypoventilation. Start warming the patient immediately.
Head trauma, CNS disease, old age, neonatal age, some systemic diseases (e.g., septicemia)	May cause a decreased sensitivity to CO_2 so RR/TV won't increase with increasing CO_2. In these patients, anticipate breathing for them from the beginning of anesthesia.

IMPORTANT POINT

Carbon dioxide is the most potent stimulator of breathing. Conscious patients and healthy patients at an appropriate anesthetic depth should increase respiratory rate and/or tidal volume in response to increased CO_2, and this increase in ventilation should return the CO_2 to normal. Figure 10-8 shows an $ETCO_2$ tracing during normal ventilation.

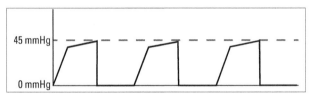

Figure 10-8. End-tidal CO_2 curves for normal ventilation. Note that the end tidal CO_2 is 45 mmHg and the base line is zero.

When/How to: Treat Hypoventilation

Hypoventilation should be treated by breathing for the patient if the end-tidal carbon dioxide (CO_2) is > 55 mmHg (the normal range is 35-45 mmHg) or the oxygen saturation is < 95% (normal is 98-100%) in a patient breathing 100% oxygen or < 90% (normal is 95-100%) in a patient breathing room air (21% oxygen). The capnograph in **Figure 10-9** shows an $ETCO_2$ curve during hypoventilation.

If CO_2 monitoring is not available in your practice, check the respiratory rate, thoracic excursions (the amount the chest wall moves when the patient breathes) and movement of the rebreathing bag. If the respiratory rate is lower than normal for that patient or the chest is barely moving or not moving with each breath, start breathing for the patient while checking for causes of hypoventilation.

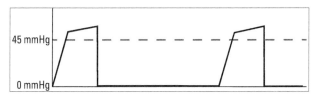

Figure 10-9. End-tidal CO_2 curves for hypoventilation. Note the slow rate and the end-tidal CO_2 of > 45 mmHg.

How to: Breathe for the Patient that is Hypoventilating

1. Close the pop-off valve or push the pop-off button.
2. Squeeze the rebreathing bag for 1 (small dogs, cats) - 2 (large dogs) seconds. The pressure delivered should be 10 (small dogs, cats) - 15 (large dogs) cmH_2O as measured on the pressure manometer on the anesthesia machine. If no pressure manometer is present, watch the thorax and deliver a breath that moves the thorax an amount similar to a normal breath if the patient was conscious.
3. OPEN THE POP-OFF VALVE.
4. Repeat this as needed to keep the CO_2 normal. In some patients, this might mean delivering only 1-2 breaths/minute or even less, while in some patients it might mean completely taking over and breathing 5-10 breaths/minute. If no CO_2 monitoring is available take over breathing if the patient is not breathing at all or breathe the number of times it takes to make the breaths you generate plus the breaths the patient generates equal a normal respiratory rate for that sized patient.
5. If a mechanical ventilator is available, see Chapter 3 for details on ventilator use.

Hyperventilation

Defined as alveolar ventilation that is too high to maintain appropriate gas exchange. Hyperventilation can be caused by an excessively fast respiratory rate or large tidal volume, or both. The capnograph in **Figure 10-10** shows an $ETCO_2$ curve during hyperventilation.

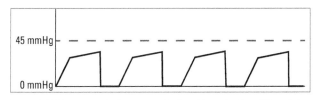

Figure 10-10. End-tidal CO_2 curves for hyperventilation. Note the fast RR and the end-tidal CO_2 of < 45 mmHg.

Most Common Causes of Hyperventilation

Hyperventilation is often due to underlying causes. It is important to identify and treat those causes since they may contribute to patient morbidity or even mortality. The main causes of hyperventilation are pain and excessively light anesthesia **(Table 10-4).**

When/How to: Treat Hyperventilation

Hyperventilation should be treated by identifying and treating the underlying cause. Treat if the CO_2 is < 25-30 mmHg. If CO_2 monitoring is not available in your practice, check the respiratory rate, thoracic excursions and movement of the rebreathing bag. If the respiratory rate is higher than normal for that patient or the chest expansion is larger than you would expect, identify the cause (Table 10-4) and start treatment.

Table 10-4
Causes and Treatment of Hyperventilation

Cause	Treatment/Comments (RR = Respiratory Rate; TV = Tidal Volume)
Pain	Very common cause of hyperventilation. Administer analgesic drugs: opioids, alpha-2 agonists, local anesthetic drugs, NSAIDs (although the slow onset of NSAIDs is not ideal for treatment of intra-operative hyperventilation).
Excessively light plane of anesthesia	Not as common as we think - more likely to be due to pain, so treat pain first! If the patient is really too light, turn up the inhalant or give a bolus of injectable anesthetic drug (e.g., propofol, ketamine, etc.).
Hypoxemia, hypercarbia, respiratory acidosis.	Oxygen delivery and acid/base status are tightly controlled by the body and will cause an increase in RR and/or TV to increase oxygen uptake. This will allow more oxygen delivery to the tissues and increased exhalation of excess CO_2 so that the pH can be maintained in a normal range. Treatment: Supplement oxygen if the patient isn't already on oxygen, breathe for the patient, decrease anesthetic depth, look for an underlying cause. THE MAIN CAUSE IS EXCESSIVE ANESTHETIC DEPTH and the hyperventilation will occur early as the patient tries to compensate but prolonged excessive anesthetic depth will lead to HYPOventilation.
Anesthetic drugs: Opioids?	Opioids can make the patient pant. They are not hyperthermic, the brain just thinks they are hyperthermic and initiates panting. No treatment necessary since this isn't technically hyperventilation and there is no change in oxygen or carbon dioxide in the blood.
Hyperthermia	If the body temperature is high enough to cause hyperventilation, start active cooling: fans, cool water baths, cooled IV fluids, etc.

Hypercarbia

Defined as a carbon dioxide tension of > 45 mmHg, as measured either by the end-tidal CO_2 monitor or by an arterial blood gas. A CO_2 of up to 55 mmHg is generally acceptable under anesthesia because some anesthesia-induced respiratory depression can be tolerated. A CO_2 > 60 mmHg is likely to cause respiratory acidosis, thus treatment should begin before $ETCO_2$ is this high. The capnograph in Figure 10-9 shows an $ETCO_2$ curve with hypercarbia occurring during hypoventilation.

Most Common Causes of Hypercarbia

There are both patient factors and equipment factors that can lead to hypercarbia.
• The most common cause of hypercarbia is hypoventilation, which can be caused by anything that impairs normal ventilation (See Table 10-3).
• Equipment factors that can cause a build-up of CO_2 in the system, resulting in rebreathing of CO_2 and a hypercarbic patient include:
  • exhausted carbon dioxide absorbent in a rebreathing system;
  • excessively low oxygen flow in a non-rebreathing system;
  • nonfunctioning one-way valves in a rebreathing system;
  • excessively long endotracheal tubes or large Y-piece on the rebreathing tubes;
  • any other equipment component that impairs the proper flow of gas in the breathing system including, plugged endotracheal tubes, kinked breathing hoses, holes in system components, etc.
• Most of these complications will cause rebreathing of $ETCO_2$ as evidenced by an end-tidal CO_2 baseline that does not return to zero **(Figure 10-11)**.

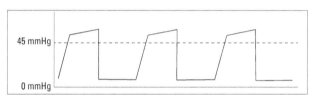

Figure 10-11. End-tidal CO_2 curves for rebreathing of CO_2. Note the normal rate, the high CO_2 and the baseline CO_2 that does not return to zero.

When/How to: Treat Hypercarbia

• Treat if either the end-tidal CO_2 ($ETCO_2$) or the arterial CO_2 obtained by a blood gas analysis ($PaCO_2$) is greater than 55 mmHg.
• Since hypoventilation is by far the most likely cause of hypercarbia, start breathing for the patient (or start mechanical ventilation).
  • Since excessive anesthetic depth is the main cause of hypoventilation, check the depth of the patient and turn down the vaporizer - or turn off the vaporizer if the patient is dangerously deep.
  • Even if the patient isn't too deep, TURN DOWN THE VAPORIZER - breathing for the patient will increase both RR and TV, which will increase the amount of inhalant gas delivered to the patient and will increase anesthetic depth.

IMPORTANT POINT

In most patients, the CO_2 will return to normal with respiratory support and decreased anesthetic depth. If the CO_2 does not return to normal, start trouble shooting using the list below. If the CO_2 does return to normal but the patient becomes hypercarbic when respiratory support is decreased, realize that this is a patient that just needs more support than other patients and keep breathing for it! This can happen with any patient but is most likely to happen with very young, old or sick patients. Ventilatory assistance can be anticipated for patients with gastric distension, pneumothorax, hemothorax, pyothorax, chylothorax, thoracic trauma and pregnancy (all of these diseases/conditions make it hard for the thorax to move so breathing is impaired).

- If the CO_2 does not start decreasing after delivery of 5-6 deep breaths, START TROUBLE SHOOTING!! Make sure that:
  - Oxygen is flowing into the machine from the oxygen source and from the machine to the patient.
  - The oxygen flow is adequate for the patient's size, especially in a non-rebreathing system. (See Chapter 3)
  - The CO_2 absorbent is not exhausted. Change the absorbent if there is any question of efficacy. (See Chapter 3)
  - The one-way (or 'flutter' or 'unidirectional') valves are moving and are not stuck closed or open (rebreathing system).
  - There are no kinks or plugs in the breathing hoses or the endotracheal tube.
  - Patient positioning is not making it difficult for the patient to breathe. Patients in dorsal recumbency (on their backs) have a harder time breathing, especially if they have pressure on the diaphragm from a distended abdomen as might occur during gastric dilatation or pregnancy.
  - The distance from the animal's incisors to the breathing system hoses (or 'breathing circuit') is not excessive. Excessive distance increases 'deadspace' which causes rebreathing of CO_2 by the patient. Common causes of this include endotracheal tubes that are too long, a large mainstream end-tidal CO_2 monitor placed at the end of the endotracheal tube, etc.
  - The patient's body temperature is normal. HYPOthermia can cause hypoventilation and HYPERthermia can cause increased CO_2 production, both can cause hypercarbia.

Hypocarbia

Defined as a carbon dioxide tension of < 35 mmHg, as measured either by the end-tidal CO_2 monitor or by an arterial blood gas. An arterial carbon dioxide tension as low as 25-30 mmHg can be tolerated but CO_2 lower than this is likely to cause respiratory alkalosis and should be treated. The capnograph in Figure 10-10 shows an ETCO$_2$ curve with hypocarbia occurring during hyperventilation.

Most Common Causes of Hypocarbia
Hyperventilation is the most likely cause of hypocarbia. Underlying causes of hyperventilation include, pain, an excessively light plane of anesthesia, hypoxia, hyperthermia, and metabolic acidosis, all of which increase ventilatory drive (i.e., the stimulus to breathe).

When and How to Treat Hypocarbia
Treat the underlying problem! It is often caused by overzealous breathing by a person or the ventilator. Be sure to use the correct ventilatory guidelines (Chapter 3).

CRITICAL TIP!
If the numbers on the $ETCO_2$ monitor have been normal and suddenly start to drop very low (Figure 10-12) or the monitor suddenly stops providing an $ETCO_2$ value at all (Figure 10-13), assess the patient IMMEDIATELY!

• Low cardiac output (as in really low blood pressure or cardiac arrest) results in a lack of CO_2 return to the lungs. If CO_2 isn't returned to the lungs, it can't be exhaled and if it can't be exhaled, the monitor can't measure it. Sudden low CO_2 is a BAD sign. Check the pulse, MM color and CRT to determine the status of the patient. If the patient is in trouble, turn the inhalant off and be prepared to start CPR.

• If the lack of a reading isn't due to low perfusion, it may be due to a disconnection between the endotracheal tube and the breathing system. So, if the patient is fine, check the connection and reconnect immediately or the patient may become hypoxemic (because of lack of oxygen delivery) or wake up (from lack of inhalant anesthetic delivery).

• Whether the problem is poor perfusion or a disconnection, you must identify the problem and fix it QUICKLY.

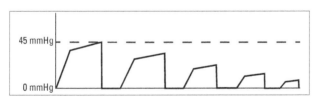

Figure 10-12. End-tidal CO_2 curves that could represent poor perfusion. Note the rapidly decreasing size of the complexes without a change in RR.

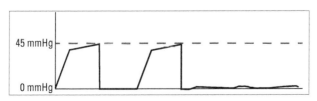

Figure 10-13. End-tidal CO_2 curves that could represent either cardiac arrest or disconnection of the patient from the breathing system or CO_2 monitor. Note the sudden cessation of the tracing.

Hypoxemia and Low Oxygen Saturation

Hypoxemia is low oxygen concentration in the blood, which is measured by arterial blood gas analysis and abbreviated PaO_2 (**Table 10-5**). Most practices don't use arterial blood gas analysis but do use pulse oximetry, which measures the amount of hemoglobin that is saturated with oxygen (abbreviated SpO_2). Although these two parameters don't measure exactly the same thing, they are related and if either is low, oxygen delivery to the tissues is decreased. Low oxygen delivery is critical because oxygen is the 'fuel' that cells need to function normally. Without oxygen, cells may experience dysfunction or may even die.

Table 10-5
Normal Values for SpO_2 and PaO_2

Patient breathing	SpO_2	PaO_2
Room Air	> 90%	80-100 mmHg
100% Oxygen	> 95%	> 300 mmHg

Most Common Causes of Low Oxygen

The most common causes of hypoxemia and/or decreased oxygen saturation are:
• Hypoventilation from all causes in Table 10-3.
• Inadequate oxygen supply (e.g., an anesthetized patient is not receiving supplemental oxygen, the oxygen flow is too low for a nonrebreathing system or the nitrous oxide delivery is too high [few practices use nitrous oxide]).
• Severe pulmonary disease (which would have been diagnosed prior to anesthesia).
• A congenital heart defect that allows blood to shunt through the heart (e.g., a patent ductus arteriosis [PDA]) without going through the lungs to pick up oxygen (which would have been diagnosed prior to anesthesia).
• Blood perfusing alveoli that aren't ventilated and don't contribute to oxygen uptake. This is called 'ventilation-perfusion' (V/Q) mismatch. An example is blood that perfuses areas of atelectatic (collapsed) lung tissue. A very common example is endobronchial intubation (the endotracheal tube is in one bronchus rather than in the trachea) since this will result in only one-half of the lung field receiving oxygen but both halves receiving perfusion.
• Hypotension (the lung is poorly perfused so oxygen is not picked up and carried to the tissues).

When and How to: Treat Hypoxemia

Treat anytime the PaO_2 or SpO_2 is below the normal range.
• Administer supplemental oxygen if the patient isn't already receiving oxygen.
• Since hypoventilation is the most likely cause of hypoxemia, start breathing for the patient (or start mechanical ventilation) while you are trouble shooting to make sure it isn't something else. Use the breathing guidelines listed under hypoventilation.
• You may need to use positive end expiratory pressure (PEEP) or use a

recruitment maneuver which is a very deep breath (40 cm H_2O on the manometer) held for 20 seconds and repeated 2-3 times with a 1-minute 'rest' between each inflation. This will help to expand the alveoli, giving more surface area for oxygen diffusion. This may also cause a momentary drop in blood pressure because of compression of the venae cava and decreased blood return to the heart.

- If none of these steps improve oxygenation, start trouble shooting:
  - Close the pop-off valve and administer a breath to evaluate the ability to expand the lungs.
  - Make sure that the oxygen flow is appropriate for the breathing system and patient size.
  - Check the oxygen supply. Is there adequate oxygen in the tank? Is the hospital line plugged in to the correct port?
  - Insure that the fresh gas port is connected to the breathing system that you are using.
  - Check for leaks in the machine & breathing system.
  - Make sure that there is no obstruction in the airway or breathing circuit.
  - Make sure that nothing is impeding movement of the thorax and/or diaphragm.
  - Manage hypotension and correct poor perfusion.
  - Administer a bronchodilator such as albuterol or terbutaline. If all of this is normal, trouble shoot the SpO_2 monitor as described in Chapter 5.

Respiratory Arrest

If the patient completely stops breathing, immediately intubate the patient (if it isn't already intubated), administer supplemental oxygen and start breathing for it using the breathing guidelines listed under hypoventilation. The causes of respiratory arrest are those listed in Table 10-3 for hypoventilation. If anesthesia related, excessive anesthetic depth is the most common cause. Severe systemic disease can also cause respiratory arrest, in which case life support and medical therapy should be instituted. Respiratory arrest can rapidly lead to cardiac arrest so work quickly!

CRITICAL POINT!
Respiratory arrest, meaning the patient has completely stopped breathing, is an EMERGENCY. Cardiac arrest is likely within a few minutes of total cessation of breathing if the patient is breathing room air (21% oxygen) and within 5+ minutes if the patient is breathing 100% oxygen. This makes monitoring of breathing EXTREMELY IMPORTANT!

CLINICAL TIP
The patient may have apnea immediately after induction to anesthesia and may not breathe during anesthesia maintenance. This is not 'respiratory arrest' and should NOT be an emergency since the apnea would be recognized, is transient and the anesthetist could breathe for the patient. Respiratory arrest as an emergency most commonly occurs in recovery when the patient isn't being as diligently monitored or supported.

Cardiac Arrest

If you suspect that the patient has had, or is near having, a cardiac arrest, the patient should be quickly assessed (don't trust the monitors without looking at the patient). Take a QUICK pulse, listen to the heart with a stethoscope, check for breathing and check mucous membrane color / capillary refill time. If arrest is confirmed or appears imminent, the anesthetic gas should be immediately turned off and the rebreathing bag should be emptied of anesthetic gas and refilled with oxygen. Begin compressions IMMEDIATELY and call for a team member - successful cardiopulmonary cerebral resuscitation (CPCR) cannot be performed alone. Unfortunately, the survival rate for patients that arrest in a veterinary hospital is very low. The CPCR success rate is slightly higher in anesthetized patients, in part because they are already intubated and receiving oxygen.

Current Guidelines for CPCR

The old recommendation for CPCR was to follow the ABCs (airway, breathing, circulation). The current recommendation, however, is to utilize the acronym CAB (circulation, airway, breathing; Fletcher et al. 2012) as depicted in **Figure 10-14**. Starting compressions immediately can be advantageous because the chest compressions not only help to initiate blood flow but may also actually help to maintain gas exchange since air may be moved in and out of the chest as the chest is compressed and then re-expands. In addition, immediately after arrest, most patients have adequate oxygen in their blood (especially those receiving supplemental oxygen like anesthetized patients) but the oxygen must be circulated - so start compressions!

(C) Circulation

Although 'C' to most people means 'compressions', it should actually mean 'circulation'. Of course improving circulation is done mainly by utilizing thoracic compressions, but may also require the administration of IV fluids to increase circulating volume and drugs that improve pump function and vascular support.

Compressions: Start compressions AS SOON AS POSSIBLE and DO NOT STOP for longer than 10 seconds at a time. If the patient is 'flat' chested (e.g., Sighthound), lay the patient on its right side and place both hands directly over the heart - which is roughly located behind the left elbow approximately at the middle of the rib-cage. If the patient is 'round' chested (e.g., bulldogs), you may want to lay the patient on its back and place both hands at the tip of the sternum. These patients can be placed in lateral recumbency but are often easier to maintain in dorsal recumbency. Regardless of body shape, in patients < 7 kg the fingers of one hand should be placed on one side of the chest and the thumb on the other and compressions should be done by gently squeezing the fingers and thumb together.

Begin compressions almost as fast as possible (80 to 100/min with a 1:1 compression time to relaxation time ratio). Compressions should move the

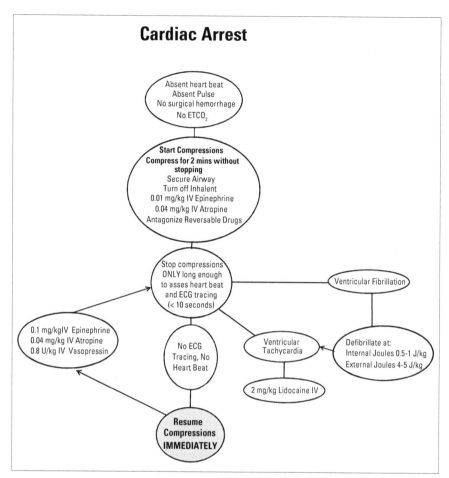

Cardiac Arrest

Absent heart beat
Absent Pulse
No surgical hemorrhage
No ETCO$_2$

Start Compressions
Compress for 2 mins without stopping
Secure Airway
Turn off Inhalent
0.01 mg/kg IV Epinephrine
0.04 mg/kg IV Atropine
Antagonize Reversable Drugs

Stop compressions
ONLY long enough
to asses heart beat
and ECG tracing
(< 10 seconds)

Ventricular Fibrillation

0.1 mg/kgIV Epinephrine
0.04 mg/kg IV Atropine
0.8 U/kg IV Vasopressin

No ECG
Tracing, No
Heart Beat

Ventricular
Tachycardia

Defibrillate at:
Internal Joules 0.5-1 J/kg
External Joules 4-5 J/kg

2 mg/kg Lidocaine IV

Resume
Compressions
IMMEDIATELY

Figure 10-14. Flow chart for CPR.

chest approximately ⅓ of its width or depth and the chest should be allowed
to completely recoil (i.e., return to normal position) during relaxation. Continue
compressions while having another team member feel for a pulse AND attach a
Doppler. If no pulse can be felt or no flow can be heard with the Doppler, compressions must be intensified. The Doppler probe can be lubricated and placed under
the eyelid for assessment of cerebral blood flow. Perform compressions for a FULL
TWO MINUTES without stopping, then QUICKLY attach the ECG leads and stop
compressions to assess the ECG tracing and listen for a heartbeat with a stethoscope and/or feel for a pulse but do not stop for longer than 10 seconds. Resume
compressions immediately if no cardiac activity is detected. Periodically switch out
the person doing the compressions as they fatigue. Don't try to be a hero - if you
are tired, switch. Ineffective compressions will not resuscitate the patient.

> **CRITICAL POINT!**
> Maintenance of blood flow is critical for CPCR success so NEVER stop compressions for longer than 10 seconds (unless you intend to completely stop CPCR) when assessing the ECG, listening to the heart or changing people doing the compressions.

ADVANCED Compressions: Consider internal compressions (opening the chest and directly compressing the heart) only in large dogs or in dogs with an open abdomen or thorax (these two situations make accessing the heart very easy). Internal compressions are much more effective than external compressions in this size patient but they must be instituted soon after the arrest to have an impact. Open chest compressions (or 'massage') are not likely to increase efficacy over closed chest compressions in small patients.

Circulating Fluid: Start IV fluids in patients that are hypovolemic but DO NOT OVERHYDRATE. Fluids may not be indicated in patients with normal hydration/ circulating volume (Fletcher et al. 2012). When fluids are indicated, balanced electrolyte crystalloids (e.g., LRS or Plasmalyte) are generally a good choice. Consider colloids or hypertonic saline if rapid volume increase is necessary. Administer blood if the cardiac arrest is due to hemorrhage. Although we have listed this in the 'C' section since fluids support circulation, rapid administration of IV fluids is not generally a critical step. Thus, IV fluids should not be started until compressions, airway and breathing are implemented.

(A) Airway
This will probably already be done if the patient is under anesthesia. If not, one team member should set up to intubate the patient while the other team member begins chest compressions. Intubation needs to be performed rapidly so that compressions don't have to be stopped for > 10 seconds. Utilize laryngoscopes, stylets or any other tool that will facilitate intubation. MAKE SURE THE TUBE IS INSERTED INTO THE TRACHEA. Insertion into the esophagus will NOT help with breathing/oxygen delivery. If intubation is not possible and the airway is compromised, prepare for a tracheotomy.

(B) Breathing
• PROVIDE OXYGEN. Anesthetized patients will probably be receiving oxygen but oxygen delivery will need to be started in all other patients.
• Deliver breaths at a NORMAL RATE (5 to 10 per minute). DO NOT HYPERVENTILATE - hyperventilation leads to respiratory alkalosis and an abnormal pH.
• Don't excessively pressurize the chest. Remember to use your pressure gauge and stay below 10 to 15 cm H_2O. If a pressure gauge is not available, watch the chest and expand it to a point that looks like a normal breath.
• Don't hold the breath too long or deliver only quick, shallow breaths. Artificial ventilation should closely mimic normal breathing and the breath should last approximately 1-2 seconds.

- If the patient is not yet intubated, ventilate the animal by closing the mouth and performing mouth-to-nose ventilations. Make sure the head and neck are straight so that the breath will flow easily through the upper airway and into the lungs.

(D) Drugs

A variety of drugs (See Figure 10-14 and Tables 10-6, 10-7) are administered during and after CPCR for everything from improved myocardial contraction to treatment of post-CPCR arrhythmias.

- Intravenous (IV) administration is the most effective route for drug delivery but some drugs can be administered intra-tracheally (IT) if no IV catheter is in place.
- For IT administration the drug dosage is generally increased over the IV dosage and the drug is diluted in 2 to 10 ml sterile water (depending on the size of the patient) and administered into the distal trachea through a long catheter (e.g., 'tomcat' catheter or small red rubber feeding tube).
- Drugs that can be safely administered IT can be remembered by the acronym 'LEAN' (lidocaine, epinephrine, atropine, naloxone). Vasopressin can also be administered IT.
- In small patients and neonates intraosseous (IO) administration can be substituted for IV administration.
- EFFECTIVE COMPRESSIONS during drug administration are imperative or the drug will not reach the target organs.

IMPORTANT POINT
In addition to the emergency drugs listed in Tables 10-6 and 10-7 administer reversal drugs for anesthetics as appropriate.

Post Resuscitation

If CPR is successful, the hard part has just begun. Post-resuscitation support includes fluid therapy, oxygen, analgesia, antiarrhythmic drugs, ventilatory support, inotropic drugs, etc. Many patients that have arrested will re-arrest so continue to monitor and support until the patient is completely stable. Very thorough guidelines have been published and should be consulted (Smarick et al. 2012).

Table 10-6
Emergency Drugs and Drugs Used for CPCR

DRUG	DOSE	COMMENTS
Epinephrine	The initial dose should be 'low dose' - 0.01 mg/kg IV or 0.03 to 0.1 mg/kg IT. If the low dose is ineffective, the 'high dose' can be administered - 0.1 mg/kg IV or IT. Repeat the dosages every 3 to 5 minutes until an effect occurs. (IT = intratracheal)	Usually the first drug administered, it improves cardiac function (beta effects) and causes vasoconstriction (alpha effects). Epinephrine may be more effective if the doses are alternated with doses of vasopressin. High dosages of epinephrine are associated with more adverse effects and should be used as a last resort.
Vasopressin	The dose is 0.2 to 0.8 U/kg IV or 0.4 to 1.2 U/kg IT. Administer every 3 to 5 minutes until an effect is noted.	This is a nonadrenergic endogenous pressor peptide that causes peripheral, coronary and renal vasoconstriction. It may be more effective if doses of vasopressin are alternated with doses of epinephrine. This drug is not commonly available in private practice.
Atropine	A dose of 0.04 mg/kg IV is repeated every 3 to 5 minutes until an effect is noted or for a total of 3 doses. Can be administered IT.	Administer if bradycardia is determined or suspected. Severe bradycardia is often a cause of cardiac arrest in animals but less likely in humans.
Lidocaine	An initial bolus of 2 mg/kg IV in dogs and 0.5 mg/kg IV in cats should be administered. May need to continue administration as a constant rate infusion (CRI) following successful resuscitation at 25 to 75 microg/kg/min IV in dogs and 10 microg/kg/min IV cats.	Administer to treat ventricular tachyarrhythmias. Can be administered IT.
Amiodarone	The dose is 5.0 mg/kg IV or IO over 10 minutes. One repeated dose (2.5 mg/kg IV) may be administered 3 to 5 minutes after the first dose.	MAY be a better choice for treatment of ventricular fibrillation if electrical defibrillation is an option. Most of us don't have - or need - amiodarone in private practice.
Dopamine or dobutamine	Administer as a CRI following successful CPR at a rate of 1 to 10 microg/kg/min (up to 15 microg/kg/min for dopamine).	Administered to improve cardiac contractility.

Other Anesthetic Complications

There are many other anesthetic complications that can occur. Appropriate monitoring and support will greatly decrease the incidence of complications. Other complications to watch for in the anesthetized patient include but are not limited to:

• Hyperthermia (See Chapter 6),
• Hypothermia (See Chapter 6),
• Anaphylaxis,
• Gastrointestinal (GI) reflux,
• Esophageal ulcers from reflux,
• Pulmonary edema,
• Aspiration pneumonia,
• Heating pad burns,
• Muscle or nerve injury from inappropriate padding or positioning (more common in horses, see Chapter 11),
• Infection at catheter sites,
• Corneal ulcers from insufficient eye lubrication, pressure on the eye or damage to the eye,
• Tracheal damage from the ET tube,
• Laryngeal damage from the ET tube.

Table 10-7
Cardiovascular Emergency Drug Dosing Chart

Drug (mg/ml)	Atropine* (0.54)	Epinephrine* (1.0) Low Dose	Epinephrine* (1.0) High Dose	Vasopressin (20 UNITS/ml)	Lidocaine (20) DOG	Lidocaine (20) CAT	Calcium Gluconate (100)
Comments	Administer first if arrest is due to bradycardia. Otherwise, use at the same time as epinephrine. If necessary, repeat dose every 3-5 minutes for a total of 3 doses.	Administer first unless bradycardia is seen to be the cause of the arrest - then use atropine first. If necessary, repeat dose every 3-5 minutes for a total of 3 doses.	Only use if low-dose epinephrine has failed to work. High dose is likely to cause arrhythmias.	If available, alternate administration of vasopressin with administration of epinephrine.	Administer to treat ventricular tachyarrhythmias. Inject slowly (over 30 seconds - 1 minute).	Administer to treat ventricular tachyarrhythmias. Inject VERY slowly (over 2-5 minutes).	Administer if arrest or arrhythmias are due to hypocalcemia or hyperkalemia.
Dose mg/kg / Dose mg/lb	0.04 mg/kg / 0.02 mg/lb	0.01 mg/kg / 0.005 mg/lb	0.1 mg/kg / 0.05 mg/lb	0.8 U/kg / 0.4 U/lb	2 mg/kg / 1 mg/lb	0.5 mg/kg / 0.125 mg/lb	10 mg/kg / 5 mg/lb
Patient Weight	DOSE TO BE ADMINISTERED in MILLILITERS (MLS) IV or INTRAOSSEOUS *Can administer intratracheally - double the dose and dilute with saline at 1:1 ratio. Rounded to nearest 0.01 mls. by volume						
2.5 kg / 5 lb	0.2	0.02	0.25	0.1	0.25	0.06	0.25
5 kg / 10 lb	0.4	0.05	0.5	0.2	0.5	0.13	0.5

7.5 kg 15 lb	0.6	0.07	0.75	0.3	0.75	0.19	0.75
9 kg 20 lb	0.8	0.09	0.9	0.4	0.9	0.23	1.0
11 kg 25 lb	0.9	0.11	1.1	0.5	1.1		1.1
14 kg 30 lb	1.1	0.14	1.4	0.6	1.4		1.4
16 kg 35 lb	1.3	0.16	1.6	0.7	1.6		1.6
18 kg 40 lb	1.5	0.18	1.8	0.8	1.8		1.8
20 kg 45 lb	1.7	0.2	2.0	0.9	2.0		2.0
23 kg 50 lb	1.9	0.23	2.3	1.0	2.3		2.3
25 kg 55 lb	2.0	0.25	2.5	1.1	2.5		2.5
27 kg 60 lb	2.2	0.27	2.7	1.2	2.7		2.7
30 kg 65 lb	2.4	0.3	3.0	1.3	3.0		3.0
32 kg 70 lb	2.6	0.32	3.2	1.4	3.5		3.2

(Table 10-7 is designed to copy and post on the wall for quick reference)

References

Fletcher DJ, Boller M, Brainard BM, Haskins SC, Hopper K, McMichael MA, Rozanski EA, Rush JE, Smarick SD; American College of Veterinary Medicine.; Veterinary Emergency and Critical Care Society. RECOVER evidence and knowledge gap analysis on veterinary CPR. Part 7: Clinical guidelines. J Vet Emerg Crit Care 2012; 22 Suppl 1:S102-31.

Smarick SD, Haskins SC, Boller M, Fletcher DJ; RECOVER Post-Cardiac Arrest Care Domain Worksheet Authors. RECOVER evidence and knowledge gap analysis on veterinary CPR. Part 6: Post-cardiac arrest care. J Vet Emerg Crit Care 2012; 22 Suppl 1:S85-101

Chapter 11
Equine Anesthesia and Analgesia

Tamara Grubb, DVM, PhD, DACVAA.

Contributions from:

Mary Albi, LVT; Shelley Ensign, LVT, CVPP;

Janel Holden, LVT, VTS (Anesthesia/Analgesia);

Shona Meyer, BS, LVT, VTS (Anesthesia/Analgesia);

Nicole Valdez, LVT, VTS (Anesthesia/Analgesia)

Introduction

As with other species, anesthesia for horses can be divided into four equally important phases: Preparation/premedication, induction, maintenance and recovery. Specific needs of the horse should be evaluated for each phase and complications that could occur in each phase should be anticipated. Although the phases are the same, the process is slightly different for horses that are anesthetized in the field for brief, elective procedures and horses that are anesthetized in-hospital for longer, more complicated procedures.

Preparation for General Anesthesia - Step by Step:

1. Decide whether the procedure should be done in the field (e.g., castration) or in the hospital (e.g., orthopedic procedures or colic surgery). If the procedure will take longer than one hour or requires advanced surgical or anesthesia techniques, it should be done in the hospital.

2. Decide whether the horse can be managed in the field. Horses that require advanced or prolonged surgical procedures, that are compromised and need physiologic support or that may have difficulty with recumbency (e.g., draft horses) are best anesthetized in the hospital.

3. Perform a thorough physical examination: Assess body condition, check mucous membrane color and capillary refill time, auscultate the heart and lungs, auscultate gastrointestinal (GI) sounds, palpate the peripheral pulse and weigh or estimate the weight of the horse.

4. Assess the area for induction. Inductions in the field should be done in a large open area that is covered with short grass, sand or soft dirt and which is free from any obstructions (like feed troughs). In-hospital inductions should be done in a padded anesthesia induction stall where appropriate restraint is possible.

5. Insure that there are enough qualified people to help - and get the rest of the people out of the way.

6. Place an IV catheter if needed. This is usually not necessary for short field procedures but is required for long procedures and all horses undergoing inhalant anesthesia **(Figure 11-1)**.

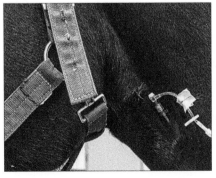

Figure 11-1. An IV catheter in a horse. Note that the catheter is placed high up in the horse's neck near the mandible. The jugular vein is the shallowest, and easiest to access, in the upper ⅓ of the horse's neck. This catheter has an extension set for easy administration of drugs.

7. Place a strong halter and lead rope on the horse. Check the buckles on the halter and the snap on the lead rope for strength **(Figure 11-2)**.

8. Choose drugs and calculate the dosages as described in the next steps.

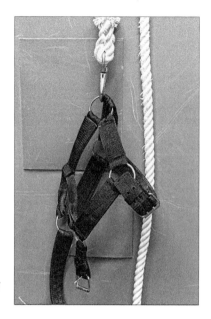

Figure 11-2. A heavy halter and lead rope with good strong snaps should be used for controlling the horse's head during induction to and recovery from anesthesia.

Premedication and Induction
Premedication Drugs
Should include both sedative and analgesic drugs. See **Tables 11-4, 11-5** and Chapter 4.

Alpha-2 Agonists
Xylazine, detomidine or romfidine should definitely be part of the protocol for equine anesthesia. Alpha-2 agonists provide dose-dependent sedation and mild to moderate analgesia. The effects of the alpha-2 agonists are reversible (although effects in horses are rarely reversed) with atipamezole, yohimbine or tolazoline.

Acepromazine
Although not a common addition to field anesthesia protocols, acepromazine ('ace') can be used in combination with an alpha-2 agonist for premedication of horses anesthetized in-hospital. Acepromazine is also used for long-term light sedation (e.g., in mares when separation from the foal is required). Acepromazine can cause priapism (extrusion of the penis) in stallions/geldings, which is generally not a problem but long term extrusion could cause penis injury, which could be an issue for breeding stallions. For this reason, ace is rarely used in stallions.

Butorphanol or Other Opioid

Opioids provide reversible analgesia and the effects are synergistic with those of the alpha-2 agonists. The fear of opioid use in horses causing ileus (GI stasis) and excessive excitement is over-rated. While these effects are common in pain-free horses receiving very high dosages of opioids, as occurs in most of the published research, they are very uncommon in painful horses receiving appropriate dosages of opioids (Clutton 2010). Opioids can be administered as a premedication with the sedatives or as part of induction. Butorphanol, an agonist-antagonist opioid, is the most commonly used opioid in horses but the use of full mu- and kappa-agonist opioids like morphine, methadone, hydromorphone and fentanyl is becoming more routine in horses that are hospitalized with surgical, medical or trauma pain.

Anti-inflammatory Drugs

Since most surgical pain is caused by INFLAMMATION, non-steroidal anti-inflammatory drugs (NSAIDs) are ideal for management of surgical pain. NSAIDs are generally administered pre-emptively but can also be administered postoperatively.

Induction Drugs

(See Table 11-5 and Chapter 4)

Induction drugs must be delivered rapidly so that the horse falls quickly and does not go through a prolonged ataxic phase, which could be dangerous to both the horse and the anesthesia personnel. Drugs are not delivered 'to effect' as they are in small animal anesthesia and there are fewer drug options available for adult horses.

Ketamine

Ketamine is the main induction drug used in horses. The of onset anesthesia following IV ketamine is 1-2 minutes and the effects last for 20 to 30 minutes, which is a perfect duration for most field procedures. Ketamine causes muscle rigidity and must be administered with or after a muscle relaxant. Alpha-2 agonists are potent muscle relaxants and are often used as both the sedative and the muscle relaxant during equine field procedures. True muscle relaxants like the benzodiazepines (diazepam, midazolam) and guaifenesin are also commonly added to the ketamine, especially for in-hospital procedures. Ketamine provides cardiovascular support through stimulation of the sympathetic nervous system and causes no respiratory depression, making it an ideal drug for anesthesia in the field, where monitoring and support are minimal at best.

Telazol (Tiletamine/Zolazepam)

Telazol is sometimes used for induction but recoveries can be VERY rough. NOT recommended for brief field procedures but may be used for longer procedures where inhalants are also used and the Telazol has time to be metabolized prior to recovery.

Propofol

Propofol is sometimes used for induction in foals but the volume required for adult horses is too large to be administered rapidly enough for a smooth induction.

Guaifenesin

Guaifenesin is a centrally-acting muscle relaxant used during induction and/or as part of injectable maintenance as 'triple drip'. It is administered as a large volume from a 0.5 or 1.0-L fluid bag. Alpha-2 agonists and ketamine are added to the guaifenesin for 'triple drip', which is described later in this chapter..

Benzodiazepines

Midazolam and diazepam are short-duration peripherally-acting muscle relaxants that are often administered with the ketamine.

Sedation and Induction Technique - Step by Step

1. Administer the Alpha-2 Agonist
   - Administer the butorphanol with the alpha-2 agonist or wait and administer with the induction drug.
   - If the horse is to be intubated, wash any loose feed and hay out of the mouth so that it is not pushed down the trachea with the endotracheal tube **(Figure 11-3)**.
   - Allow the alpha-2 agonist adequate time to provide appropriate sedation (5 to 10 minutes). An adequately sedated horse should stand with its head down, the ears and lower lip should be 'droopy' and the horse should be relatively insensitive to sound **(Figure 11-4)**.

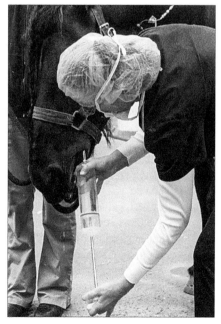

Figure 11-3. Wash any loose feed and hay out of the horse's mouth before intubation.

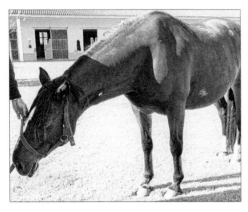

Figure 11-4. A horse that is deeply sedated and can be induced to anesthesia. Note the lowered head and 'droopy' ears and lower lip.

- If adequate sedation does not occur, administer more alpha-2 agonist and wait another 5 to 10 minutes.
- If sedation is still inadequate, insure that the dose is correct, that the correct drug is being administered and that the injection is delivered IV. Try one more dose and include the butorphanol if it was not previously included.
- If adequate sedation does not occur, do not induce the horse as dangerous ataxia and excitation can occur. It is better to come back another day, reduce distractions for the horse (like other horses, noise) and try again for sedation.

CRITICAL TIP!
DO NOT induce the horse unless it is adequately sedated.

2. Once the horse is adequately sedated, administer the induction drug +/- benzodi-azepine or guaifenesin and +/- butorphanol
3. Step to the head of the horse.
4. Control the head at induction so that the horse falls as smoothly as possible.
- The method of head control will generally depend on the location of induction (field vs hospital). In the field, anesthesia personnel will control the head by gently pulling on and lifting the halter rope to steady the horse's head **(Figure 11-5)**. In the hospital, anesthesia personnel may elevate the horse's head by placing the halter rope through a strong metal ring placed high in the wall.
- Be careful to keep fingers from being caught in the halter and keep far enough in front of the horse so that the legs of the person on the head do not become entangled with the horse's forelegs.
- Keep the horse's head elevated as much as possible so that the horse falls backward on its hindquarters rather than forward on its head.
5. Once the horse is down (or 'recumbent'), the vital signs (heart rate, respiratory rate, mucous membrane color, capillary refill time) should be quickly checked.
6. For horses in the field, immediately after vital signs are assessed, check positioning to make sure that the horse is not laying on any objects, pull the 'down' leg forward, place a towel over the eyes and use the towel to pad any areas where the halter is touching the head. Alternatively, the halter can be removed but we

recommend leaving it in place just in case the horse unexpectedly moves, in which case immediate control of the head would be necessary.

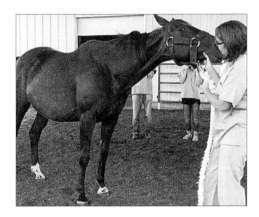

Figure 11-5. Supporting the head for field anesthesia.

CRITICAL TIP!
Pull the 'down' foreleg (the foreleg that the horse is laying on) forward to take the weight off of the radial nerve (Figure 11-6). Make sure that the 'down' eye is closed and insure that the halter is not pressing on the facial nerve.

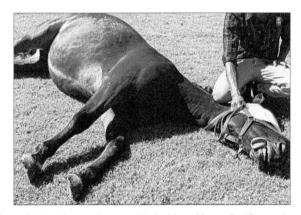

Figure 11-6. Horse in lateral recumbency with the 'down' leg pulled forward and a towel covering the eye and padding the halter.

7. For horses anesthetized in-hospital, positioning will be important when the horse is moved into the operating room but is not critical for the short duration that the patient will be in the induction stall. The horse should now be intubated. Intubation is blind in the horse (meaning you can't see the endotracheal tube enter the airway) but, as in other species, the tube will be placed between the arytenoid cartilages ('vocal cords') into the trachea
  • Place a 'gag' in the horse's mouth to hold it open **(Figure 11-7)**. Choose the appropriate sized endotracheal tube **(Table 11-1)**.

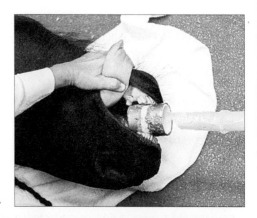

Figure 11-7. A mouth gag is placed between the horse's teeth to facilitate placement of the endotracheal tube through the mouth and into the trachea.

Table 11-1
Endotracheal Tube Size for Horses of Different Body Size. The Designation 'id' is for Internal Diameter.

HORSE SIZE	TUBE SIZE
Adult draft horses and large warmbloods	30 mm id
Most adult horses	24 to 26 mm id
Small adult horses	20 to 24 mm id
Ponies (depends on size of pony)	14 to 20 mm id
Foals (depends on size of foal)	10 to 14 mm id

TIP
Horses that weigh roughly 500 kg can generally be intubated with a 26 mm id tube.

• Extend the head and neck straight out as far as possible - this creates a straight path for the tube to go through the mouth and enter the trachea. A flexed head and neck will increase the likelihood that the tube will enter the esophagus instead of the trachea.

• Gently insert the endotracheal tube through the mouth gag and the mouth, being careful not to tear the tube's cuff on the horses' teeth.

• Once past the slight resistance that will occur at the base of the tongue, the next resistance will be the arytenoids.

• Don't force the tube through the arytenoids. Instead, very gently 'bump' the arytenoids with the tube and try to stimulate them to open.

   • If the tube doesn't slide easily (meaning that the arytenoids did not open), pull the tube back 4-6 inches, rotate it 90 degrees (this is to change the position of the bevel on the end of the tube - it may pass more easily in a different position), reinsert the tube and gently bump the arytenoids again.

- Keep repeating this process until the tube slides easily into the trachea. If the tube does not slide easily, it is likely in the esophagus.
- If the tube doesn't slide into the trachea within 6 to 8 tries, consider trying a smaller tube.

IMPORTANT POINT
Don't try to force the tube between the arytenoids. The tube will most likely slide into the esophagus instead and may cause trauma to the arytenoids.

TIP
If the horse is known to have upper airway dysfunction or if the tube continues to meet resistance even with the head/neck extended and the proper sized-tube selected, consider using an endoscope to visualize the arytenoids and to guide the tube into the trachea.

Anesthesia Maintenance

Anesthesia can be maintained with either injectable or inhalant drugs. This phase of anesthesia should include provision of analgesia and physiologic monitoring/support.

Injectable Anesthesia
- The original induction dose of alpha-2 agonist + ketamine is generally adequate for maintenance for short field procedures like castrations.
- For procedures that will take slightly longer, inject ¼ to ½ of the original dose of both the alpha-2 agonist and the ketamine if the horse is inadequately anesthetized. This can be safely repeated two times.
- If the surgery is predicted to last > 30 minutes, consider **'triple-drip' (Table 11-5)**.
  - 'Triple drip' is a combination of 1000mg ketamine and 500 mg of xylazine in 1-L of guaifenesin. This is the most common combination but other combinations are also used.
  - The triple drip should be administered 'to effect'. The delivery rate is roughly 2 ml/kg/hr. This equates to 2 drops/second for a 250 kg (550 lb) or 4 drops/second for a 450 kg (1000 lb) horse when a 15 drop/ml infusion set is used. Boluses (100 to 300 ml delivered rapidly) of the combination can be used if the horse is not adequately anesthetized.
  - Total anesthesia time should be kept to < 60 minutes since monitoring and support of the anesthetized patient is difficult in the field and complications are more likely to occur as the duration of recumbency increases.

Inhalant Anesthesia
- The horse should be carefully positioned on a thick pad with the weight distributed evenly across the dependent ('down') muscle masses. Proper positioning is critical for the prevention of myopathy and neuropathy **(Figure 11-8)**.

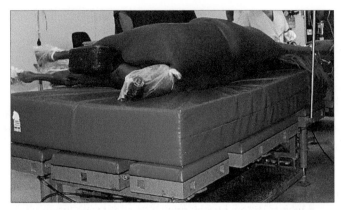

Figure 11-8. A horse anesthetized in-hospital should be placed on a very thick pad with the weight of the horse evenly distributed over the muscle masses that are in contact with the table. For this horse in lateral recumbency, that primarily means the shoulders and the lateral thigh/hip. For horses in dorsal recumbency, weight should be evenly distributed on both gluteals ('rump' muscles).

Important Definition
Myopathy is pathology or damage to the muscles and neuropathy is pathology or damage to the nerves. Improper positioning and hypotension are major contributors to myopathy and neuropathy in anesthetized horses. These conditions can result in severe pain and impairment or loss of function of the affected limb.

• The horse should be intubated and maintained with sevoflurane or isoflurane delivered in oxygen.
  • The MAC of sevoflurane in the horse is 2.3 and the MAC of isoflurane is 1.3. Surgical anesthesia usually occurs at approximately 1.5 x MAC.

Reminder
'MAC' is the 'Minimum Alveolar Concentration required to keep patients asleep. It is basically the 'dose' of the inhalant anesthetic.

• Eye lubricant must be applied to both eyes and a towel may need to be placed around the 'down' eye to prevent scrub solution, sweat, etc., from contacting the eye.
• A catheter should be placed in the facial or metatarsal artery **(Figure 11-9)** for measurement of arterial blood pressure, ECG leads should be placed on the thorax and a SpO_2 probe should be placed on the tongue.
• IV fluids should be started at 5 to 20 ml/kg/hr depending on the patient's needs.
• Intermittent positive pressure ventilation (IPPV) is necessary for most horses anesthetized with inhalant anesthetics. IPPV is most effective at maintaining normal gas exchange if started as soon after induction as possible.

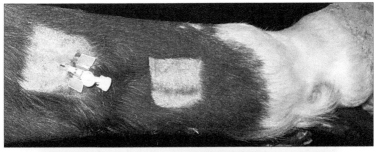

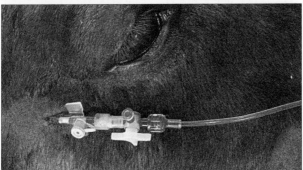

Figure 11-9. Arteries that can be catheterized in the horse include the metatarsal *(top)* and the transverse facial *(bottom)*.

Intraoperative Analgesia

(See Chapter 7)

Maintenance of anesthesia is much easier and safer if analgesia is provided prior to the painful stimulus. Most anesthetic drugs, including the anesthetic gases, block the brain's response to pain but don't actually block pain itself. If the pain is severe enough, the brain can still respond and make the animal appear to be inadequately anesthetized. The result is often that the vaporizer is turned up and the brain ceases to respond, but the patient is now too deeply anesthetized and can be at a very dangerous physiologic plane since the adverse effects of inhalants are dose-dependent. A more appropriate response is to decrease the pain with analgesic drugs and maintain anesthesia at a light, safe depth.

Opioids

Specific drugs

Butorphanol (agonist-antagonist), and buprenorphine (partial agonist) provide mild to moderate analgesia. Buprenorphine provides longer-duration analgesia than the other opioids. Morphine, hydromorphone, methadone and fentanyl (full agonists) provide profound analgesia. Tramadol efficacy is questionable.

Advantages

Provide mild to profound analgesia for surgical, medical, trauma and chronic pain. Opioids have a high safety margin, their effects are reversible, many are inexpensive and all are versatile (can be administered PO, IM, IV, SQ, in the epidural space, in the intra-articular space).

Disadvantages

Opioids can cause excitement in horses and the fear of excitement has limited the use of opioids in this species. However, excitement is common in non-painful, healthy horses, which is the group of horses in which most of the research is done, but very uncommon in painful horses, which is the group of horses that need opioids (Clutton 2010). Slowed GI motility is also a concern but this effect is also less likely to occur in painful horses and, in general, is unlikely to have a clinical impact when it does occur (Sellon et al. 2004; Andersen et al. 2006; Love et al. 2006). Pain also causes slowed GI motility.

Clinical Use

Butorphanol is the most commonly used opioid in horses but morphine use is increasing. Morphine is more potent, has a longer duration of action and is a lot cheaper than butorphanol. The duration of morphine (roughly 4 hours) makes it very appropriate for in-hospital surgeries but may be too long for field procedures (could lead to excitement in recovery). Buprenorphine is expensive for use in adult horses but has been used in foals. Butorphanol, morphine or fentanyl constant rate infusions (CRIs) are commonly used during in-hospital procedures and butorphanol is used in conjunction with alpha-2 agonists for standing procedures and as a CRI for postoperative pain. Fentanyl patches have also been used in both adult horses and foals.

Local Anesthetic Drugs

Specific Drugs

Lidocaine provides approximately 1.5 hours, mepivacaine (Carbocaine®) provides 2-3 hours and bupivacaine provides roughly 4 hours of analgesia. Liposome-encapsulated bupivacaine (NOCITA®) provides 72 hours of analgesia.

Advantages

Local anesthetics are inexpensive, easy to administer and very effective. They decrease the response to painful stimulus AND decrease the overall sensation of pain even beyond the expected duration of the local anesthetic drug. Local anesthetics should be included in every painful procedure if possible (See Chapter 7).

Disadvantages

Almost none if dosed correctly, which is true of all drugs.

Clinical Use

There is a long list of local anesthetic blocks that can be used in horses including: incisional or wound blocks, testicular blocks, ophthalmic blocks, dental/oral blocks, epidurals, a large number of blocks on the legs, etc. The blocks on the legs are often used for lameness diagnosis and should also be used to prevent/ treat surgical pain. Lidocaine is also commonly used as a constant rate infusion, especially in horses with colic.

> **NOTE**
> USE LOCAL ANESTHETIC DRUGS! They are cheap, easy and very effective.

Alpha-2 Adrenergic Agonists

Specific Drugs

Xylazine, detomidine and romifidine are commonly used in horses. Medetomidine and dexmedetomidine are occasionally used for analgesia.

Advantages

Alpha-2 agonists provide dose-dependent analgesia and sedation. The effects of the drugs are reversible although reversal is rarely used in horses unless an adverse reaction occurs. Reversing sedatives in an excitable or nervous horse can lead to a horse that is even more excited or nervous and potentially hard to control.

Disadvantages

Alpha-2 agonists cause vasoconstriction which increases cardiac work. This can be detrimental to patients with cardiovascular compromise, but this is an uncommon occurrence in horses and horses with cardiovascular disease are rarely anesthetized.

Clinical Use

Xylazine, detomidine and romifidine are used for sedation/analgesia prior to painful procedures and can be used as low-dose boluses or CRIs to maintain sedation/ analgesia during the procedure. This is common for standing procedures but should also be considered for horses receiving inhalant anesthesia if an appropriate plane of anesthesia is difficult to maintain. Medetomidine and dexmedetomidine are expensive for use in adult horses and are not used routinely. However, they provide more profound analgesia than the other alpha-2 agonists and are occasionally used as a CRI during surgery.

Ketamine (NMDA Receptor Antagonist)

Ketamine is commonly used as an anesthesia induction drug but can also be used for pain management when administered as a sub-anesthetic dose CRI. Ketamine antagonizes the receptors (the N-methyl-D-aspartate or 'NMDA' receptors) in the spinal cord that are partly responsible for central sensitization (also called 'wind-up'). Central sensitization should be prevented or treated if at all possible because it results in an amplification of the pain signal so the patient experiences more intense pain. Pain from central sensitization is very difficult to treat (see Chapter 7).

Advantages
Used to prevent or treat central sensitization; inexpensive.

Disadvantages
None at the CRI dose.

Clinical Use
Induction to anesthesia, CRI during surgery. Ketamine CRIs should also be considered for treatment of laminitis pain and other chronic pain conditions.

Monitoring and Support: General Comments
Diligent monitoring of anesthetized patients is critical for prevention of anesthesia-related morbidity and mortality. Anesthesia can cause adverse effects in all organ systems and the degree of these effects is based on the type of drug chosen, the health of the patient, and the invasiveness and duration of the surgical procedure. Adverse effects in the central nervous system (CNS), cardiovascular and respiratory systems are the most immediately life threatening so monitoring is focused on these systems.

Monitoring for Field Anesthesia
Monitoring is generally done by watching the horse breathing and noting bleeding at the surgery site. If surgery is prolonged, consider taking a pulse oximeter and Doppler along. These are particularly useful when anesthetizing foals in the field but generally aren't necessary for most routine field surgery in adult horses. The CNS should be at least briefly checked as described below for in-hospital anesthesia.

Monitoring for In-Hospital Anesthesia
Monitoring the Central Nervous System
There are no advanced monitoring techniques for the CNS so one of the most important systems in the body must be monitored by using routine, but extremely important, techniques such as assessment of palpebral reflex, eye position and response to surgery/pain.

> **TIP**
> The presence of nystagmus (eye movement) in anesthetized horses is a fairly accurate indicator of an excessively light plane of anesthesia (commonly seen in horses at induction and recovery). If the horse is exhibiting nystagmus, anticipate that it might be about to move! Increase the inhalant concentration or administer a bolus of ketamine and/or an alpha-2 agonist.

TIP

Lacrimation (or 'tearing') may indicate a light surgical plane of anesthesia in horses, although this is not consistent.

Monitoring the Cardiovascular System

(See Chapter 5)

Most anesthetic drugs cause some degree of cardiovascular compromise. Basic monitoring techniques should be combined with advanced techniques for effective monitoring.

Basic Monitoring Techniques

These include assessment of mucous membrane color (pink vs pale), capillary refill time, pulse strength and heart rate (Table 11-2).

Table 11-2
Normal Values For Physiologic Parameters In Anesthetized Horses

Physiologic Parameter	Expected normal value
Eye Position & Responses	Centered, light or absent palpebral reflex, no nystagmus
Heart Rate	28-45 beats/min in adult horses; 40-60 in ponies; 60-80 in foals, maybe lower in juvenile foals
Mucous Membrane Color	Pink, horses may have a slight yellow tint
Capillary Refill Time	< 2 seconds
Systolic Arterial Blood Pressure	Maintain at > 90 mmHg all horses
Mean Arterial Blood Pressure	Maintain at > 70 mmHg adult horses; > 60 mmHg ponies and foals
Diastolic Arterial Blood Pressure	Maintain at > 40 mmHg all horses
Respiratory Rate	Based on body size, 5-10 breaths/min in adult horses and 10 to 15 breaths/min in ponies and foals
Tidal Volume	10 to 15 ml/kg
Oxygen-hemoglobin saturation (pulse oximeter; SpO_2)	>95%
End-tidal CO_2	35-45 cmH$_2$0, up to 55 cmH$_2$0 acceptable
Arterial blood gas: PaO_2	200 to 500 mmHg on 100% oxygen
Arterial blood gas: $PaCO_2$	35-45 cmH$_2$0, up to 55 cmH$_2$0 acceptable
Arterial blood gas: pH	7.3- 7.4

Advanced Monitoring Techniques

These include measurement of blood pressure and assessment of the electrocardiogram (ECG).

Blood Pressure Measurement: This should be the gold standard of monitoring in all practices that utilize inhalant anesthesia in horses. Blood pressure measurement is not necessary for brief, field anesthesia in healthy horses. Hypotension in the anesthetized horse is defined as a MAP < 70 mmHg. This is higher than the minimal MAP recommended in small animals because the sheer weight of the horse causes collapse of the vessels supplying blood to the muscles, potentially causing myopathies. There is evidence that a mean arterial blood pressure of 70 mmHg or greater helps to prevent this collapse. In ponies, foals, and miniature horses, a mean arterial pressure of 60mmHg or greater (like in small animals) is probably adequate. Systolic arterial blood pressure should be >90 and diastolic arterial blood pressure > 40 mmHg in all horses (See Table 11-2).

• Direct measurement of blood pressure by placement of a catheter in an artery should be required for all adult large animals undergoing inhalant anesthesia. Catheters can be placed in the metatarsal artery or in various branches of the facial artery (See Figure 11-9).

• Indirect measurement using an inflatable cuff over the artery at the base of the tail or on a limb is appropriate for foals, small ponies and for very short procedures in adult large animals. Either the Doppler, which uses amplification of the sound of blood flow through the arteries, or the oscillometric unit, which uses detection of oscillations caused by changes in blood flow, can be used.

ECG: The ECG should be evaluated throughout the procedure. In horses, a 'biphasic' (two peaks) P wave and an inverted (upside down) QRS complex are normal **(Figure 11-10)**.

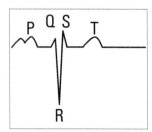

Figure 11-10. In horses, a 'biphasic' (two peaks) P wave and an inverted (upside down) QRS complex are normal.

Supporting the Cardiovascular System

(See Chapter 6)

HORSES ARE EXTREMELY PRONE TO HYPOTENSION-INDUCED MYOPATHIES AND NEUROPATHIES and hypotensive patients must be treated. To support blood pressure:

• Turn the inhalant gas to the lowest effective dose (turn the vaporizer down). The addition of analgesia to the protocol (opioid boluses or local anesthetic blockade) will allow a lower inhalant dose.

- Increase the rate of administration of IV fluids.
- Administer colloids or hypertonic fluid if necessary.
- Utilize positive inotropic drugs, which increase myocardial contractility, like dopamine or dobutamine. Dosages are in Table 11-5. Horses anesthetized with inhalant anesthetics are very likely to need positive inotropic drugs for blood pressure support.

Monitoring the Respiratory System
(See Chapter 5)
Most anesthetic drugs cause some degree of respiratory compromise. Basic monitoring techniques should be combined with advanced techniques for effective monitoring.

Basic Respiratory Monitoring Techniques
These include respiratory rate, tidal volume (watch thoracic excursions and movement of the rebreathing bag carefully) and mucous membrane color (pink vs blue). The normal respiratory rate in anesthetized patients should be based on body size. Guidelines are 5 to 10 breaths/min in adult horses and 10 to 15 breaths/min in ponies and foals. Tidal volume should be approximately 10 to 15 ml/kg body weight (See Table 11-2).

Advanced Respiratory System Monitoring Techniques
These include measurement of oxygen-hemoglobin saturation and end-tidal carbon dioxide as well as assessment of arterial blood gases (See Table 11-2).

Measurement of Oxygen-Hemoglobin Saturation: The pulse oximeter (SpO_2) is a good basic monitor because it provides some information regarding both the respiratory and cardiovascular systems. However, because of the shape of the oxygen-hemoglobin dissociation curve (see Chapter 5), this is NOT a true respiratory monitor - especially in patients on 100% oxygen. A normal saturation in anesthetized patients on 100% oxygen is 98-100%.

Measurement of End-Tidal Carbon Dioxide ($ETCO_2$): This is a true respiratory monitor because it measures carbon dioxide. Normal $ETCO_2$ in anesthetized patients is 35 to 45 mmHg but up to 55 mmHg is acceptable in horses in which ventilation is difficult (e.g., colic horses with distended abdomen). Horses commonly develop ventilation/perfusion (V/Q) mismatch under anesthesia, which means that some alveoli are ventilated and some are perfused but that both ventilation/perfusion may not occur (are not 'matched') at all alveoli. This will adversely affect the accuracy of the $ETCO_2$ monitor and arterial blood gases will need to be assessed.

Measurement of Arterial Blood Gases: This is the ideal method for assessing respiratory function and should be utilized in all large animals anesthetized with inhalant anesthetics. It is not practical or necessary for brief periods of field anesthesia (no inhalants) in healthy horses. Normal values for anesthetized patients are a $PaCO_2$ of 35 to 55 mmHg, PaO_2 of 200 to 500 mmHg (ideal is 5 x the percent of O_2 in inspired air) and a pH of 7.3 to 7.4.

Supporting the Respiratory System
(See Chapter 6)

Horses frequently require positive pressure ventilator support during anesthesia. Ventilation/perfusion (V/Q) mismatch is common in anesthetized horses (**Table 11-3**), and both anesthetic drugs and surgical positioning contribute to impaired ventilation and perfusion. Horses in dorsal recumbency have greater respiratory impairment than horses in lateral recumbency. Once V/Q mismatch occurs, adequate ventilation may be difficult, thus initiating ventilation immediately following induction should be considered.

Table 11-3
Tips on Using Positive Pressure Ventilation in Horses

- Ventilator settings are generally 6 to 10 breaths/min, 10 to 15 ml/kg tidal volume with 20 to 30 cmH_2O peak inspiratory pressure (PIP) and an I:E (inspired to expired) ratio of no less than 1:3.
  - NOTE: The I:E (inspired:expired) ratio determines how much time is spent in inspiration and how much time is spent in expiration. Adequate expiratory time is necessary to reduce the time of positive pressure in the thorax and allow normal venous return. Some ventilators have a fixed I:E ratio (Drager ventilators), making extreme changes in respiratory rate more difficult, while some ventilators have an infinite I:E ratio (the Mallard Medical and Hallowell ventilators) allowing greater control over respiratory rate.
- Patients with abdominal distension are better ventilated with a faster rate and lower PIP.
- Positive end-expiratory pressure (PEEP) allows the alveoli to stay slightly inflated during exhalation and decreases the incidence of atelectasis. A low PEEP (5 to 10 cm H_2O) is generally effective. A PEEP higher than this may cause decreased cardiac filling due to prolonged positive pressure in the thorax.
- Initiation of positive pressure ventilation often causes a decrease in cardiac return and a decrease in cardiac output and arterial blood pressure. This is caused by compression of the vena cavae. The compromise is worse when patients are hypovolemic so rapid volume expansion is necessary. Cardiac support with positive inotropes may also be required.

Recovery from Anesthesia: Step by Step

Now comes the tough part! Recovery is the most critical phase of anesthesia for horses. Horses tend to get excited and have rough recoveries. Some tips for a smooth recovery include:

1. Use sedative/analgesic drugs to keep the horse calm and comfortable. Anesthetic procedures in the field are extremely short and the alpha-2 agonist/opioid administered at premedication/induction is usually sufficient to provide sedation and analgesia in recovery. Conversely, horses that have been anesthetized with inhalants for longer procedures very commonly need a dose of an alpha-2 agonist, and

sometimes an opioid, to facilitate a comfortable, calm recovery. Horses that were really excited prior to anesthesia will wake up the same way so those horses will definitely need a dose of an alpha-2 agonist in recovery after inhalant anesthesia.

2. For horses recovering from inhalant anesthesia provide respiratory support (keep intubated until the patient swallows, provide oxygen) as necessary.

3. In-hospital keep the patient on a padded floor or mat. In the field keep the patient on soft dirt or grass.

4. In-hospital keep the recovery stall lights dim and sound to a minimum. In the field keep the eyes covered with a towel and try to minimize stimulus (noise from tractors, other horses, etc.).

5. In-hospital the horse can either be left to quietly recover on its own or can be assisted with ropes placed on the head and the tail **(Figure 11-11)**. In the field (all horses) and in the hospital (horses trying to stand up before they have totally regained consciousness) keep the horse from standing too soon by holding its head down **(Figure 11-12)**, then support the head as it stands.

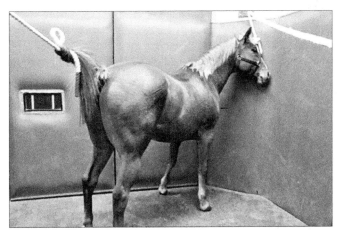

Figure 11-11. Horses recovering from inhalant anesthesia are often assisted to a standing position with ropes placed on the head and the tail.

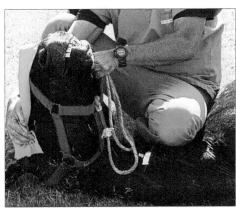

Figure 11-12. Horses that try to stand immediately after the end of anesthesia are often dangerously ataxic and may even fall. If the horse is attempting to stand before it appears to be ready, it should be held down by placing the handler's weight at the top of the horse's neck and pulling the horse's nose up in the air.

How to Anesthetize a Horse: Quick Tips for Horse Inhalant Anesthesia from a Fellow LVT

Shelley Ensign, LVT, CVPP

The examples below are for an average sized-horse of 1129 lbs (513 Kgs).

Premedication

- **Xylazine** — 1 mg/kg (0.5 mg/lb) will be administered IV right before induction
  - Quick Calculation: Take the horse's weight in kg, divide in half (or take the weight in lbs and divide by 4.2 - in most cases 4.0 will be fine) and round up to the nearest 50 mg increment. That number is the number of mgs of xylazine to start with.
    - **Example: 513 kg horse divided by 2 = 265, round up to 300 mg of xylazine. In lbs, an 1129 lb horse divided by 4 = 282, again, round up to 300.** THAT'S THE MINIMUM depending on: 1) How much drug the horse has already received, AND 2) the level of sedation required.
    - Increase xylazine using 50 mg to 100 mgs boluses as needed to achieve adequate sedation.
- Walk the horse into the induction stall and administer butorphanol 0.01-0.022 mg/kg IV.
  - Quick Calculation: For horses from 409-513 kg (900-1000 lbs) administer 10 mg of butorphanol.
    - Calculate the dose (rather than automatically administering 10 mg) for small horses, ponies or miniatures.
  - For all horses, you can re-dose every 45 minutes as needed for intraoperative pain.

Table 11-4
Pharmacology of Equine-Specific Anesthetic Drugs

Alpha-2 agonists used in horses include xylazine, detomidine and romifidine (See Chapter 4 for xylazine and for general alpha-2 information).

- **Detomidine Hydrochloride**
  - **Alpha-2: Alpha-1 binding:** 260:1
  - **FDA approval:** Horses only
  - **Species:** Primarily horses but can be used in other large animals
  - **Routes of administration:** IV, IM, epidurally
  - **Dose:** 0.05 to 0.04 mg/kg (generally low end of dose for premedication)
  - **Onset of action:** 2 to 4 minutes IV; 3 to 5 minutes (up to 10 minutes) IM
  - **Duration of action:** 60 to 120 minutes depending on dose
  - **KEY POINTS**
    - **Very potent, commonly used for preoperative sedation in more difficult to manage horses and used for standing sedation as a bolus or infusion.**

Table 11-4 continued

- **Romifidine**
  - **Alpha-2: Alpha-1 binding:** 340:1
  - **FDA approval:** Horses only
  - **Species:** Primarily horses but can be used in other large animals
  - **Routes of administration:** IV, IM
  - **Dose:** 0.04-0.12 mg/kg
  - **Onset of action:** 2 to 4 minutes IV; 3 to 5 minutes (up to 10 minutes) IM
  - Duration of action: 60 to 120 minutes depending on dose
  - **KEY POINTS**
    - **May cause less ataxia than other alpha-2 agonists.**

Muscle relaxants commonly used in horses include the benzodiazepines (See Chapter 4) and guaifenesin guaiacolate.
- **Guaifenesin guaiacolate**
  - **Classification:** Central muscle relaxant
  - **DEA Class:** Not controlled
  - **FDA approval:** Horses only
  - **Routes of administration:** IV
  - **Dose:** Dose 'to effect' (muscle relaxation), usually 75 to 150 mg/kg
  - **Onset of action:** 2 to 4 minutes
  - **Duration of action:** Muscle relaxation for 15 to 25 minutes
  - **Clinical use:** Primarily horses and other large animals for muscle relaxation as part of induction and as a carrier for injectable drugs for maintenance of anesthesia, like in 'triple drip' (guaifenesin, ketamine and xylazine).
  - **Metabolism/Clearance:** Hepatic
  - **Reversal drugs:** None
  - **Effects:** Muscle relaxation
  - **Adverse Effects:** Causes ataxia (because of the muscle relaxation) in the standing horse.
  - **Precautions:** Be prepared for ataxia.
  - **Absolute contraindications:** None, but not ideal for horses that cannot be easily controlled during induction or recovery.
  - **KEY POINTS**
  - **Administered 'to effect' and the desired effect is muscle relaxation, which will be recognized as slight ataxia. Once the horse is relaxed (1 to 4 minutes after beginning administration), administer the bolus of induction drug.**
  - **Guaifenesin usually comes as a concentrated solution. It should be diluted to a 5% solution. More concentrated solutions can cause hemolysis and local irritation with potential thrombus formation at the site of injection.**
  - **ADMINISTER THROUGH A CATHETER. Extravascular guaifenesin can cause tissue reaction.**

Induction

- Induction begins after the horse's lips and ears are droopy
- **Ketamine** — 2 mg/kg (1 mg/lb) IV
  - Quick Calculation: Take the horse's weight in pounds and round up to the nearest 100. Administer 100mg of ketamine for every 100 lbs of horse.
    - **Example: 1129 lb horse gets 1200 mgs of Ketamine (100 mg/ml). For kgs, multiply by 2.2, so a 513 kg horse x 2.2 = 1129. Thus the dose is again 1200 mg.**
- **Diazepam or midazolam** — 0.1 mg/kg IV combined with the ketamine
  - Quick Calculation: Administer 2 mls less of the diazepam or midazolam than ketamine
  - **Example: If a horse receives 12 mls of ketamine, it would receive 10 mls of diazepam or midazolam (5 mgs/ml)**
- Mix the ketamine with the diazepam or midazolam and give as a rapid bolus IV.
- Once the horse falls, place a mouth gag between the incisors, extend the neck and pull the tongue to the side for intubation. If resistance occurs when passing the endotracheal tube, pull the tube back 4-6 inches and rotate the tube ¼ turn, repeat until the tube passes smoothly into the trachea.
  - **Endotracheal Tube Sizes:** Most horses between 900-1500 lb (409-682 kg) will need a 26 id tube, but a 24 id tube should be ready in case the 26 doesn't fit. Pressure check the tube cuffs and place the adapter that connects the tube to the breathing system on the end of the tube before anesthetizing the horse.
  - Tape around the end of the tube and then around the nose to secure the tube.
- Lubricate the eyes.

Maintenance

- Start the isoflurane or sevoflurane. Isoflurane is most commonly used.
- Lidocaine CRIs are generally started if the patient is painful (e.g., horses with colic) as soon as possible.
  - Start with a bolus of 1 mg/kg (0.5 mg/lb) of lidocaine administered over 10 minutes, then start CRI at 25 mcg/kg/min.
    - **Bolus Example: 513 kg horse times 1 mg/kg dose divided by 20 mg/ml lidocaine concentration = 25 mls of lidocaine.**
  - The lidocaine dose can be increased as needed up to 50 mcg/kg/min.
  - Lidocaine provides analgesia and lowers MAC requirements. Keeping inhalant dose as low as possible helps maintain normal blood pressure.
  - Lidocaine also supports normal GI motility, which is especially useful in patients with colic.
- Check the blood pressure. If the mean arterial blood pressure is < 70 mmHg start a dobutamine drip 'to effect'. To make/deliver the drip:
  - Add 62.5 mg dobutamine to a 250 ml bag of saline. This is 5 ml of the standard 12.5 mg/ml solution.
  - Start with 1 drop every other second using a 60 drop/ml drip set.
  - Increase to 2 drops per second or as needed to increase blood pressure.
  - Other drugs used to treat hypotension:

- Calcium chloride (100 mg/ml) 500 mg total dose over 3 minutes, followed by another 500 mgs 10 minutes later if needed.
- Vetstarch: Administer up to 20 ml/kg (or more depending on patient needs).
- Crystalloid fluids: LRS can be delivered as rapidly as possible. One liter of hypertonic saline can be administered if not administered prior to anesthesia.
- If hypertension (> 95 mmHg mean blood pressure) occurs, increase the inhalant dose if the patient is light. Increase the lidocaine CRI and redose butorphanol or give a dose of a more potent opioid (eg, morphine) if the patient is painful.

- **Ventilation**
  - Most horses receiving inhalant anesthesia will need mechanical ventilation.
  - Start with 20 cm of water inspiratory pressure (measured by the pressure manometer) and 4 liters in the ventilator bellows.
  - Check an arterial blood gas to assess the adequacy of ventilation.
    - Ideal PaO_2 is above 300 mmHg oxygen and $PaCO_2$ between 40-50.
  - If oxygen is lower than 100 mmHg, administer 10 puffs of albuterol into the endotracheal tube.
  - If CO_2 is high increase ventilation if possible. The starting point is usually 7 breaths per minute at 1:3.5 I:E ratio (See definition in Chapter 3). Sometimes the only thing that will improve ventilation is opening the abdomen to relieve pressure on the diaphragm so the horse can breathe.

Recovery

- Oxygenate for at least 5 minutes in the recovery stall. If the horse is not breathing on its own give 1 breath every minute with a demand valve until the horse starts breathing.
- Stuff cotton in both ears and place a towel over the eyes to keep the environment quiet and dark.
- Squeeze phenylephrine nasal spray 2 times in each nostril to decrease nasal edema. The phenylephrine spray is the over-the-counter spray used in humans.
- Administer xylazine 100 mg or 10 mgs of romifidine IV.
  - Not typically administered to foals or sick horses.
- Extubate when the horse swallows or is breathing normally. A good sign that the horse is ready for extubation is when it takes one big breath followed quickly by 1 or 2 small breaths.
- If breathing isn't adequate, place an 11 or 12 id endotracheal tube in one nostril and tape it in place. Leave as long as needed to keep the nostril open.

Table 11-5
Drugs Used for, or in Conjunction with, Equine Anesthesia

DRUG CLASS	Dose (mg/ kg unless stated)	Route	Dosing Interval	Comments
ALPHA-2 AGONISTS				**Used for sedation and analgesia.** For all alpha-2 agonists, use low end of dose for light sedation and high end of dose for deeper sedation. High end of dose is generally necessary for induction to anesthesia in patients that will be maintained on injectable anesthesia.
Detomidine	0.005-0.04 0.02-0.04 0.06	IV IM PO	q2-4hr	Approved as a sedative / analgesic in US.
	0.15-0.3 µg/kg/min	IV	CRI	Loading dose 6 to 10 µg/kg; adjust CRI to achieve desired sedation.
Romifidine	0.04-0.120	IM, IV	q2-4hr	Approved as sedative / analgesic and as a preanesthetic in US.
Xylazine	0.25-1.0 1.0-2.2	IV IM	q2-4hr	Approved as a sedative / analgesic in US.
	0.17	Epidural		Generally added to lidocaine.
Medetomidine	0.005-0.007	IV	q2-4hr	More commonly used in small animals for sedation and in horses only for analgesia.
	3-5 µg/kg/hr	IV	CRI	Used as a CRI for analgesia. Loading dose 5 µg/kg.
Dexmedetomidine	1-4 µg/kg/hr	IV	CRI	Used as a CRI for analgesia in horses. Loading dose 1-2 µg/kg.
INDUCTION DRUGS				
Ketamine-		IV	Once	Most commonly used equine induction drug.

Diazepam or Midazolam	0.1	IV	Once	Used with ketamine for muscle relaxation.
Guaifenesin	To effect, usually 75-150	IV	Once	Muscle relaxant used for induction & maintenance.
MAINTENANCE				
'Triple drip' Guaifenesin, ketamine, alpha-2 agonist	Most common: Add 1000 mg ketamine & 500 mg xylazine to 1 liter of 50 mg/ml guaifenesin	IV	As needed to maintain anesthesia	Administer at an average of 2 ml/kg/hr, which is roughly 2 drops/second for a 250 kg (550 lb) or 4 drops/second for a 450 kg (1000 lb) horse when a 15 drop/ml infusion set is used. Bolus 100-300 mls if the horse gets light.
Isoflurane	1-3%	Inhaled	As needed to maintain anesthesia	Causes dose-dependent cardiovascular and respiratory depression. Keep dosages as low as possible.
Sevoflurane	2-4%	Inhaled	As needed to maintain anesthesia	Causes dose-dependent cardiovascular and respiratory depression. Keep dosages as low as possible.
OPIOIDS				
Morphine	0.05-0.1 / 0.1-0.3	IV / IM	q3-4hr	Used for analgesia
				Inject slowly if administered IV. Horses may have excitatory response so administer sedative first.
	0.1-0.2	Epidural	Q12-24hr	qs to 10 to 30 mls with sterile saline.
	0.1	Intra-articular	Once, intra-op	qs to 5 to 10 mls with sterile saline or local anesthetic.
	0.1 mg/kg/hr	IV	CRI	Loading dose 0.15 mg/kg IV.

Table 11-5 continued

Methadone	0.05-0.1	IM, IV	q3-4hr	Loading dose 0.15 mg/kg IV.
Fentanyl	0.1 mg/kg/hr	IV	CRI	Does not seem to cause excitement so administration of concurrent sedation is not generally necessary.
	2 of the 100 microg patches/450 kg	Trans-dermal	Change patches at 48 hours	
Butorphanol	0.02-0.1	IM, IV	q2-3hr	Approved for the relief of pain (in some countries).
	23.7 µg/kg/ min (0.013 mg/kg/hr)	IV	CRI	Loading dose 0.02 mg/kg.
Buprenorphine	0.01-0.03 (up to 0.06)	IV, IM, SQ		Moderate analgesia. Useful in foals. Currently too expensive for use in adult horses.
Tramadol	2	PO		Analgesic effects unknown. Maybe not effective.
LOCAL ANESTHETICS				
Lidocaine	4-6 mg/kg total	Tissue infiltration	Once	Blocks pain at surgery site for 1.5-2 hours.
Mepivacaine (carbocaine)	3-5 mg/kg total	Tissue infiltration	Once	Blocks pain at surgery site for 2-3 hours.
Bupivacaine or Ropivacaine	1-2 mg/kg total	Tissue infiltration	Once	Blocks pain at surgery site for 4-6 hours. NOCITA is a liposome-encapsulated bupivacaine that provides analgesia for 72 hours. See Chapter 7.
CONSTANT RATE INFUSIONS				
Lidocaine CRI	0.05 mg/kg/min	IV	CRI	Commonly used for GI pain but good for all pain.
Ketamine CRI	0.4-1.2 mg/kg/hr	IV	CRI	Prevents or treats central sensitization (or 'wind up') at the NMDA-receptors.

		IV	CRI	
Alpha-2 agonists & opioids	Various	IV	CRI	See specific drugs in the alpha-2 agonist and opioid sections.
NSAIDS				Anti-inflammatory drugs used for analgesia
Phenylbutazone	2-4	PO, IV	q12hr	Approved for use in some countries; reduce dose to 2 mg/kg on second day; used most commonly for musculoskeletal pain.
Flunixin meglumine	1	PO, IV, IM	q12hr or 24hr	Approved for use in some countries. Used most commonly for GI pain and treatment of endotoxemia.
Ketoprofen	2-3	IV	q24hr	Approved for use in some countries.
Firocoxib	0.1	PO	q24hr	Approved for use (in some countries) for up to 14 days for the control of pain and inflammation associated with equine osteo-arthritis.
Diclofenac sodium	5 inch ribbon of cream	Topical, over painful joint	q12hr	Approved for the treatment of joint pain and inflammation for up to 10 days in some countries.
Carprofen	0.7	IV	q24hr	Approved for horses in some countries (not US).
Meloxicam	0.6	IV	q12hr	Approved for horses in some countries (not US).
SUPPORT				
Dopamine	1-15 mic/kg/min	IV	CRI	Positive inotrope with alpha & beta effects.
Dobutamine	1-10 mic/kg/min	IV	CRI	Positive inotrope with primarily beta effects.
Ephedrine	0.03-0.06 mg/kg IV	IV	Once, can repeat in 45-60 mins	Alpha agonist that increases BP by causing vasoconstriction. May decrease tissue blood flow.
Hetastarch	20 ml/kg/24hr (total dose)	IV	1-2 boluses or CRI	Colloid used for increasing blood pressure. Can administer as repeat boluses of 5 ml/kg or use as a CRI.

Table 11-5 continued

Hypertonic Saline	5 ml/kg; start with 1 liter total & assess effect	IV	1-2 boluses	Increases blood pressure by pulling fluid from the tissues into the intravascular space. Must run crystalloids concurrently.
Albuterol	2-10 puffs' from the nebulizer	In airway	1-2 series of ' puffs'	Used for bronchodilation in hypoxemic horses.
Phenylephrine	2-5 'puffs' from the nebulizer	In nostrils	1-2 series of ' puffs'	Used for intranasally vasoconstriction to decrease edema in patients that have edematous nostrils post-operatively.
MISCELLANEOUS				
Gabapentin	10-40 mg/kg starting dose	PO	Q6-12hr	Used to treat pain from myopathies, neuropathies and laminitis. May need to increase the dose in patients that are severely painful.

References

Andersen MS, Clark L, Dyson SJ, Newton JR. Risk factors for colic in horses after general anaesthesia for MRI or nonabdominal surgery: absence of evidence of effect from perianaesthetic morphine. Equine Vet J. 2006;38(4):368-74.

Clutton RE. Opioid analgesia in horses. Vet Clin North Am Equine Pract. 2010;26(3):493-514.

Love EJ, Lane JG, Murison PJ. Morphine administration in horses anaesthetized for upper respiratory tract surgery. Vet Anaesth Analg. 2006; 33 (3):179-88.

Sellon DC, Roberts MC, Bilkslager AT, Ulibarri C, Papich MG. Effects of continuous rate intravenous infusion of butorphanol on physiologic and outcome variables in horses after celiotomy. J Vet Intern Med. 2004;18 (4):555-63.

Chapter 12
Anesthesia and Analgesia for Pocket Pets

Introduction

Small 'exotic' mammals or 'pocket pets' can be difficult to anesthetize, in large part because little information is available for many of these species. Because of their small body size, drug dosing can be difficult and drugs often have to be diluted prior to administration. Standard anesthesia equipment like breathing systems for inhalant gas delivery, if useful at all, may need to be adapted for the patient and monitoring equipment may not be able to accurately detect/measure physiologic parameters. Furthermore, complications like hypothermia, hypoglycemia and abnormal circulating volume (e.g., hypovolemia from dehydration or hemorrhage; volume overload from excess fluid administration) are common. All of these factors add up to a risk of anesthesia-related mortality that is much higher than the risk in dogs and cats (Brodbelt 2009) **(Table 12-1)**. This risk can be minimized with: 1) stabilization of the patient prior to anesthesia; 2) selection of appropriate anesthetic/analgesic drugs and drug dosages; and 3) continuation of monitoring and support of the patient throughout the entire perioperative period. 'Pocket pets' include rabbits, ferrets, rats, mice, gerbils, hamsters, and many other species. Not all species are covered in this chapter.

Table 12-1
Anesthesia and Sedation-Related Deaths in Small Animals
(Brodbelt 2009)

Species	Risk of anesthesia-related death
Dog	0.17%
Cat	0.24%
Rabbit	1.39%
Rat	2.01%
Chinchilla	3.29%
Hamster	3.66%
Guinea Pig	3.80%

General Comments on Drugs
Drug Dosages

For all drugs, patients with high metabolic rates (most all of the very small mammals) will require increased dosages of sedative/anesthetic/analgesic drugs when compared to dogs and cats.

Routes of Drug Administration

Subcutaneous (SQ) injection of most sedative/anesthetic/analgesic drugs is not recommended in larger species since the uptake of drugs from the SQ tissue is slow, resulting in a long delay in onset of effects and a lower serum concentration of the drug, which results in drug-induced effects that are not as profound as expected/desired. However, in many of the very small species, the muscle mass is too small to allow IM injections, thus SQ injections are necessary. In larger patients like many rabbits and ferrets, IV injections are possible and are generally preferred for induction to anesthesia since drugs can be more easily titrated 'to effect' when administered IV **(Figure 12-1)**. In some of the very smallest patients intraperitoneal (IP) injections are utilized, but rarely in clinical practice.

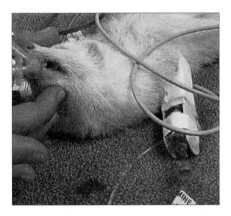

Figure 12-1. IV catheter in a ferret. Tongue depressors were used to stabilize the leg, which decreases the likelihood that the catheter will be accidentally kinked or pulled out of the vein. *(Photo courtesy of Dr. Tania Perez, WSU)*

Analgesia

Analgesia should be provided for all patients, including small mammals. These patients do feel pain and pain causes adverse effects like delayed healing, GI dysfunction (eg, slowed motility, ulceration), immune system suppression, anorexia, catabolism, insomnia, etc. Patients that receive adequate analgesia can be expected to heal faster and to have fewer stress-related (pain is the stressor) complications. Furthermore, analgesia will allow lower dosages of induction and maintenance anesthetic drugs, which improves anesthetic safety since the adverse effects from these drugs are generally DOSE DEPENDENT. Analgesia may also prevent death in some species. It is the authors' experience that anesthetic deaths in rabbits have decreased since analgesia has become a standard part of anesthetic protocols. In addition to pain prevention, pain assessment should be standard care for all patients that might experience pain. Typical signs of pain in pocket pets are listed in **Table 12-2** (Goldberg & Shaffran [2015] and Gaynor & Muir [2014]).

Analgesic Drugs

Analgesic drugs useful in small mammals include the opioids, alpha-2 agonists, local anesthetics and non-steroidal anti-inflammatory drugs. Although outside the scope of this chapter, treatment of chronic pain may include gabapentin and joint health modifiers. Dosages for analgesic drugs are presented in **Table 12-3**.

Opioids
Opioids are commonly used in small mammals and should be considered anytime that patients experience pain, especially moderate to severe pain. As in other

Table 12-2
Signs of Pain in Small Mammals
(Goldberg & Shaffran [2015] and Gaynor & Muir [2014])

	Rabbit	Ferret	Rat/Mouse/Gerbil/Hamster	Guinea Pig
Behavior	Not interactive, faces back of cage. Depending on degree of pain, dull & withdrawn or aggressive	Often aggressive, biting or teeth baring	Depending on degree of pain, dull & withdrawn or aggressive;	Not interactive. Usually dull & withdrawn but can appear agitated
Posture	Hunched	Hunched	Hunched, rigid	Hunched
Movement	Inactive - abnormally still - but may have bouts of excessive locomotion	Prefers to stay curled in tight ball	Inactive to excessive - running in circles often described	Inactive, may drag hindlegs
Facial Changes	Grimace scale validated	Eyelids squinted	Grimace scale validated in rat & mouse	Not validated but obvious
Vocalization for Acute Pain	'Piercing' squeal	High pitched vocalization or grunting	High pitched squeals, often inaudible to human ear	Repeated high pitched squeals
Other	Anorexic or hyporexic; bruxism common	Often shiver, even if not cold; focal muscle fasciculations; 'bristle tail' (looks like pipe cleaner)		

Table 12-3
Anesthetic and Analgesic Drugs Commonly Used in Small Mammals.

(Muir & Hubbell, 2012; Carpenter, 2013; Gaynor and Muir, 2014)
All Abbreviations Are Common Except For OTM (Oral Transmucosal Or Buccal).
All Dosages Are In Mg/Kg. Blank Squares = No Data Available; ?=Minimal Or Anecdotal Data.

Drug	Rabbit	Ferret
OPIOIDs		
Buprenorphine[+]	0.03-0.1 IM, SQ, IV, OTM?* q6-12h	0.01-0.05 IM, SQ, IV, OTM?* q6-12h
Butorphanol	0.1-0.5 IM, SQ, IV q2-4h	0.05-0.4 IM, SQ, IV q2-4h
Fentanyl	0.005-0.01 IV; CRI 0.005-0.03 mg/kg/hr; ½ small fentanyl patch for > 3 kg rabbit	0.001-0.003 IV; CRI 0.002-0.02 mg/kg/hr; ½ 25 microg/hr patch for average adult
Hydromorphone	0.3-1.0 IM, SQ, IV q2-6h	0.1-0.2 IM, SQ, IV q2-6h
Methadone	0.3-1.0? IM, SQ, IV q2-6h	0.3-0.5 IM, SQ, IV q2-6h
Morphine	0.5-2.0 SQ, IM q2-6h	0.1-0.3 IM, SQ q2-6h
Oxymorphone	0.05-0.2 IM, SQ, IV q2-6h	0.05-0.2 IM, SQ, IV q2-6h
NSAIDs		
Carprofen	2.0-4.0 SQ q24h 1.0-5.0 PO q12h	1.0 -5.0 SQ, PO q12-24h
Meloxicam	0.1-1.0 SQ, IM, PO q12-24h	0.1-0.3 SQ, IM, PO q12-24h
LOCAL ANESTHESIA		
Lidocaine	2.0-4.0 tissue infiltration	2.0-4.0 tissue infiltration
Bupivacaine	1.0-2.0 tissue infiltration	1.0-2.0 tissue infiltration

Table 12-3 continued

SEDATIVES

Acepromazine	0.25-1.0 SQ, IM	0.02-0.25 SQ, IM
Dexmedetomidine	0.02-0.1 (up to 0.25) SQ, IM, IV	0.008-0.01 (up to 0.04) SQ, IM, IV
Medetomidine	0.04-0.2 (up to 0.5) SQ, IM, IV	0.015-0.02 (up to 0.08) SQ, IM, IV
Xylazine	1.0-3.0 (IV); 5.0 (IM)	1.0 SQ, IM
Midazolam	0.5-2.0 SQ, IM, IV; 3.0-5.0 intranasally, intraperitoneally (IP)	0.3-1.0 SQ, IM, IV
Diazepam	0.5-5.0 IV, IM/SQ?	0.5-2.0 IV, PO, IM/SQ?

ANESTHETICS

Ketamine	10-20 IV; 20-50 IM#	2.0-5.0 IV; 10-20 IM#
Alfaxalone	2.0-5.0 IV following premed, IM dose for sedation 1.0-5.0; IM for anesthesia 5.0-10.0?	2.0-5.0 IV following premed, IM dose for sedation 0.5-1.0; IM dose for anesthesia 5.0-10.0?
Propofol	2.0-5.0 (up to 10.0 if no premed) IV	2.0-5.0 (up to 10.0 if no premed) IV

*OTM=oral transmucosal. Little to no data are available for use in these species. If trying this route, use the high end of the dosing range since absorption is lower after OTM administration than after IV or IM administration.

+More current dosages listed here are higher than older dosages.

Dose depends on degree of sedation/anesthesia desired and on degree of sedation from premeds.

species, opioids can cause sedation, which is generally a positive effect when opioids are used as premedicants. Opioids can also cause mild respiratory depression and slowed GI motility, but rarely to a clinically significant degree. Respiratory depression can be countered by delivering supplemental oxygen to the patient. Slowed GI motility is most common in rabbits and Guinea pigs and should be treated with fluids and oral syringe feeding of high fiber diets if it is clinically significant. REMEMBER that pain can also cause slowed GI motility and the need for treatment like fluids and special diets! If opioid-mediated adverse effects are clinically significant, they can be reversed using naloxone or partially reversed using butorphanol. Buprenorphine, an opioid partial agonist, is the most commonly used opioid in small mammals and it may have a lower incidence of adverse effects than full opioid agonists. It is, however, less potent and should be used as part of a multimodal protocol or reserved for mild pain. The full opioid agonists (morphine, hydromorphone, oxymorphone, methadone, and fentanyl) are also used in pocket pet species, as is butorphanol (an opioid agonist-antagonist) which is a good sedative but has a short duration of analgesia.

Alpha-2 Agonists
Alpha-2 agonist drugs (medetomidine, dexmedetomidine, xylazine) provide sedation AND analgesia and are an excellent addition to most anesthetic protocols. Safety of this drug class is enhanced by the fact that the drug effects can be reversed with an alpha-2 antagonist, like atipamezole.

Local Anesthetic Drugs
Local anesthetic drugs (lidocaine, bupivacaine, ropivacaine) are potent, easy to use, inexpensive and safe (when used at the correct dose) and should be considered for use in ALL patients in which a specific nerve or a 'region' (e.g., skin with an incisional block; abdomen and rear limbs of the patient with an epidural; etc.) can be desensitized with a local/regional anesthetic block. **Figure 12-2** shows an epidural injection in a rabbit.

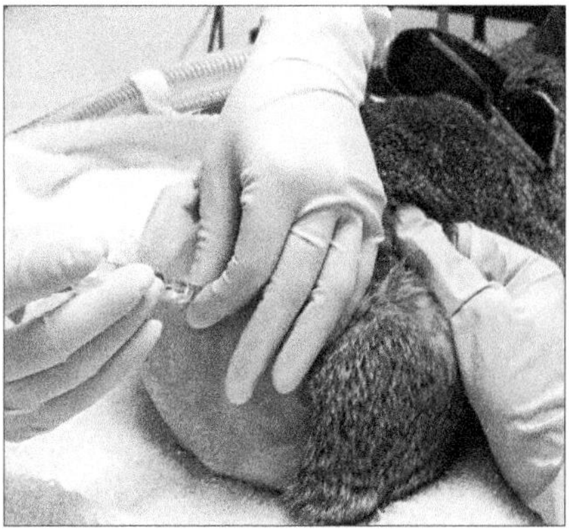

Figure 12-2. Epidural administration of opioids and local anesthetic drugs to a rabbit. Epidurals are fairly easy to do in rabbits and ferrets. (Photo courtesy of Dr. Tania Perez, WSU).

Nonsteroidal Anti-inflammatory Drugs

NSAIDs are frequently used in pocket pets and are very effective since most pain is caused, at least in part, by inflammation. Meloxicam and carprofen are the most commonly used NSAIDs in these species.

Anesthesia

As with other species, all four phases of anesthesia (preanesthesia/premedication, induction, maintenance, recovery); (See Figure 1-1) should be addressed as equally important. The goals of anesthesia should include:
• Provision of adequate analgesia.
• Utilization of short acting and/or reversible drugs so that recovery can be rapid. Long recoveries contribute to hypothermia and hypoglycemia (since the patient isn't eating).
• Delivery of supplemental oxygen whether the patient is anesthetized with inhalant or injectable drugs.
• Support of normal body temperature - these patients get cold FAST.

Preanesthesia/Premedication

• To the extent possible without causing undue stress, every patient should have a thorough physical examination.
• The patient should be as healthy as possible prior to anesthesia and diseases should be stabilized or cured (if possible). 'Stabilization' can include anything from administration of antibiotics for days/weeks prior to anesthesia to administration of supplemental fluids and pain meds for minutes/hours prior to anesthesia. As an example of the importance of stabilization, sick rabbits are more than 7 times more likely to die than healthy rabbits (Brodbelt 2009; risk factor for death 7.37% if ASA III-V and 0.73% if ASA I-II). If patients can be stabilized with subsequent improvement in health status, the risk of death decreases with each decrease in ASA (American Society of Anesthetists) risk level (See Table 1-1).
• Unlike dogs and cats, fasting is neither necessary nor recommended in rabbits and small rodents since they do not vomit. Furthermore, fasting can cause hypoglycemia and can contribute to abnormal gastrointestinal motility, especially in rabbits and Guinea pigs. Fasting does not eliminate the food that Guinea pigs store in their 'cheek pouches'. Ferrets can vomit and a short fast (3-4 hours) is recommended. Water should never be withheld from any species.

IMPORTANT POINT

Ferrets should be fasted for a few hours prior to anesthesia but no other pocket pet should undergo fasting as it can cause detrimental hypoglycemia. All species should have access to water right up until the time of premedication.

Drugs
(See Table 12-3)
• An opioid should be chosen from the list under the 'analgesia' section above and administered as a premedicant. In sick patients, this may be enough to decrease the dose of other anesthetic drugs, although the addition of a benzodiazepine may be necessary for adequate sedation. In healthy patients, a sedative (alpha-2 agonist, acepromazine or benzodiazepine) should be added to the opioid.
• Alpha-2 agonists (eg, medetomidine and dexmedetomidine) are potent sedative/analgesic drugs and their effects are reversible. Many dosages are listed for medetomidine in the literature, remember that dexmedetomidine dosages would be one-half of the medetomidine dosage as calculated by **mg**/body weight but, the VOLUME of dexmedetomidine as calculated by **ml**/kg is the same as the volume of medetomidine. Xylazine is used occasionally.

EXAMPLE of Medetomidine vs Dexmedetomidine Dosing
You want to sedate a 2-kg rabbit in your practice with 0.2 mg/kg medetomidine, which is 1 mg/ml.
  • **2 kg x 0.1 mg/kg = 0.2 mg 0.2 mg divided by 1 mg/ml = 0.2 ml**
  • Then you realize that all you have in your practice is dexmedetomidine. You look up the dose and it is 0.05 mg/kg and the concentration of dexmedetomidine is 0.5 mg/ml
  • **2 kg x 0.05 mg/kg = 0.1 mg 0.1 mg divided by 0.5 mg/ml = 0.2 ml**
• Benzodiazepines - Midazolam is often added to an opioid as a premedicant because it is predictably absorbed after IM administration (diazepam is not predictably absorbed when administered IM). Midazolam can also be administered intranasally in rabbits and other species with nares large enough to deliver the drug by this route. Although not potent sedatives, pre-treatment with a benzo-diazepine will often make the patient calm enough for catheter placement, IV administration of other drugs, mask induction, etc. Benzodiazepines should not be used alone in aggressive or excited patients as they may make the patient more aggressive and/or excited.
• Acepromazine provides long-duration calming, which is a benefit in nervous patients, but it may cause prolonged non-reversible sedation, which can delay recovery. The drug is more commonly used in rabbits than in other small mammal species. Acepromazine does not provide analgesia.
• Alfaxalone is an IV induction drug that can also be administered IM as part of a sedation protocol. Alfaxalone does not provide analgesia and the effects are not reversible. Following IM administration the effects last 20-45 minutes (depending on dose). Sedation is unpredictable with alfaxalone alone, thus combination with an opioid is recommended.
• Anticholinergics (atropine, glycopyrrolate) are really support drugs not anesthetic/analgesic drugs and should be administered any time that bradycardia is contributing to hypotension. They are included here because they are also commonly administered as premedicants to pocket pet species to maintain heart rate and to decrease the volume of salivary and respiratory secretions produced

by the patient. This is rarely necessary in larger patients like dogs and cats but the small size of the endotracheal tube used in pocket pets means that occlusion by these secretions is more likely than it is in larger patients. Furthermore, ketamine is commonly used in pocket pets for induction and ketamine tends to cause increased production of salivary and respiratory secretions. Either atropine or glycopyrrolate is acceptable in most species but most rabbits make the enzyme atropinase which can render atropine ineffective so glycopyrrolate is the better choice for rabbits.

> **IMPORTANT POINT**
> **IN RABBITS, glycopyrrolate should be used for treatment of bradycardia and maintenance of adequate heart rate since approximately 50% of all rabbits make an enzyme (atropinase) that makes atropine ineffective.**

Induction
Inhalant induction is often used in pocket pets. While this can be acceptable following adequate sedation, injectable induction, especially in larger patients like rabbits and ferrets, is generally preferred.

Drugs
(See Table 12-3):
• Ketamine is often used to induce small mammals to anesthesia and adminis-tration of the drug is extremely easy since it can be administered IV but is also well-absorbed following IM injection. Ketamine should be combined with drugs that provide sedation and muscle relaxation (e.g., benzodiazepines and alpha-2 agonists) along with those that provide analgesia (e.g., alpha-2 agonists, opioids).
• Propofol is an ideal induction drug in patients in which a rapid recovery is desirable, like most pocket pets. However, the use of propofol is limited by venous access and is thus reserved for larger small mammals like rabbits and ferrets. In order to alleviate dose-dependent propofol-mediated adverse effects, premedi-cation with sedative/analgesic drugs should be used and/or a dose of a benzodi-azepine or fentanyl should be administered immediately prior to the administration of the propofol. Because propofol can cause some respiratory depression, preoxy-genation for 3-5 minutes prior to induction is recommended.
• Alfaxalone can be administered either IV or IM for induction of anesthesia. For larger patients (medium-sized cats and up), the volume of alfaxalone is generally too large for IM induction of anesthesia but the volume is appropriate, although still somewhat large, for pocket pets. Even in larger patients, a lower dose of alfaxalone can be administered IM with an opioid for premedication or sedation. Alfaxalone causes physiologic effects that are very similar to those caused by propofol, thus the guidelines for use (premedicate or combine with a sedative, administer oxygen, etc.) are the same as those for propofol.
• Inhalant induction with sevoflurane or isoflurane delivered by mask or chamber may be necessary if IV access is not possible and IM induction is not appropriate. Although pocket pets can be induced to anesthesia by mask delivery of inhalant anesthetic drugs used alone, this is not always the safest option since the dose of

inhalant drug required to reach an induction plane of anesthesia if no other drugs are administered is quite high, and adverse effects from inhalant anesthetic drugs are dose-dependent. Furthermore, struggling by the patient increases the amount of drug required to induce anesthesia and this, combined with the excessive amount of catecholamines (excitatory neurotransmitters) released during fear and struggling, adds to the danger of inhalant induction. In dogs, cats and horses, anesthetic risk is significantly increased when inhalant drugs are used alone for both induction and maintenance of anesthesia (Brodbelt 2009). The same is likely true for all mammals. A dose of a sedative drug should be administered prior to mask or chamber induction - or analgesic drugs administered immediately after induction but prior to a painful stimulus. This will allow a decrease in the dose of inhalant drugs needed to maintain anesthesia, which will increase anesthetic safety and promote normotension, normoventilation, normothermia AND faster, smoother recoveries. A very brief exposure to inhalants can be used for sedation when injectable drugs are not indicated/desired. Some specific tips:

- Rabbits tend to breath-hold and inhalant administration may need to be stopped if the breath-holding is prolonged. Sevoflurane tends to cause less breath-holding.
- Masks for very small mammals can be made using syringe cases covered with a latex glove with a small hole cut into it to seal the 'mask' around the patient's nose/muzzle and the opposite end of the casing opened up to connect to the breathing system. Insure that the mask is not pressing on the patient's eyes.

Maintenance
Drugs
Depending on the duration & invasiveness of the procedure and the species & health of the patient, maintenance anesthesia can be achieved with either injectable or inhalant anesthetic drugs. For injectable anesthesia, ketamine is most commonly used to provide maintenance anesthesia since it can be administered IM. IV maintenance can be provided by ketamine, propofol or alfaxalone. For inhalant anesthesia, both isoflurane and sevoflurane are appropriate.

Techniques
Medium to large rabbits can be intubated using a blind technique or a stylet can be placed with visualization of the larynx using an otoscope. Laryngeal masks like those made for humans are available for rabbits **(Figure 12-3)**. Ferrets can be intubated using the same techniques as used for cats **(Figure 12-4 A&B)**. Larger rats can be intubated using an otoscope for visualization of the larynx for stylet placement. For most other pocket pets, maintenance by mask delivery of inhalants is necessary.

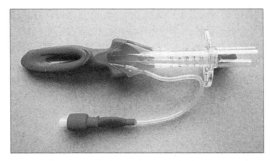

Figure 12-3. Laryngeal mask airways (LMAs) fit right over the larynx instead of advancing into the trachea like endotracheal tubes. They are very easy to place in rabbits and there are LMAs that are specifically made for rabbits. This view shows the opening of the LMA (purple area on the left of the photo) that would fit over the larynx.

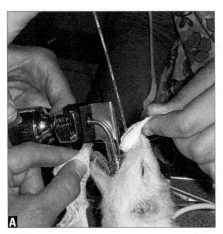
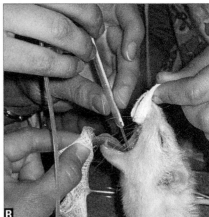

Figure 12-4. Ferrets are intubated much like cats. **A:** Use a laryngoscope to place a stylet through the larynx; **B:** With the laryngoscope removed, place the tube over the stylet. Gently rotate the tube to get it through the larynx. The laryngoscope could be used throughout the entire intubation but it can get in the way since the ferret's mouth is very small.

Monitoring

As with all anesthetized patients, monitoring is critical.

• Monitoring response to surgery, mucous membrane color, capillary refill time, respiratory rate, and heart rate should be routine for all patients.

• The pulse oximeter will work in many small patients. The tongue is a good location for the oximeter probe in larger patients like rabbits and ferrets but in smaller patients placing the probe over the entire paw often works. Placing the probe on the lip, vulva, prepuce, or a fold of skin - like the skin on the caudal-ventral abdomen in front of the stifle (the 'flank') or the fold at the base of the tail, may work. Reflectance probes are often more useful in very small patients (more information in Chapter 5).

• A Doppler is an excellent choice and will work in almost all patients (blood pressure cannot be obtained in all patients but blood flow will be audible). Sites for probe placement include the ventral side (or 'under' side) of the carpus or tarsus, ventral side of the tail or over the femoral artery on the inside of the thigh. The hair at the probe site should be shaved in most species, but the fur on rabbit metatarsals (hind feet) should not be shaved as this can cause skin irritation.

• Blood pressure can be determined by Doppler or oscillometric units but the smallest blood pressure cuff is a size 1. This will work in most rabbits and many ferrets but not in smaller species. The width of the blood pressure cuff should be 40% of the circumference of the limb (or tail) on which the cuff will be placed. A cuff that is too large will cause the blood pressure unit to display a falsely low pressure.

• An ECG is useful in most patients but the 'alligator clips' on the ECG leads tend to cause excessive tissue trauma in small patients with thin skin. Thus, a needle (very small - like 25-G 0.75 inch) or a small loop of wire suture should be inserted through the skin and the alligator clips attached to the needle or wire **(Figure 12-5)**.

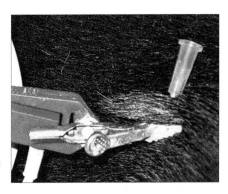

Figure 12-5. Needle inserted through the skin for attachment of alligator clips.

• Because of the small tidal volume and high respiratory rate, the $ETCO_2$ monitor will not be accurate in most very small patients. However, the monitor may provide information on the CO_2 trend. An adapter that extends into the endotracheal tube **(Figure 12-6 A&B)** will improve the accuracy of $ETCO_2$ results. The ET tube must be a size 4.0 or larger or the adapter may occupy too much of the tube lumen.

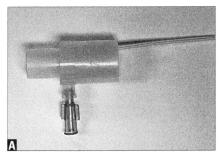
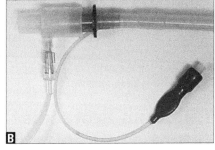

Figure 12-6. Adapter for more accurate measurement of $ETCO_2$. The adapter is made from a 'tom cat' or large IV catheter or polypropylene tubing. The free end on the right extends down into the trachea for collection of CO_2 samples deeper in the trachea **(A)**. The end on the endotracheal tube adapter hooks to a side-stream $ETCO_2$ monitor sampling line **(B)**.

Support

As with all anesthetized patients, support is critical.

- Every action should be performed with <u>body temperature support</u> in mind:
  - The patient should be wrapped in warm towels during all phases of anesthesia. Covering the patients with bubble or plastic wrap also helps to maintain body temperature.
  - The surgery room should be warm if possible and the recovery room should definitely be warm or a warm cage or incubator should be used for recovery.
  - The surgical scrub solution should be warm and the amount used on the patient should be minimal so as not to drench the whole patient in fluid.
  - The IV (or SQ) fluids should be warm and/or delivered through an IV fluid line warmer placed as close to the catheter as possible (so the fluid stays warm as it gets to the patient).
- Fluids should be administered IV or intraosseus (in the bone) if possible or SQ if these routes are not practical.
  - Fluids with glucose may be necessary since hypoglycemia is common in these patients however, glucose containing fluids should not be administered SQ as they can cause tissue necrosis.
- Oxygen should always be provided even in patients that are sedated but not anesthetized since this group of species has a high metabolic rate with subsequent high oxygen consumption.
- Eye protection is important - especially for rodents and other species with large protruding eyes. In addition, ketamine often causes the eyes to remain open with no blinking so the cornea is likely to become too dry. Frequent application of eye lubricant is important.

Recovery

Keep all patients WARM and quiet (especially rabbits since they are more likely than the other species to experience excitement or dysphoria in recovery). Readdress analgesia.

IMPORTANT TIP

In recovery, don't forget to evaluate the duration of analgesic drugs that have been administered pre- and intra-operatively. If the patient has undergone a painful procedure, consider administering another dose of the analgesic drug if the end of the expected duration is close, especially if no other analgesic drugs have been administered.

Common Protocols

Common Protocol for Healthy Rabbits

- Buprenorphine 0.03-0.05 mg/kg (or butorphanol 0.3-0.5 mg/kg); dexmedetomidine 0.02 OR medetomidine 0.04 mg/kg; and ketamine at 10-20 mg/kg all combined in the same syringe and administered IM.

- Dosages in the lower range of the protocol = deep sedation; higher dosages = light anesthesia.
  - Can be administered SQ but will not generally provide surgical anesthesia by this route.
- Large rabbits can be intubated and all smaller rabbits can be maintained using mask delivery of inhalant anesthetic drugs.
- The alpha-2 agonist can be reversed at the end of the procedure if necessary, but both sedation AND analgesia will be reversed so the patient may experience pain unless analgesia has been provided by other drugs (e.g., opioids or NSAIDs).

Common Protocol for Unhealthy Rabbits
- 0.03-0.05 mg/kg buprenorphine (or 0.3-0.5 mg/kg butorphanol) combined with 0.5-1.0 mg/kg midazolam and administered IM.
  - Lower end of the dosage range if REALLY sick, higher end of the dosage range if mild-moderate disease.
- Propofol or alfaxalone can then be administered in the brachial vein or the ear vein of large rabbits.
- If IV access is not possible, patients can be induced to anesthesia using inhalant drugs delivered by mask at low dosages.

Common Protocol for Ferrets
- Use the same protocols that you use in cats, healthy or sick.
- Premedication: 0.03 mg/kg buprenorphine or 0.1 mg/kg hydromorphone PLUS 0.01 mg/kg dexmedetomidine if healthy. Change dexmedetomidine to 0.2 mg/kg midazolam in unhealthy ferrets.
  - Add 5-10 mg/kg ketamine to the opioid and dexmedetomidine and administer IM to healthy ferrets. This is especially useful for fractious ferrets.
- Alternatively propofol, alfaxalone or ketamine/benzodiazepine can be administered IV following sedation with dexmedetomidine/opioid.
- Ferrets can be intubated and maintained on inhalant anesthetics.

CRITICAL POINT!
FOR ALL patients, additional analgesia must be provided. Opioids, and NSAIDs are all appropriate for small mammals as are local anesthetic blocks - don't forget to use blocks!

Species Specific 'Issues'
There are numerous species specific 'issues' to consider when anesthe-tizing small animals. Examples include the tendency of rabbits to kick violently backwards and injure their backs when restrained inappropriately and the tendency of guinea pigs to retain large amounts of food in the pharynx. These issues are too numerous to present in this chapter and they should be investigated in pocket pet specific references.

References

Brodbelt D. Perioperative mortality in small animal anaesthesia. The Vet J 2009; 182:152; 161.

Carpenter JW. Exotic Animal Formulary, 5th edition. Elsevier 2018.

Muir WW, Hubbell JAE. Handbook of Veterinary Anesthesia, 5th edition. Mosby, 2012

Gaynor J, Muir WW. Handbook of Veterinary Pain Management, 3rd ed. Elsevier 2014.

Goldberg ME, Shaffran N. Pain Management for Veterinary Technicians and Nurses. Wiley-Blackwell 2015.

Recommended Readings

Allweiler S. How to improve anesthesia and analgesia in small mammals. Vet Clin Exot Anim 2016:19:361-377.

Barter LA. Rabbit analgesia. Vet Clin Exot Anim 2011; 14:93-104.

Cantwell SL. Ferret, rabbit and rodent anesthesia. Vet Clin Exot Anim 2001; 4(1):169-192.

Egger CM, Love L, Doherty T. Pain Management in Veterinary Practice 1st Edition. Wiley-Blackwell, 2013.

Flecknell PA. Analgesia of small mammals. Vet Clin Exot Anim 2001; 4(1):47-56.

Johnston MS. Clinical approaches to analgesia in ferrets and rabbits. Sem Avian and Exot Pet Med 2005; 14(4):229-235.

Glossary and Abbreviations

agonist. A drug that activates a receptor specific for that drug. Examples include morphine, which is an opioid agonist, and dexmedetomidine, which is an alpha-2 agonist.

agonist-antagonist. A drug that activates a receptor specific for that drug while simultaneously antagonizing ('blocking') another drug-specific receptor. Butorphanol is an example. It is an agonist at the kappa-opioid receptor and an antagonist at the mu-opioid receptor.

alpha-2 agonist. A group of drugs that work by activating the alpha-2 receptors. Examples include dexmedetomidine, medetomidine, detomidine, romifidine and xylazine.

allodynia. A sensation of pain in response to a stimulus that should NOT have been nonpainful.

antagonist. A drug that blocks or reverses the effect of another drug by antagonizing the activity of the drug at a receptor specific for that drug. Examples include naloxone, which is an opioid antagonist, and atipamezole, which is an alpha-2 antagonist.

anticholinergic drug - a drug that blocks the action of the neurotransmitter acetylcholine. Anticholinergic drugs, like atropine and glycopyrrolate, are used to prevent or treat bradycardia by blocking acetylcholine at the vagus nerve.

APL. Adjustable pressure limiting valve, also called a 'pop-off' valve.

apnea. Cessation of breathing.

ASA. American Society of Anesthesiologists. The ASA risk chart is used to determine a patient's risk for anesthetic adverse events.

atelectasis. collapse of alveoli ('air sacs') in the lungs.

bain mount or block. A small apparatus designed to allow use of an airway pressure manometer, APL valve and scavenging connection with a nonrebreathing system.

balanced anesthesia. Using a combination or 'balance' of drugs to provide anesthesia. This technique, which includes premedicants, induction drugs, and maintenance drugs, is safer than using just one anesthesia drug because a combination allows decreased dosages of each drug, thereby reducing dose-dependent side effects.

barotrauma. Damage to the lungs from excessive intrapulmonary (inside the lung) pressure. This can occur when the pop-off valve (APL) is left closed or with any occlusion in the expiratory limb of a rebreathing or circle system.

benzodiazepine. A group of drugs that are used for muscle relaxation and calming. Examples include diazepam (Valium) and midazolam (Versed).

brachycephalic. Dogs and cats with short ('brachy') noses. These patients often have a variety of upper airway abnormalities that can make breathing difficult.

bradycardia. Slower than normal heart rate.

bradypnea. Slower than normal respiratory rate.

cardiac output. The amount of blood ejected by the heart over time. The formula for cardiac output is heart rate x stroke volume.

caudal. Toward the tail of the animal.

central sensitization. Amplification of a pain signal secondary to a variety of pain pathway changes, primarily the activation of receptors (particularly NMDA receptors) in the spinal cord. This is also called 'windup'.

CNS. Central Nervous System, includes the brain and spinal cord.

cranial. Toward the head or front of the animal.

CRI. Constant rate infusion, used to administer analgesic drugs as a slow infusion over time. (See Chapter 7).

CRT. Capillary refill time. The time it takes blood to return to an area that has been blanched by digital (finger) pressure.(See Chapter 2).

denitrogenation. Removing nitrogen from the lungs by using a high oxygen flow. (See Chapter 3).

dorsal. Toward the 'top' (top of the back or head) of the standing or sternal animal.

dysphoria. A state of confusion that often occurs in the recovery phase of anesthesia. It can be fairly brief or can be profound and the patient can appear highly agitated. Pain can cause or exacerbate dysphoria. Patients experiencing moderate to profound dysphoria or dysphoria that lasts > 1 minute should be treated with analgesic and sedative drugs.

emetic. A drug that causes vomiting.

emesis. Vomiting.

ET. Endotracheal.

ETCO$_2$. End-tidal carbon dioxide. This is measured by a capnometer.

ETT. Endotracheal tube.

fresh gases. Any gas that enters the breathing system from the anesthetic machine and has not yet been breathed by the patient. It is usually a mix of oxygen and inhalant gas but can be oxygen alone.

gas exchange. The process of inhaling oxygen and exhaling carbon dioxide.

hyperalgesia. The sensation of excessive pain in response to a stimulus that should be only mildly painful.

456

hypercalcemia. Abnormally high serum calcium.

hyperkalemia. Abnormally high serum potassium.

hypercarbia/hypercapnia. These terms are often used interchangeably, although they are technically slightly different. Both mean abnormally high carbon dioxide (CO_2) but hypercarbia indicates high CO_2 in the blood (measured by analysis of an arterial blood gas sample) and hypercapnia indicates high CO_2 in the exhaled air (measured by a capnometer). The CO_2 values obtained by both methods should be very close to equal.

hyperpnea. Panting.

hypertension. Blood pressure higher than normal.

hyperventilation. Gas exchange higher than normal. This can be caused by increased respiratory rate or tidal volume.

hypocarbia/hypocapnia. These terms are often used interchangeably, although they are technically slightly different. Both mean abnormally low carbon dioxide (CO_2) but hypocarbia indicates low CO_2 in the blood (measured by analysis of an arterial blood gas sample) and hypocapnia indicates low CO_2 in the exhaled air (measured by a capnometer). The CO_2 values obtained by both methods should be very close to equal.

hypoglycemia. Abnormally low concentration of serum glucose.

hypotension. Blood pressure lower than normal.

hypoventilation. Gas exchange lower than normal. This can be caused by decreased respiratory rate or tidal volume.

hypovolemia. Low circulating fluid volume. Usually caused by dehydration, hemorrhage or excessive vasodilation.

hypoxia/hypoxemia. These words are often used interchangeably but there is a slight technical difference. Both mean abnormally low oxygen concentration but hypoxia means low oxygen in the tissues and hypoxemia means low oxygen in the blood. Since we only measure oxygen in the blood (using an arterial blood gas), hypoxemia is the more correct term for the parameter that we can actually measure.

I:E ratio. Inspired:Expired ratio. Describes the setting on a ventilator that controls the time a patient spends in inspiration and the time spent in expiration. For example, an I:E ration of 1:3 means that the patient spends ⅓ of the respiratory cycle in inspiration and ⅔ in expiration. See Chapter 3.

IPPV. Intermittent positive pressure ventilation. Means that breaths are being delivered to the patient, either using a ventilator or a person squeezing the breathing bag.

lumbosacral. The space between the lumbar and sacral vertebrae through which an epidural needle is inserted for a lumbosacral epidural injection of analgesic drugs.

minute ventilation. The amount of air moved through the alveoli in a minute. It is calculated as respiratory rate x tidal volume.

multimodal analgesia. Using more than one drug or treatment to provide pain relief, which generally improves both efficacy and safety of therapy. Multimodal analgesia is required to control moderate to severe pain. Examples include opioids + NSAIDs + local blocks for acute pain and NSAIDs + gabapentin + acupuncture for chronic pain.

myocardium. Heart muscle.

neurotransmitter. A chemical 'messenger' that is used to send a signal between locations in the body. An example is a neurotransmitter that crosses a synapse (junction) between nerves to send a signal, like a pain signal, along the nerve.

NMDA. N-Methyl-D-aspartate. NMDA receptors are in the CNS and activation of the receptors results in central sensitization. Ketamine can be used to antagonize the NMDA receptors, which decreases the pain from central sensitization.

nociceptor. Pain receptor.

opioids. A group of drugs that provide analgesia by activating opioid receptors, primarily mu and kappa receptors. Examples include morphine, hydromorphone, methadone, fentanyl, buprenorphine and butorphanol.

OTM. Oral transmucosal. Describes the route of drug delivery achieved by applying a drug to the mucosa of the oral cavity, which allows absorption of the drug into the blood stream. An example of a drug that can be delivered in this manner is buprenorphine, which is commonly delivered OTM to cats and small dogs (the volume is too large for adequate absorption in big dogs).

oxygen delivery. The process of providing oxygen to cells, which they use as fuel. Adequate oxygen delivery requires normal function of both the cardiovascular and respiratory systems.

partial agonist. A drug that partially activates a certain receptor. Buprenorphine is an example. Buprenorphine is a partial agonist at the mu opioid receptor.

pathologic pain. Pain that serves no protective purpose and causes decreased quality of life. Acute pain in excess of that necessary to be protective and most causes of chronic pain are examples of pathologic pain.

PEEP. Positive end expiratory pressure. The pressure in the lungs at the end of exhalation. This is normally zero but may be increased accidentally by the machine (which can lead to barotrauma if excessive) or intentionally by the anesthetist (to help maintain alveolar inflation).

peripheral sensitization. Amplification of a pain signal secondary to activation of a variety of processes, including inflammation, at the site of the tissue damage.

physiologic pain. This is normal pain after an injury or surgery. It is also called protective pain because it causes the patient to limit activities that would cause more injury. However, a patient should still receive analgesic drugs to treat pathologic pain. Most of the analgesic drugs we use allow treatment of pathologic pain without elimination of protective pain.

PIP. Peak inspiratory pressure. This is the highest pressure that should be delivered when giving a patient a breath. This is measured by the airway manometer on the anesthesia machine.

positive inotrope or inotrope. A drug used to increase contractility of the heart muscle. Examples include dopamine and dobutamine.

PSI. Pounds per square inch. Used to designate the pressure in gas (like oxygen) tanks.

respiratory acidosis. Abnormally low blood pH due to hypoventilation

respiratory alkalosis. Abnormally high blood pH due to hyperventilation.

SpO_2. The percent of hemoglobin that is saturated with oxygen. This is measured by a pulse oximeter.

stroke volume. The amount of blood ejected by the heart with each beat.

vagal tone. Describes the level of activity from the vagus nerve. High vagal tone often causes bradycardia, which would require treatment with an anticholinergic if the bradycardia resulted in hypotension.

vasoconstriction. Constriction of the blood vessels.

vasodilation. Dilation of the blood vessels.

ventral. Toward the 'bottom' (the most ventral would be the paws) of the standing or sternal animal.

waste anesthetic gas. Inhalant anesthetic that was exhaled from the patient or was never inhaled and just circulated through the breathing system. This gas needs to be scavenged.

Recommended Readings

Books

Our book provides a comprehensive overview of many topics in anesthesia and analgesia. If you need more information, we recommend the following books:

Duke-Novakovski T, de Vries M, Seymour C. BSAVA Manual of Canine and Feline Anaesthesia and Analgesia. BSAVA British Small Animal Veterinary Association, 2016

Egger C M, Love L, Doherty T (editors). Pain Management In Veterinary Practice, 1st Edition. Wiley-Blackwell, 2013.

Flecknell PA. Analgesia of small mammals. Vet Clin Exot Anim 2001; 4(1): 47-56.

Gaynor JS, Muir W W. Handbook of veterinary pain management, 3rd Edition. Mosby, 2014.

Goldberg ME, (Editor), Shaffran N (Consulting Editor). Pain Management For Veterinary Technicians And Nurses, 1st Edition. Wiley-Blackwell, 2014.

Grimm Kurt, Tranquill William, Lamont Leigh. Small Animal Anesthesia, 2nd Edition, 2011, John Wiley and Sons, Inc.

Mathews K. Veterinary Emergency and Critical Care Manual, 3rd Edition. Life Learn, 2017

Mathews K, Sinclair M, Steele AM, Grubb T. Analgesia and Anesthesia for the Ill or Injured Dog and Cat. Wiley-Blackwell, 2018

Web Site Links

AmericanAnimalHospitalAssociation(AAHA):https://aaha.org/professional/resources/painmanagement.aspx.

The International Veterinary Academy of Pain Management: https://ivapm.org/.

The World Small Animal Veterinary Association (WSAVA): http.//www.wsava.org/guidelines/global-pain-councilguidelines .

Appendices

Handy Calculations
Basic Conversions
Converting kilograms (kgs) to pounds (lbs): Multiply the body weight in kg by 2.2
Converting pounds to kilograms: Divide the body weight in lbs by 2.2
Converting Celsius to Fahrenheit: Multiply degrees in Celsius by 1.8, then add 32.
Converting Fahrenheit to Celsius: Subtract 32 from the degrees in Fahrenheit, then multiply the resulting number by 0.55.

Drug and Fluid Calculations
Basic Dosage Calculations
(See Chapter 8)
Take the dose of the drug in milligrams (mgs per body weight) and multiply by the patient's weight (generally pounds [lbs] or kilograms [kgs] but may be grams [gms] in very small patients like pocket pets). Then divide that number by the concentration of the drug (look at the bottle!). The result will be the milliliters (mls) to administer to the patient.

Example
A painful patient 15 kg needs a dose of 0.5 mg/kg of morphine (15 mg/ml)

$$15 \text{ kg} \times 0.5 \text{ mg/kg} = 7.5 \text{ mg}$$
$$7.5 \text{ mg} \div 15 \text{ mg/ml} = 0.5 \text{ ml}$$

Tip
If the drug dose is in micrograms (microg), it is often easiest to convert it to mgs before starting the calculation. All you have to do is divide the dose in micrograms by 1000.

Example
A patient you are working on needs a dose of 5 microg/kg.

$$5 \text{ microg} \div 1000 = 0.005 \text{ mg}$$

Calculations for Diluting Drugs
A 0.7 kg ferret in your clinic needs 0.05 mg/kg acepromazine (10 mg/ml). This would be 0.7 kg x 0.05 mg/kg divided by 10 mg/ml = 0.0035 ml, which is hard to accurately draw up.

Ace Dilution
Draw up 0.1 ml of the 10 mg/ml acepromazine. This will be 1 mg of acepromazine. Dilute this with 0.9 ml sterile water. Now the solution is 1 mg/ml and the volume for the ferret is 0.035, which can accurately be drawn up in a tuberculin (TB) syringe.

Basic Fluid Rate Calculations
(See Chapter 8)
Decide on the appropriate fluid rate (mls/kg/hour or mls/lb/hour) for your patient and multiply it by the patient's body weight (in kgs or lbs). Then choose the appropriate sized drip set (drips/ml - usually 60 or 15). You can plug those numbers into the formula:

Weight x rate x drip set ÷ 3600 = drops/min

The 3600 is determined by the fact that the calculation should result in drops/second and fluid rate is usually defined as mls/hour. So 60 seconds in a minute x 60 minutes in an hour = 3600 seconds.

Example
A 25-kg dog needs a fluid rate of 5 ml/kg/hour using a drip set of 15 drops/ml

(25 kg x 5 ml/kg/hr x 15 drops ml) / 3600 = roughly 0.5 drops/second (round to 1 drop every 2 seconds to make it easier to administer).

Example
A 4-kg cat needs a fluid rate of 3 ml/kg/hour using a drip set of 60 drops/ml

(4 kg x 3 ml/kg/hr x 60 drops ml) / 3600 = roughly 0.2 drops/second (round to 1 drop every 5 seconds to make it easier to administer).

Calculations for Constant Rate Infusions
(See Chapter 7)

Method 1
Drugs that don't need to be diluted and can be administered from a syringe pump.

Quick calculation for a 50-ml syringe-pump infusion of lidocaine/ketamine or lidocaine/ketamine/morphine:
1. DRAW 42.2 ML SODIUM CHLORIDE INTO A 60 ML SYRINGE.
2. ADD 7.5 ML (150 MG) of 20 mg/kg LIDOCAINE
3. ADD 0.3 ML (30 MG) of 100 mg/kg KETAMINE
4. IF YOU CHOOSE TO ADD MORPHINE, ADD 0.8 ML (12MG) of 15 mg/ml MORPHINE
   • For accuracy, subtract another 0.8 mls of saline at the start (total saline in the syringe would be 41.4 mls so that the total final volume of saline + drugs will be 50 mls. This isn't critical but does increase precision of the concentration of the infusion.
ADMINISTERED AT 1 ML/KG/HR, THIS WILL DELIVER LIDOCAINE 50 MCG/KG/MIN; KETAMINE 10 MCG/KG/MIN; MORPHINE 4 MCG/KG/MIN

Method 2
Drugs that will be diluted in a volume of fluid.

Plug everything into the formula:
- A = desired dose in microg/kg/min* (look up the dose)
- B = patient body wt in kg
- C = Diluent volume in mls (for example, a 250 ml bag of fluids or 60 ml syringe)
- D = Desired fluid rate in mls/hr (for example, 1 ml/kg/hr)
- E = Drug concentration in mg/ml (look at the bottle!)

A x B x C x 60 / D x E x 1000 = mls of drug to add to diluent (the fluid bag or syringe)
NOTE: If the dose at A is in mg/kg/hr, the two conversion factors in the formula (60 in the numerator and 1000 in the denominator) should be removed from the formula and the mg/kg/hr dose be used instead of the microg/kg/min dose. In this case the formula is A x B x C / D x E.

Calculations for Making Glucose Solutions
Start with a 50-ml bottle of 50% (500 mg/ml) dextrose. Decide the fluid that you will put the dextrose into (usually LRS or Plasmalyte), the final concentration of dextrose that you want to make and the total volume that you would like to administer to the patient.

Multiply the new concentration that you want to make in MG/ml by the final volume you want to obtain and divide that by the 500 mg/ml of the 50% dextrose.

Example
To make 20-ml of a 2.5% dextrose solution:

2.5% = 25 mg/ml

25 mg/ml x 20 ml divided by 500 mg/ml = 1 ml of 500 mg/ml dextrose added to 20 mls of LRS or Plasmalyte.

Another way to do this is to use the formula V1 x C1 = V2 x C2
V=volume and C=concentration
Rearrange to:
V1 (the volume you need to know) = (V2 x C2) divided by C1
Using the numbers in the example:
V1=(20 ml x 25 mg/ml) divided by 500 mg/ml = 1 ml

Table for Making 2.5% Dextrose Solutions	
MLS of Solution to Administer	**MLS of 50% Dextrose to Add**
10	0.5
20	1.0
30	1.5
40	2.0
50	2.5
100	5.0
500	25.0
1000	50.0
5000	250.0

Equipment Calculations

Calculation for Determining Rebreathing Bag Size

The rebreathing bag volume should be 4 to 6 times the patient's tidal volume (10 to 15 ml/kg), or approximately 60ml/kg of patient body weight.

Example

A 12 kg dog will need a rebreathing bag of (12 kg x 60 ml/kg) 720 mls. Since there is no rebreathing bag of this size, you would round UP to a 1-liter bag.

Calculation to Determine Oxygen Flow in Rebreathing Systems

The average oxygen flow for rebreathing systems is 30 ml/kg/min, or roughly 15 ml/lb/min (range 20 to 40 ml/kg/min). Multiply this by the patient's body weight.

Example

A 35 kg patient would need an oxygen flow of 30 ml/kg/min x 35 kg = 1050 ml/min.

Remember

Sometimes this calculation results in a very low oxygen flow that is appropriate for the patient but may not be for the vaporizer. Vaporizers are often inaccurate at oxygen flows less than 500 ml/min so this should always be the minimum flow.

Calculation to Determine Oxygen Flow in Nonrebreathing Systems

The average oxygen flow for nonrebreathing systems is 200 ml/kg/min, or roughly 90 ml/lb/min (range 150-300 ml/kg/min). Multiply this by the patient's body weight.

Example
A four kg patient would need an oxygen flow of 200 ml/kg/min x 4 kg = 800 ml/min.

Calculation to Determine the Amount of Oxygen Remaining in the Oxygen Cylinder
Multiply the pressure seen on the cylinder gauge by 3 for the H (wall) tanks and by 0.3 for the E (anesthesia machine) tanks.

Example
The cylinder gauge reads 200 psi on the small E tank on your anesthetic machine
200 x 0.3 = 60 liters of oxygen remaining in the tank

How to: Set-Up for Anesthesia

ITEM OR TASK	Check!
Patient	
Do a good physical exam	
Weigh the patient	
Complete and assess blood work or other necessary diagnostics	
Machine and breathing system set-up	
Inhalant levels full	
Oxygen connected and adequate amount available	
Rebreathing system set for patients over 5 kg	
Bain circuit (non-rebreathing system) for patients under 5 kg	
Carbon dioxide absorbent checked/changed	
Breathing system pressure checked	
Pressure relief valve (pop-off valve) open	
IV catheter set-up	
Catheter: Cats and toy dogs 22-gauge; Small, medium, large dogs 20-gauge; Very large and giant dogs 18 gauge	
Clippers, scrub & alcohol	
Injection cap or injection port ('T-port')	
Saline or heparinized saline for flushing the catheter	
Dry sponges to dry skin, tape to secure catheter. Secure it well!	
Supplies for premedication	
Anesthetic record with appropriate patient information and drug dosages	
Choose and calculate dosages for premedication drugs; Draw up drugs	
Supplies for induction	
Anesthesia mask for pre-oxygenation	
Choose and calculate dosage for induction drugs; Draw up drugs	
Laryngoscope	
Endotracheal tube • palpate trachea and use your best judgment, also have a tube one size smaller and one size larger at your station • Inflate the cuff of the tube, **leave inflated for about 15 minutes** to really test the cuff	
Sterile lube to LIGHTLY lube the endotracheal tube before insertion into the trachea. Be careful not to occlude the 'Murphy eye' or the end of the tube with lube!	
Stylet for ET tubes under 5.0 mm	

466

Lidocaine for cats (1 to 2 drops on each arytenoid)	
Dry gauze sponge to hold the tongue	
Tube tie. Be sure to secure the tube to the patient's head!	
Ophthalmic ointment. Be sure to lube the eyes well!	
Supplies for maintenance	
Choose maintenance drugs (usually isoflurane or sevoflurane)	
Turn on a heating pad and place a towel or blanket on the pad. Never place a patient directly on a heating pad!	
Fluid supplies	
Choose the appropriate fluid and warm it	
Connect the appropriate sized drip set (15 drops/ml for medium to large patients; 60 drops/ml for cats, toy-sized dogs, kittens, puppies)	
Attach an extension if necessary	
Monitoring Equipment	
Turn on all monitoring equipment	
Attach the blood pressure cable and choose the correct size blood pressure cuff	
Attach the ECG leads to the monitor and set out alcohol or lube to wet the leads where they attach to the patient	
Attach the pulse oximeter probe, make sure it works by placing it on your own finger	
Attach the end-tidal CO_2 probe (mainstream) or tubing (side-stream) and blow through it to make sure it works	
Attach the temperature probe or set a thermometer out	
Supplies for recovery	
Prepare a warm, quiet place to recover	
Have a syringe to deflate the ET tube cuff	
Have a thermometer to take body temperature	
Anticipate the need for analgesic or sedative drugs	
Anticipate the need for supplemental oxygen and/or IV fluids	
Use a pain scoring system to evaluate the patient's pain level	

Index

A

Abdominal blocks, 259-274

Abdominal radiography/ultrasound, preanesthesia, 12

Abdominocentesis, preanesthesia, 13

Acepromazine
for castration protocol, 347
for hypertension, 388
for postoperative pain, 335
in premedication
for dogs and cats, 93
for horses, 411
precautions for, 85-86
in recovery phase, 114, 116
for renal disease protocol, 360
for small mammals, 444, 447

Acupuncture, 233

Adjunctive analgesics, with local anesthetics, 246

Adverse effects, 73

Airway pressure manometer, 40, 203

Albuterol, for horses, 436

Alfaxalone, 4
in cesarean section, 349
for healthy cats, 343
for hepatic disease protocol, 357
in hypoventilation, 391
in induction phase, 97-98, 105, 106
infusions, in maintenance phase, 112-113
in maintenance phase, 109
in premedication, 94
for rabbits, 453
for renal disease protocol, 360
for seizure protocol, 362
for small animals, 444, 447, 448
titration of, 311

Alfaxan®, 97-98

Alpha-2 adrenergic agonists, 231, 431

Alpha-2 agonists, 236
administered concurrently with induction drugs, 104
causing bradycardia, 185
clinical use of, 87-88
in CRIs, 281, 435
in diabetes protocol, 352
effects and adverse effects of, 87
for horses, 432, 433

administering, 413-417
in CRIs, 435
for induction, 413
with ketamine in anesthesia maintenance, 417
with opioids in recovery, 426-427
premedication, 411-412
ketamine and, 111
key points for, 89
with local anesthetics, 246
in pale mucous membrane color, 133
for postoperative pain, 335
precautions for, 88
in premedication, 86-89
in recovery phase, 114, 116
for renal disease protocol, 360
reversal of, 118, 335
side/adverse effects of, 86-87
in sinus bradycardia, 379, 380
for small animals, 445, 447
specific drugs, 89-90
systemic vasoconstriction with, 132
for trauma patients, 365

Alpha-2 antagonists, in alpha-2 agonist reversal, 118

American Society of Anesthesiologists (ASA) physical status scores, 8, 344
increasing or decreasing, 13

Amiodarone, for emergencies and CPCR, 403, 404

Analgesia
for brachycephalic airway disease and upper respiratory dysfunctions, 345
in cesarean section, 340
four phases of, 234-235
goal of, 213-214
for healthy cats, 341-342
for healthy dogs, 340
for heart disease protocol, 355
for hepatic disease protocol, 357
importance of, 2-3, 212
for intraoperative pain, 183
multimodal, 224
perioperative protocols for, 236-241
for postoperative pain, 335
preemptive, 223
principles of, 3

Blood pressure monitoring, 147-150
  invasive, 152
    troubleshooting, 156-157
  noninvasive
    Doppler, 150-153
    oscillometric, 151-156
  for small animals, 451
Blood pressure monitors
  invasive, 149
  noninvasive, 19, 148
    setting up, 149-151
Blood pressure support, 183-184
  circulating fluid volume, 189-198
  heart rate, 184-189
Blood smear, preanesthesia, 13
Blood transfusion, procedure for, 389
Blood work, preanesthesia, 12
Body fluids, 191
  distribution of, 191-192
Body temperature
  monitoring, 177
    abnormalities in, 177-178
    normal values for, 177
  preanesthesia, 11
Body temperature support, 204
  for hyperthermia, 208
  for hypothermia, 204-208
Body weight, preanesthesia, 9
Bounding pulse, 135
Brachial plexus block, 275-278
  for trauma patients, 365, 366
Brachycephalic airway disease, 158
  protocol for, 343-346
Brachycephalic airway syndrome, 199, 201
Brachycephalic patients
  endotracheal tube sizes for, 307
  extubation of, 334, 335
  increased vagal tone and bradycardia in, 185
  inhalant induction contraindicated in, 103
  in recovery, 333, 346
  respiratory compromise in, 299
  upper airway abnormalities in, 344, 391, 456
Bradycardia, 130-131, 184-185
  anticholinergic drugs for, 186-188
  common perioperative causes of, 185
Bradypnea, 159
Breathing
  irregular, 161
  preanesthesia, 11

Breathing hoses, 33-34, 43
Breathing systems, 16, 30
  choosing, 45-49
  coaxial, 42, 43
  non-rebreathing, 42-45
  pressure checking, 49-52
  rebreathing, 17, 30-42
  troubleshooting leaks in, 52-54
Bupivacaine, 243, 244
  for hepatic disease protocol, 357
  for horses, 420-421, 434
  in sacrococcygeal epidural, 273
  for seizure protocol, 362
  for small mammals, 443
  for trauma patients, 366
Buprenorphine, 226-227
  for diabetes protocol, 352
  for ferrets, 453
  for healthy cats, 343
  for horses, 434
    intraoperative, 419-420
  ketamine and, 111
  for lumbosacral epidural analgesia, 263
  for postoperative pain, 119
  in premedication, 77-78
  for rabbits, 452, 453
  in recovery phase, 115, 116
  for renal disease protocol, 361
  in reversal of opioid effects, 75, 84
  reversibility of, 72
  for small mammals, 443
Buretrol device, 198
Butorphanol, 226
  in CRIs, 279-280
    dosages in cats, 288
    dosages in dogs, 286
  for horses, 434
    intraoperative, 419-420
    in premedication, 412
  ketamine and, 111
  in opioid reversal, 117
  in premedication, 79, 84
  for rabbits, 452, 453
  in recovery phase, 115
  in reversal of opioid effects, 74-75
  reversibility of, 72
  for small mammals, 443
  Telazol® and, 112

C

Calcium, adding to IV fluid, 320
Calcium channel blockers, 379, 381
Calcium chloride, 431
Calcium gluconate, 406-407
Capillary refill time (CRT), 133
  abnormalities of, 133-134
  assessing, 133
  preanesthesia, 9-11
Capnographic waves, normal and abnormal, 168
Capnometer, 164
  main stream, 165-166
  side stream
    advantages and disadvantages of, 166-167
    setting up, 167
Carbocaine® (mepivacaine), 244
  for horses, 420-421, 434
Carbon dioxide abnormalities, 167-168
Carbon dioxide absorbent granules and canisters, 34-37
Carbon dioxide elimination, 158, 202
  inadequate, 161
Carbon dioxide monitoring, for hypoventilation, 392
Carbon dioxide tension, low, 396-397
Carbon monoxide poisoning, 133
Cardiac arrest, 170, 400
CPCR guidelines for, 400-404
  lidocaine causing, 385
  postoperative, 366-367
  respiratory arrest and, 399
Cardiopulmonary cerebral resuscitation (CPCR), 400
  airway, 402
  breathing, 402-403
  circulation in, 400-402
  current guidelines for, 400-404
  drugs for, 403, 404
  post resuscitation, 403
Cardiovascular emergency drug dosing chart, 406-407
Cardiovascular system, 128
  complications and emergencies of, 375-389
  monitoring of, 128
    advanced, 139-157
    basic but essential, 128-138
    for horses, 423-425

Cardiovascular system support
  of blood pressure, 183-184
    circulating fluid volume, 189-198
    heart rate, 184-189
  for horses, 423-425
Carprofen
  for horses, 435
  for small animals, 443
Castration, protocol for, 346-347
Catheter, choosing correct size of, 301
Catheterization
  approaches to, 301-302
  of horses, 418-419
  placement of
    step by step, 302-306
    tips for, 306-307
  procedure for, 300-307
  veins to use in, 298-299, 300
Cats
  anesthesia and sedation-related deaths in, 440
  healthy, protocols for
    inhalant drug based, 341-342
    injectable drug based, 342-343
Caudal maxillary block, 252-255
Central nervous system (CNS)
  complications and emergencies of, 374-375
  monitoring of, 124
    advanced, 127-128
    basic but essential, 124-127
    for horses, 422-423
  support for, 182-183
Central nervous system (CNS) disease, in hypoventilation, 392
Cerenia® (maropitant), premedication, 95, 96
Cesarean section protocol, 347-348
  anesthetic plan in, 349-351
  concerns and plan in, 348-349
  drug contraindications in, 349
  recovery from, 350-351
Chinchillas, anesthesia and sedation-related deaths in, 440
Circle rebreathing system, 40
Circulating fluid volume support, 189
  fluids for, 190-196
    based on patient needs, 197-198
  monitoring fluid therapy in, 198
  reasons for fluid therapy in, 189
  routes of fluid administration in, 190
  volume of fluids to administer in, 196-197